Lymphatic Filariasis

Trilok Chandra Goel • Apul Goel

Lymphatic Filariasis

Springer

Trilok Chandra Goel
Department of General Surgery
King George's Medical University
Lucknow
India

Apul Goel
Department of Urology
King George's Medical University
Lucknow
India

ISBN 978-981-10-2256-2 ISBN 978-981-10-2257-9 (eBook)
DOI 10.1007/978-981-10-2257-9

Library of Congress Control Number: 2016957157

Printed on acid-free paper

This Springer imprint is published by Springer Nature
The registered company is Springer Science+Business Media Singapore Pte Ltd.
The registered company is 152 Beach Road, #22-06/08 Gateway East, Singapore 189721, Singapore

Foreword I

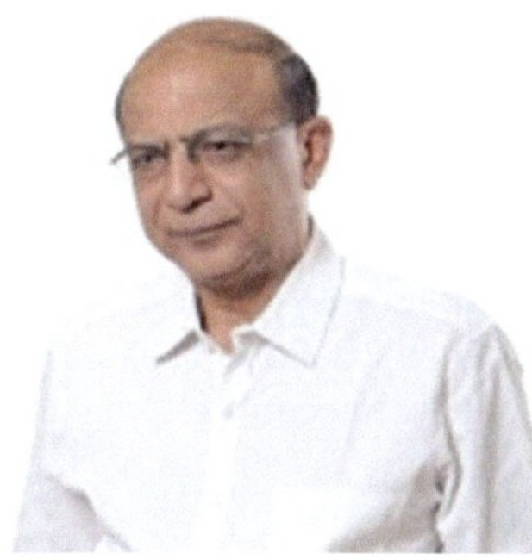

Filaria is a disease of the impoverished. A full text on filariasis could not have been written outside Indian subcontinent or Africa in 2015. In colonial times, such monographs were written in English language by foreigners who worked in the continents of Asia or Africa. These enriched the tropical disease departments in Europe and America. Times have changed since. Several technological developments have taken place in surgery.

Surgical care – a lucrative business from a purely commercial perspective – can be seen as two types of procedures: those with highly predictable outcomes in gallbladder or kidney stones, through laparoscopic or robotic procedures, and those surgical anomalies that require multiple surgical procedures with not-so-happy outcomes, for example, bladder exstrophy, epispadias, and filarial elephantiasis and chyluria.

You need a rich surgeon to write a full text on filariasis. "Will he esteem thy riches? No, not gold, nor all the forces of strength (King James' version of parallel verses, Bible)." You need the richness of mind as filaria has a difficult pathogenesis to understand. Richness of surgical technicianship must be there for filarial surgery requires persevering with multiple and seemingly endless procedures. You need to be rich because your patients with elephantiatic limbs and scrotum and ram-horn penis are a poor lot seen on the banks of *Ganges* in *Haridwar*, *Prayag*, and *Varanasi*. It had to be a production that comes from a public sector experience.

Writing a book on filariasis as opposed to books on laparoscopy, recent advances, MCQs, and illustrative Atlas, I beg to draw a corollary, is like a *Prasar Bharati* telecast of classical music against a parallel light music channel. I reiterate that it requires a rich surgeon to be investing his time on a subject with likely poor commercial dividends.

And surely this book on filariasis is *richie-rich* in content and nonetheless a full and a complete text in one place, never seen before, assembled in 40 chapters. It will enrich those who read it. In this era of surgical education loaded with technology-oriented teaching, this is a refreshing text for surgeons of my generation who entered the portals of surgical education four decades ago and worked in public sector hospitals. It would open a whole new vista of knowledge for the new *genre* of surgeons, of a hitherto neglected surgical disease. For surgical examiners, this will be an ever-enriching journey to brush their mustache while framing questions from the knowledge acquired from this book. It is not too uncommon to find one such patient in the galaxy of stealthily called "clinical material" in India.

I enjoyed reading it. It has given me an edge in my surgical package of knowledge. If it can entice you to treat a few with elephantatic limbs or save people from developing a crippling illness by a simple prescription of diethylcarbamazine or *ivermectin*, it would serve its purpose. It is the richness of this pharmaceutical – ivermectin – that earned a Nobel Prize to Dr. William C. Campbell from Dublin. Dr. Campbell delivered his Nobel lecture on 7 December 2015 at Aula Medica Karolinska Institutet, Stockholm, Sweden. This simple ivermectin 6–12 mg pharmaceutical has the capability of eradicating the scourge of filariasis from humankind, and Dr. TC Goel's book is surely an instrument toward this.

Dr. Sandeep Kumar
MS FRCS (Edinburgh) PhD (Wales) MMSc (Newcastle)
Consultant Surgeon, Scientist, and Epidemiologist
Professor of Surgery Ex King George's Medical University
Founder Director AIIMS Bhopal
M: +91 93352 40880
E: profsandeepsurgeon@gmail.com

Foreword II

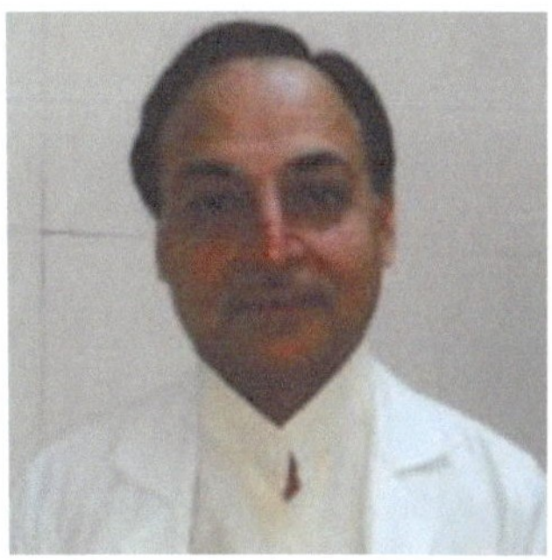

Going through the contents of this book gives a feeling of searching a pearl in the ocean of knowledge. For centuries, filariasis has been termed a tropical disease of the poor, so it could get a value of only a footnote in surgical books. As a result, there has been little contemporary research on this topic as compared to other diseases. But now, in changing times, filariasis has been recognized as a crippling disease affecting millions of people. The swollen penis, scrotum, and limbs have made the life of millions of patients miserable. Investigators including basic scientists, physicians, microbiologists, and surgeons are trying to understand the disease process to better treat these patients.

The authors have covered every aspect of this disease and brought it under one cover. With comprehensive coverage of all facets of this disease, I am sure this book will be of interest to readers working in this field.

I am confident that readers will find this book useful.

I wish all the best to Prof. TC Goel and pray to God to keep him healthy so that he can contribute to such works in the future also.

Dr. AC Dwivedi
Head, Department of Surgery
Dr. Ram Manohar Lohia Combined Hospital
Lucknow

Preface

I started my surgical career with filariasis when I did my first operation, i.e., eversion of sac in a scrotal hydrocele in 1963, during my internship in surgery. Most of the hydroceles around Lucknow are filarial. Hence, it must be a filarial hydrocele.

Then when I worked as chief resident of Professor SC Misra, Head of the Department of Surgery in January 1966 and later as Lecturer in Surgery from April 1966 onward, I found extensive clinical research work going on the management of chronic lymphedema–elephantiasis, especially of the lower extremity in his surgical unit. Hence, I had an experience on a variety of lymphangioplasties including subcutaneous implantation of nylon threads, stainless steel wire, and polythene tubes, Thompson and Charles operation, and omental transposition.

After the retirement of Professor SC Misra in 1969, his place was taken over by Professor PC Dubey, and I continued to do clinical work on filariasis. Then we had a patient of chyluria. After a discussion, he did a cystoscopy and found chylous eflux from the right ureter. Hence, he asked me to do pyelolymphatic disconnection on the right kidney. During the exploration of the right kidney, I found the renal pedicle and renal hilum studded with a crowd of varicose lymphatics. They were all excised. The patient was relieved and went home happy. My interest in lymphatic filariasis problem has continued till today. Hence, this book is the result of a long experience of studying, treating, writing, and teaching about lymphatic filariasis.

In spite of the Global Programme to Eliminate Lymphatic Filariasis (GPELF), filariasis is still a major clinical problem in our country.

I wrote this book in 2005 but I could not get it published due to my illness. After recovery, I revised the whole book and made it up to date. Now it is in front of you for studying deficiencies and efficiencies, giving suggestions for further improvement.

This book will be of help to undergraduate medical students; postgraduates in general surgery, urology, general medicine, and plastic and reconstructive surgery; and medical officers in various government medical services.

Lucknow, India

T.C. Goel

Acknowledgments

We are grateful to the following for their help and encouragement:

King George's Medical University, Lucknow

1. Professor Ravi Kant, Vice Chancellor
2. Professor PK Agarwal, Former Professor of Pathology
3. Professor Sandeep Kumar, Former Professor of Surgery and Former Director of All India Institute of Medical Sciences, Bhopal, MP
4. Professor D Dalela, Former Head of Department of Urology
5. Professor Ashish Wakhlu, Department of Pediatric Surgery
6. Professor JD Rawat, Department of Pediatric Surgery
7. Professor AA Sonkar, Head of Department of General Surgery
8. Professor SN Sankhwar, Head of Department of Urology
9. Professor Sandeep Tewari, Department of General Surgery
10. Professor Vinod Jain, Department of General Surgery
11. Professor Arshad Ahmad, Department of General Surgery
12. Professor Anand Mishra, Department of General Surgery
13. Professor Shally Awasthi, Head of Department of Medical Education
14. Professor Pallavi Aga, Department of Radiodiagnosis
15. Professor Vishwajeet Singh, Department of Urology
16. Professor Brijesh Mishra, Department of Plastic Surgery
17. Professor Divya Narain, Department of Plastic Surgery

Other Institutions

1. Professor Rajiv Agarwal, Head of Department of Plastic Surgery and Burns, Sanjay Gandhi Postgraduate Institute of Medical Sciences, Lucknow
2. Professor IP Jain, Former Head of Department of Pharmacology GSVM Medical College, Kanpur – Antifilarial drugs

Private Clinics and Diagnostic Centers, Lucknow

1. Dr. SS Sarkar, Sarkar Diagnostics
2. Dr. RK Mishra, SIPS
3. Dr. Surajit Bhattacharya, Plastic and Reconstructive Surgeon

4. Dr. Ashutosh Pandey, Pediatric Surgeon, Vivekananda Polyclinic
5. Dr. MK Srivastava, Surgeon, Mayo Medical Centre
6. Dr. S.K. Vaish and Dr. Miti Gupta

Special thanks to my wife Aruna who looks after many of my daily needs and requirements at the site where I am working (like Bhamati). I thank my dear daughter Alpana for the help and encouragement.

I am very grateful to Dr. KN Singh and Mrs. Madhulika Singh, Mayo Medical Centre, Gomti Nagar, and Dr. Satyavan, Dr. (Mrs.) Satyaprabha Satyavan, and Dr. Saurabh Baiswar of Satya Shiv Hospital, Mahanagar Extension, Lucknow, where I have done a part of writing work.

Mr. Mohammad Affan and Mr. Shyam Kashyap have done computer work excellently well, and my driver Mr. Ram Sagar made me reach these people regularly once a week – I thank all of these three gentlemen.

TC Goel
Emeritus Professor of Surgery
King George's Medical University
Lucknow

Contents

About the Authors

Trilok Chandra Goel After graduating from King George's Medical College (India) with distinction, Dr. Trilok Chandra Goel completed his training in Surgery in 1965 with the award of best surgical postgraduate of the year. He has been teaching since 1966 and was appointed as Emeritus Professor of Surgery by King George's Medical University, India, in 2015. On the occasion of Teacher's Day (2014), Dr. Goel was honored with the first "Life-time Achievement Award" by King George's Medical University. He has published more than 60 research papers and 11 books.

Apul Goel Dr. Apul Goel finished his graduate training (MBBS) in 1989 from King George's Medical College, Lucknow, India, with honors in surgery, medicine, and forensic medicine. He completed his postgraduation in surgery (MS) from the same college in 1993. After his specialization in urology (MCh) from All India Institute of Medical Sciences, New Delhi, he joined King George's Medical University where he is currently working as Professor in the Department of Urology. He had more than 150 publications to his credit and is an Associate Editor of *Indian Journal of Urology*. He has contributed eight chapters in three medical books and has coauthored four medical books including one *Textbook of Surgery* in Hindi. He is a reviewer for many prestigious medical journals.

Part I

Parasitology Including General Discussion

History

1

Lymphatic filariasis is caused by microscopic round worms where the adult worms live in the lymphatic system and cause disease. Hence, it is known lymphatic filariasis.

As there is no written record, the ancient history of the lymphatic filariasis is not known exactly. There are some ancient artifacts available in the Nile river region as early as 2000 years BC. A statue of Pharaoh Mentuhotep II depicts swollen limbs, i.e., elephantiasis, which is an important chronic manifestation of filariasis. Some artifacts of Nok civilization of West Africa around 500 AD show scrotal swelling, another important feature of lymphatic filariasis. The first written account of this disease is available in Greek and Roman literature. They differentiated the symptoms of leprosy from those of filariasis and described leprosy as "elephantiasis graecorum" and lymphatic filariasis as "elephantiasis arabum" (Addiss et al. 2010).

Filariasis was known to ancient Chinese, Indian, Persian, and Arabic physicians. Sushruta (600 BC) described one of its major manifestations, i.e., elephantiasis of leg as "shleepada" (श्लीपद) where "shli" means elephant and "pada" means leg (Bhishagratna 1963). It was also recognized by Persian physicians Rhazes and Avicenna. Madhavakara in the seventh century described the signs and symptoms of filariasis in his book *Madhavanidan* (माधवनिदान). Similarly, chyluria is described in old Ayurvedic books as "payasmeha" (पायसमेह).

The first reliable written record of lymphatic filariasis was found in Goa between 1588 and 1592 (Narain and Bhatia 2010). During his trip, Jan Huygen Linschoten described about the people, "all born with one of their legs and one foot from the knee downwards as thick as an elephant's leg" (Addiss 2010).

In 1841, William Prout described chyluria caused by lymphatic filariasis which appeared in the book written by him titled *On the Nature and Treatment of Stomach and Renal Diseases* as secretion of fat from blood through kidneys.

Jean-Nicolas Demarquay (1863) in Paris was the first person to demonstrate the larval forms of *Wuchereria bancrofti* (microfilariae) in the hydrocele fluid of a man from Cuba, and Otto Wucherer (1868) in Brazil detected them in chylous urine. However, the connection between the two discoveries was not found until Timothy

T.C. Goel, A. Goel, *Lymphatic Filariasis*, DOI 10.1007/978-981-10-2257-9_1

Lewis (1872) in India found these parasites both in blood and urine. Lewis also proposed the association between these findings and elephantiasis for the first time (Chandy et al. 2011).

Joseph Bancroft (1878) in Brisbane (Australia) recognized the adult female worms, and Bourne in 1888 discovered the adult male worm (Babu and Nutman 2005). The name filaria bancrofti was proposed by Cobbold in 1877 and the generic name Wuchereria was given in 1878.

Sir Patrick Manson, the distinguished pioneer of tropical medicine, while working in Amoy in China, contributed a lot to the understanding of the biology of *W. bancrofti*. In 1877, he studied the development of parasite in mosquitoes fed on the blood of his microfilaremic gardener and speculated that the parasite was transmitted by mosquitoes. He also observed that the microfilariae were not found all the time in the blood of infected persons. By serial blood examination every few hours, he found the nocturnal periodicity of microfilariae. Later work by George Carmichael Low (1900) discovered the microfilariae in the proboscis of mosquito, demonstrated the mode of transmission, and described the morphological changes undergone by microfilariae in the intermediate host.

The Brugia malayi was first detected by Lichtenstein (1927) in its microfilarial form in the blood films of the natives of Northern Sumatra, but Brug (1927) described it as a new species. The adult males and females were first described by Rao and Maplestone (1940) from India.

Later, a lot of work was done in defining various manifestations of filariasis but still the information of the lymphatic filariasis is not complete. Hence further research is needed which is being done in many countries in the world (Chandy et al. 2011).

References

Addiss DG. Global elimination of lymphatic filariasis: addressing the public health problem. PLoS Negl Trop Dis. 2010;4(6), e741.

Addiss DG, Louis-Charles J, Roberts J, Leconte F, Wendt JM, et al. Feasibility and effectiveness of basic lymphedema management in Leogane, Haiti, an area endemic for bancroftian filariasis. PLoS Negl Trop Dis. 2010;4, e668.

Babu S, Nutman TB. Lymphatic filariasis. In: Cox FEG, Wakelin D, Gillespie SH, Despommier DD, editors. Topley & Wilson's microbiology & microbial infections. Parasitology. 10th ed. London: Hodder Arnold; 2005. p. 769–80.

Bancroft J. Cases of filarious disease. Trans Path Soc Lond. 1878;29:406–19.

Bhishagratna KKL. An English translation of Shusruta Samhita based on the original Sanskrit text, vol. 2. Varanasi, India: Chowkamba Sanskrit Series Office; 1963. p. 439–49.

Bourne AG. A note on Filaria sanguinis hominis: with a description of a male specimen. Br Med J. 1888;1(1429):1050–1.

Brug SL. Filaria malayi n. Sp. parasitic in man in Malaya Archipelago. Far Eastern Association Trop Med Transactions. 7th Congress Volume 3, 1927.

Chandy A, Thakur AS, Singh MP, Manigauha A. A review of neglected tropical diseases: filariasis. Asian Pac J Trop Med. 2011;4(7):581–6.

Cobbold TS. Discovery of the adult representative of microscopic filariae. Lancet. 1877;2:70–1.

Demarquay JN. Gaz Med Paris. 1863;18:665–7.

George Carmichael Low, 1900: Quoted by Anish Chandy et al., A review of neglected tropical disease filariasis. Asian Pac J Trop Med. 2011;4(7): 581–6.

Lewis TR. On a haematazoon inhabiting human blood, its relation to chyluria and other diseases. Lancet. 1872;1:889–90.

Lichtenstein A. Geneeskunde Tijdschriftvoor Nederland seh India. 1927; 67:742.

Manson P. Filaria sanguinis hominis. Med Rep Imperial Maritime Customs China. 1877;13:30–8.

Narain JP, Bhatia R. The challenge of communicable diseases in the WHO South-East Asia Region. Bull World Health Organ. 2010;88(3):162.

Prout W. On the nature and treatment of stomach and urinary diseases. 3rd ed. London: Churchill; 1841. p. 120.

Rao & Maplestone, 1940: Quoted by Chatterjee KD. Parasitology. 2nd ed. Calcutta: Published by Author; 1959. p. 162.

Wucherer OEH. Noticiapreliminarsobre vermes de umaspecieaindanaodescripta, encontradsonaurina de doentes de hematuria intertropical no. Brazil Gaz Med Bahia. 1868;3:406–19.

Epidemiology 2

Globally, there are nearly one billion people, i.e., 20 % of the world's population living in areas endemic for lymphatic filariasis that are exposed to the risk of infection (Michael and Bundy 1997). Among the debilitating vector-borne tropical diseases, the lymphatic filariasis is next only to malaria (WHO report 1995).

More than 120 million people are affected with filarial infection in 83 tropical and subtropical countries, in five endemic regions, i.e., Southeast Asia, Africa, Eastern Mediterranean, Western Pacific, and Americas including the Caribbean countries and Central America (DeVries 2002). See the table given below (Table 2.1).

These regions embrace practically the whole of the area lying between the Tropic of Cancer and Tropic of Capricorn (Macfee 1925).

All over the world, 40 million people are disfigured and about 1 million new persons, mainly children, are infected yearly. Hence, it is one of the most important infections worldwide. One third of people infected with this disease live in India, one third in Sub-Saharan Africa, and the rest in Southeast Asia, Western Pacific, and parts of Central and South America. It is further estimated that over 27 million men are thought to suffer with filarial hydrocele, and 15 million people most of whom are women have chronic lymphedema–elephantiasis of the leg (Haddix and Kestler 2000). There are 83.63 million microfilariae carriers (Michael et al. 1996). Filariasis is a disease of poor people and is a cause and effect of poverty (Pani et al. 2005). Most of its victims live in villages.

This disease is caused by three filarial nematodes, i.e., *Wuchereria bancrofti*, *Brugia malayi*, and *Brugia timori* (Das et al. 2002). *W. bancrofti* causes about 90 % of lymphatic filarial disease, the rest being the brugian disease (Pani et al. 2005). *Brugia timori* filariasis consists of only a few thousand patients and limited to the island of Timor in Indonesia.

Nigeria is thought to have the highest disease burden of lymphatic filariasis in Sub-Saharan Africa being the third most endemic country in the world after India and Indonesia (Michael et al. 2001; Lindsay and Thomas 2000). About 70 % of the infected patients in the world are in India, Bangladesh, Indonesia, and Nigeria (Okon et al. 2010; Chandy et al. 2011). The incidence in Papua New Guinea is 72 %

T.C. Goel, A. Goel, *Lymphatic Filariasis*, DOI 10.1007/978-981-10-2257-9_2

Table 2.1 Endemic regions and countries affected by lymphatic filariasis (DeVries 2002)

Southeast Asia (SEARO)	Africa (AFRO)	Eastern Mediterranean (EMRO)	Western Pacific (WPRO)	Americas (AMRO)
Bangladesh Myanmar India Indonesia Maldives Sri Lanka Thailand	Angola Benin Cameroon Cape Verde Chad Comoros Congo Ethiopia Gambia Ghana Kenya Liberia Madagascar Malawi Mali Mauritius Mozambique Nigeria Rwanda Senegal Seychelles Sierra Leone Tongo Uganda Tanzania Zambia Zimbabwe	Egypt Oman Pakistan Somalia Sudan Yemen	American Samoa Brunei darussalam Cambodia China Cook islands Fiji French Polynesia Malaysia Marshall islands New Caledonia Papua New Guinea Philippines Samoa Solomon islands Korea Tonga Vietnam Wallis & Futuna	Barbados Brazil Costa Rica Cuba Dominica Dominican republic French Guyana Guyana Haiti Panama Puerto Rico St Kitts & Nevis St Lucia Suriname Trinidad & Tobago Venezuela Virgin islands

Table 2.2 Prevalence of lymphatic filariasis in main four endemic countries/regions (Michael et al. 1996)

Country/region	Population (million)	Microfilaremic persons (million)	Scrotal hydrocele (million)	Lymphedema (million)
India	849	31.26	12.88	7.44
China	1134	7.54	1.63	0.84
Sub-Saharan Africa	512	27.87	10.20	4.64
South America and Caribbean	441	0.32	0.057	0.03
Other Asian countries and islands (Indonesia)	793	16.40	1.9	3.00
World	4119	83.95	26.79	16.01

and in Republic of Tongo 48 %. Latin America and Egypt have the lowest prevalence (de Almeida and Freedman 1999) (See Table 2.2).

In Nepal, 60 out of 75 districts are endemic and more than 25 million individuals are at risk. Prevalence rate above 20 % is present in 11 districts (with the highest rate of 40 %), 6–19 % in 15 districts, and 0.1–5 % in seven districts (Adhikari et al. 2015).

The lymphatic filariasis is endemic in 32 of the world's 38 least developed countries (Chu et al. 2010; Utzinger et al. 2010).

2.1 Bancroftian Filariasis

The bancroftian filariasis is widely distributed in tropics and subtropics of both the hemispheres including India, West Indies, Puerto Rico, Southern China, Japan, North Australia, West and Central Africa, South America and Pacific Islands. Its natural vector is *Culex fatigans* in urban settings and *Anopheles* and *Aedes* in rural areas. Its parasite has two forms – the nocturnally periodic microfilariae are scarce in the peripheral blood during the day and increase during the night, and sub-periodic microfilariae that are present in the peripheral blood all the time and reach at the maximum levels in the afternoon. It infects exclusively the human hosts.

2.2 Brugian Filariasis

The infection by *Brugia malayi* is common in South India, Sri Lanka, Southeast Asia, South China, and northern coastal areas of China and South Korea. This parasite also has two forms – the nocturnally periodic microfilariae are transmitted in areas of coastal rice fields, while the sub-periodic form is found in forests. Apart from men, it infects cats and monkeys naturally (Table 2.3).

2.3 Filariasis Problem in India

India contributes to approximately 40 % of total global burden and accounts for about 50 % of the people at risk of infection. There are 554 million people at risk of infection, 27 million asymptomatic microfilariae carriers, and 21 million symptomatic lymphatic filariasis patients (Sebasan et al. 2000). The people exposed to the risk of infection consist of 39.0 %, and patients with asymptomatic microfilaremia, with hydrocele, and with lymphedema consist of 37.9 %, 48.1 %, and 46.4 %, respectively (Michael et al. 1996).

An epidemiological study reported in 1995 demonstrated that out of 25 states and union territories of India (before the bifurcation of Bihar, Madhya Pradesh, Uttar Pradesh, and Andhra Pradesh), 22 were found endemic for this disease, and nine states, i.e., Andhra Pradesh (including Telangana), Bihar (including Jharkhand), Gujarat, Kerala, Maharashtra, Odisha, Tamil Nadu, Uttar Pradesh (including Uttarakhand), and West Bengal contributed to about 95 % of total burden (Pani et al. 2005) (Table 2.4).

Bancroftian Filariasis A survey done in 2001 revealed that there are about 473 million people exposed to the risk of bancroftian filariasis, and of these, approximately 125 million live in urban areas and 348 million in rural areas. About 31 million people are estimated to harbor microfilariae and more than 23 million have filarial manifestations. The state of Bihar has the highest endemicity (over 17 %)

Table 2.3 Epidemiology of lymphatic filariasis

People living in filarial endemic areas – one billion or 20 % of world's population
Second vector-borne debilitating disease after malaria
Number of tropical and subtropical countries affected – 83
Total number of people affected – 120 million
Bancroftian infection – 90 %
Brugian infection – 10 %
Five main endemic regions
1. Southeast Asia including India (SEARO)
2. Africa (AFRO)
3. Eastern Mediterranean (EMRO)
4. Western Pacific and Americas including the Caribbean countries (WPRO)
5. Central America (AMRO)
One third of infected people live in India, one third in Sub-Saharan Africa, and one third in Southeast Asia, Western Pacific, and parts of Central and South America (India 45.5 million, Sub-Saharan Africa 40 million)
Most endemic countries in the world – India, Indonesia, and Nigeria
70 % of total infected people in the world – India, Nigeria, Bangladesh, and Indonesia
Prevalence rates
Papua New Guinea – 72 %
Republic of Tongo – 48 %
Sub-Saharan Africa – 8 %
Ethiopia – 7.8 % (fourth highest burden country in Sub-Saharan Africa, with 30 million people at risk)
India – 5 %
Low prevalence countries – Egypt, Latin America
Number of patients with genital disease (hydrocele) – 25 million
Number of patients with chronic lymphedema–elephantiasis – 15 million
Number of people with preclinical damage to lymphatics and renal system – 76 million (Michael et al. 2001, 1996; Yimer et al. 2015)

Table 2.4 Epidemiology of lymphatic filariasis in India

Most endemic country – 40 % of total global burden with 5 % prevalence rate
1. *W. bancrofti* infection – 98 %, predominantly urban
2. *B. malayi* infection – 2 %, predominantly rural
One-third of infected people of world live in India
People at risk of infection – about 50 %, i.e., 554 million
Asymptomatic filariasis – 21 million
Asymptomatic microfilariae carriers – 27 million
Bihar has highest endemicity rates (over 17 %) followed by Kerala (15.7 %) and Uttar Pradesh (14.6 %)
Districts – 257 districts endemic out of 289 districts

(Das et al. 2006) followed by Kerala (15.7 %) and Uttar Pradesh (14.6 %). Andhra Pradesh and Tamil Nadu have approximately 10 % endemicity. Goa has the lowest endemicity (less than 1 %) followed by Lakshadweep (1.8 %), Madhya Pradesh above 3 %, and Assam about 5 %. The seven states, i.e., Bihar, Andhra Pradesh, Kerala, Odisha, Uttar Pradesh, Tamil Nadu, and West Bengal have more than 86 % of microfilariae carriers and 97 % clinical cases of filariasis (WHO 2005).

Das et al. (2006) studied the occurrence of filariasis in two contiguous villages of Patna district of Bihar known for filarial endemicity. Of the 1872 persons examined, 8.4 % had asymptomatic microfilaremia. Acute and chronic filariasis was found to be 0.5 % and 9 %, respectively. Microfilaremia was found in 10 % of acute and 11.2 % of chronic filarial patients. The microfilaria rate was found to be 9.9 % in males and 9.0 % in females and the parasitic species identified was *W. bancrofti*. The most prevalent vector species identified was *Culex quinquefasciatus* (93 %). The infection rate in the vector was found to be 14 % and infectivity rate 8 %.

Brugian Filariasis The nocturnal periodic infection of *Brugia malayi* is prevalent in the states of Kerala, Tamil Nadu, Andhra Pradesh, Odisha, Madhya Pradesh, Assam, and West Bengal. The only largest tract of this type of filariasis lies along the west coast of Kerala consisting of districts of Trichur, Ernaculum, Alleppey, Kottayam, Quilon, and Tiruananthapuram stretching over an area 1800 km^2. The infection in other six states is confined to a few villages only. Recent surveys have shown marked reduction of the infection in many areas (Agrawal and Sashindran 2006). Hydrocele is not seen in areas affected by brugian filariasis.

The lymphatic filariasis is endemic all over the country except Jammu and Kashmir, Himanchal Pradesh, Punjab, Haryana, Delhi, Rajasthan, Nagaland, Manipur, Tripura, Meghalaya, Sikkim, Arunachal Pradesh, Mizoram and Dadra, and Nagar Haveli (Park 2007).

The *W. bancrofti* infection is seen in the cities while the distribution of *B. malayi* infection is predominantly rural. The former type of infection in seen in the crowded center of the city (centripetal), while the latter prevails in the outskirts of the city (centrifugal) where the stagnant water of the city collects.

With rapid urbanization the *B. malayi* infection (clear water mosquito infection) is gradually being replaced by *W. bancrofti* infection (stagnant water mosquito infection) and now filariasis is being detected in towns and cities previously free from this disease.

The relative magnitude of lymphatic filariasis between global and Indian occurrence is given in the following Table 2.5.

2.4 Age and Sex

The prevalence of filarial infection and disease is markedly high in males than in females (Pani et al. 1994; Michael et al. 1994). Young adults between 15 and 44 years of age had the highest prevalence of infection (Sasa 1976). This group

Table 2.5 Relative magnitude of filariasis between Global and Indian occurrence (Michael et al. 1996)

Parameters	Global occurrence		Indian occurrence		Indian/Global occurrence	
	W. bancrofti (million)	*B. malayi* (million)	*W. bancrofti* (million)	*B. malayi* (million)	*W. bancrofti* (million)	*B. malayi* (million)
Microfilaria carriers	73.3	10.4	29.5	1.8	40.2	17.3
Scrotal hydrocele	26.8	–	12.9	–	48.1	–
Chronic lymphedema	13.2	2.8	6.9	0.9	52.3	32.1

Brugia malayi infection does not result in a scrotal hydrocele

constitutes the predominant age class in the population. Globally, this group contributes to 58.5 % of all microfilaremics, 58.3 % of hydrocele patients, and 47.2 % of lymphedema patients (Michael et al. 1996). Children and young adults less than 20 years of age reveal a high incidence of infection detected by newer tools of diagnosis. The incidence of infection in these persons varied between 6.74 % in south India to 7.70 % in Ghana (Addiss 1995), but it does not exhibit in peripheral blood smear.

The prevalence of chronic filarial disease increases from young age to reach peak level in old age. It is due to cumulative effect as these patients rarely die due to filariasis (Michael et al. 1996; Pani and Srividya 1992). The incidence of acute dermatolymphangitis (ADLA) attacks shows a similar age pattern as that of chronic disease as ADLA attacks usually occur in patients with severe chronic disease (Ramaiah et al. 1996). This problem is more in males because of the occurrence of hydrocele. The problem of hydrocele may be as high as 50 % in people above 45 years of age. But as the total number of males in the age group of 15–44 years is the highest this most productive age accounts for 15.62 out of a total 26.79 million patients of hydrocele in the world (Michael et al. 1996).

2.5 Effect of Global Programme to Eliminate Lymphatic Filariasis

Some countries that have strictly followed this program of elimination of lymphatic filariasis have stopped transmission of infection of this disease permanently (Molyneux 2003). They include China, Japan, Korea, Thailand, and Solomon Islands. Sri Lanka has eliminated Brugian filariasis. Smaller foci in Brazil, Malaysia, Costa Rica, Suriname, and Trinidad and Tobago have also been cleared of filariasis.

Awareness, i.e., knowledge and perception about this disease, is a must for the success of this program of elimination of filariasis (Rath et al. 2006) as the majority of people are least aware about the cause of hydrocele and lymphedema.

2.6 Socioeconomic Burden

The lymphatic filarial disease is characterized by serious social and economic consequences in terms of physical disfigurement, loss of self-esteem, decreased job prospects, interference in sexual function, and family discord. Poor marriage prospects and social stigma are other common problems. The extent of stigma depends on the severity and visibility of filarial lesions. It results in significant psychosocial stress on the sufferer and his/her family members, especially men afflicted with scrotal hydrocele or chronic peno-scrotal lymphedema–elephantiasis and women with chronic lymphedema–elephantiasis of breast or vulva.

The economic loss to the India due to this disease is estimated be about 840 million–1.5 billion dollars annually as shown by recent studies (Pani et al. 2005).

- Microfilaria rate (Mf rate) – It is defined as percentage of population shown to be having microfilaria in the blood.
- Disease rate – It is the percentage of people living in an area suffering with disease considered to be filariasis including hydrocele, elephantiasis, lymphangitis, and chyluria.
- Microfilarial density rate – It is defined as microfilarial count per mL of blood.
- Endemicity rate – It is the percentage of people who have signs of filarial infection either as disease or microfilaremia.

Considered together, these rates give a picture of lymphatic filarial infection in a community or geographical area (Manson-Bahr and Apted 1982).

2.7 Endemic Normals

This group includes a large number of people who live in endemic areas and are exposed to the filarial infection to the same degree as the rest of the people (uninfected but exposed persons). They have asymptomatic microfilaremia. The prevalence of such people in a population varies from 0 (Day et al. 1991) to 50 % (Steel and Nutman 2003) in various endemic areas. However, newer methods of study should be employed to find the true prevalence of endemic normals. There may be many mechanisms by which an endemic normal phenotype is attained as described below.

1. Insufficient exposure to filarial infection
2. Low-grade or occult infection not detected by available methods
3. Pre-latent infection at the time of survey
4. Natural burning out of infection
5. True immunological resistance to the causative parasite

Clinical filariasis usually takes many months to develop. The people living or staying for a long time in endemic tropical or subtropical areas are at the highest risk. The short-term travelers have very little risk (Hotez and Ehrenberg 2010; Utzinger et al. 2010).

References

Addiss DG. Clinical, parasitological and immunologic observations of patients with hydrocele and elephantiasis in an area endemic with lymphatic filariasis. J Infectious Dis. 1995;171:755–8.

Adhikari RK, Sherchand JB, Mishra SR, et al. Health seeking behaviors and self-care practices of people with filarial lymphedema in Nepal: a qualitative study. J Trop Med. 2015;2015:260359.

Agrawal VK, Sashindran VK. Lymphatic filariasis in India: problems, challenges and new initiatives. Med J Armed Forces India. 2006;62(4):359–62.

Chandy A, Thakur AS, Singh MP, Manigauha A. A review of neglected tropical diseases: filariasis. Asian Pac J Trop Med. 2011;4(7):581–6.

Chu BK, Hooper PJ, Bradley MH, McFarland DA, Ottesen EA. The economic benefits resulting from the first 8 years of the Global Programme to Eliminate Lymphatic Filariasis (2000–2007). PLoS Negl Trop Dis. 2010;4(6), e708.

Das PK, Pani SP, Krishnamoorthy K. Prospects of elimination of lymphatic filariasis in India. ICMR Bull. 2002;32(5 & 6):41–54.

Das VNR, Siddiqui NA, Kumar N, et al. A pilot study on the status of lymphatic filariasis in rural community in Bihar. J Commun Dis. 2006;38:169–75.

Day KP, Gregory WF, Maizels RM. Age-specific acquisition of immunity to infective larvae in a bancroftian filariasis endemic area of Papua New Guinea. Parasite Immunol. 1991;19: 277–90.

de Almeida A, Freedman DO. Epidemiology and immune-pathology of bancroftian filariasis. Microbes Infect. 1999;1:1015–22.

DeVries CR. The role of the urologist in the treatment and elimination of lymphatic filariasis worldwide. BJU Int. 2002;89 Suppl 1:37–43.

Haddix A, Kestler A. Lymphatic filariasis: economic aspects of the disease and programmes for its elimination. Trans R Soc Trop Med Hyg. 2000;94:592–3.

Hotez PJ, Ehrenberg JP. Escalating the global fight against neglected tropical diseases through interventions in Asia Pacific Region. Adv Parasitol. 2010;72(C):31–53.

Lindsay SW, Thomas CJ. Mapping and estimating the population at risk from lymphatic filariasis in Africa. Trans Roy Soc Trop Med Hyg. 2000;94:37–45.

MacFee WF. Filarial lymphatic varix of the breast. New York Surg Soc Philadelphia Acad. 1925;135–9.

Manson-Bahr PEC, Apted FIC. Filariases. In: Manson's tropical diseases. 18th ed. London: Bailliere Tindal; 1982. p. 148–80.

Michael E, Bundy DAP. Global mapping of lymphatic filariasis. Parasitol Today. 1997;13:472–6.

Michael E, Grenfell BT, Bundy DAP. The association between microfilaremia and disease in lymphatic filariasis. Proc Roy Soc Lond, Series B. 1994;256:33–40.

Michael E, Bundy DAP, Grenfell BT. Reassessing the global prevalence and distribution of lymphatic filariasis. Parasitol. 1996;112:409–28.

Michael E, Simonsen PE, Malecela M, et al. Transmission intensity and the immuno-epidemiology of bancroftian filariasis in East Africa. Parasite Immunol. 2001;23:373–88.

Molyneux D. Lymphatic filariasis (elephantiasis) elimination: a public health success and development opportunity. Filaria J. 2003;2:13.

Okon OE, Iboh CI, Opara KN. Bancroftian filariasis among the Mbembe people in Cross River State. Nigeria J Vector Borne Dis. 2010;47(2):91–6.

Pani SP, Dhanda V. Natural history and dynamics of progression of clinical manifestations of filariasis. In: Tropical disease: Molecular biology and control strategies. 1994. p. 1. Quoted in Epidemiology of lymphatic filariasis with special reference to urogenital manifestations. Pani SP, Kumaraswami V, Das LK. Indian J Urol. 2005;21:44–9.

Pani SP, Srividya A. Clinical manifestations of bancroftian filariasis with special reference to lymphedema grading. Indian J Med Res. 1992;102:114–8.

Pani SP, Kumaraswami V, Das LK. Epidemiology of lymphatic filariasis with special reference to urogenital manifestations. Indian J Urol. 2005;21:44–9.

Park K. Lymphatic filariasis. In: Park's textbook of preventive and social medicine. 19th ed. Jabalpur: M/s Banarasidas Bhanot Publishers; 2007. p. 220.

Ramaiah KD, Ramu K, Vijaya Kumar KN, Guyatt H. Epidemiology of acute filarial episodes caused by Wuchereria bancrofti infection in two rural villages in Tamil Nadu, South India. Trans Roy Soc Trop Med Hyg. 1996;90:639.

Rath K, Neth N, Mishra et al. Knowledge and perceptions about lymphatic filariasis: a study during the programme to eliminate lymphatic filariasis in an urban community of Orissa, India. Tropical Biomedicine. 2006;23:156–62.

Sasa M. Human filariasis. A global survey of epidemiology and control. Tokyo: University of Tokyo Press; 1976. p. 336.

Sebasan S, Palaniyandi M, Das PK, Michael E. Mapping of lymphatic filariasis in India. Ann Trop Med Parasitol. 2000;94:591–606.

Steel C, Nutman TB. CTLA-4 in filarial infections implication for a role in diminished T-cell reactivity. J Immunol. 2003;179:1930–8.

Utzinger J, Bergquist R, Olveda R, Zhou XN. Important helminth infections in Southeast Asia diversity, potential for control and prospects for elimination. Adv Parasitol. 2010;72 C:1–30.

World Health Organization. Global program to eliminate lymphatic filariasis: progress report for 2004. Wkly Epidemiol Rec. 2005;80:202–12.

World Health Organization. Bridging the gaps. Geneva: World Health Report; 1995.

Yimer M, Hailu T, Mulu W, Abera B. Epidemiology of elephantiasis with special emphasis on podoconiosis in Ethiopia: a literature review. J Vector Borne Dis. 2015;52:111–5.

Etiology 3

Lymphatic filariasis is an ancient parasitic disease caused by three filarial tissue nematodes of the Filarioides family, i.e., *Wuchereria bancrofti*, *Brugia malayi*, and *Brugia timori* which are transmitted from person to person contact by mosquitoes. The *Brugia timori* infection is least common and does not occur in India. The discussion here is confined to the first two types of nematodes which are the cause of filariasis in most of the countries in the World (Edesen 1962).

3.1 *Wuchereria bancrofti*

- *Adult worm* – The adult worms are long, hair-like, creamy white, transparent and have a filiform shape with both ends tapering (Figs. 3.1, 3.2, and 3.3).
  The male worm measures 2.5–4 cm × 0.1 mm, and the female 8–10 cm × 0.2–0.3 mm. The posterior end of male worm is curved ventrally and has two spicules of unequal length, but that of female worm is straight. The male and female worms remain coiled together and it is difficult to separate them.
  The female worm is viviparous (nematodes which give birth to larvae) and gives birth to ensheathed embryos (microfilariae) in the lymphatics from where they find their way into the blood (microfilaremia).
- *Microfilariae* – The microfilariae are colorless and transparent microworms having a blunt head and pointed tail. Each microfilaria measures 245 × 295 μm × 7.5–10 μm and covered by a hyaline sheath which is longer (359 μm) than the length of microfilaria. It can move both ways inside the sheath. The central axis of microfilaria has somatic cells or nuclei appearing as granules which are absent at places. The tail tip does not have nuclei (Fig. 3.4).

T.C. Goel, A. Goel, *Lymphatic Filariasis*, DOI 10.1007/978-981-10-2257-9_3

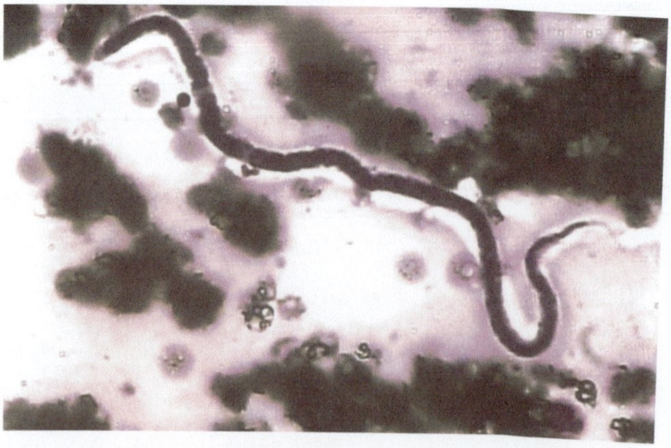

Fig. 3.1 Adult filarial worm in pleural fluid (Courtesy – Dr Miti Gupta)

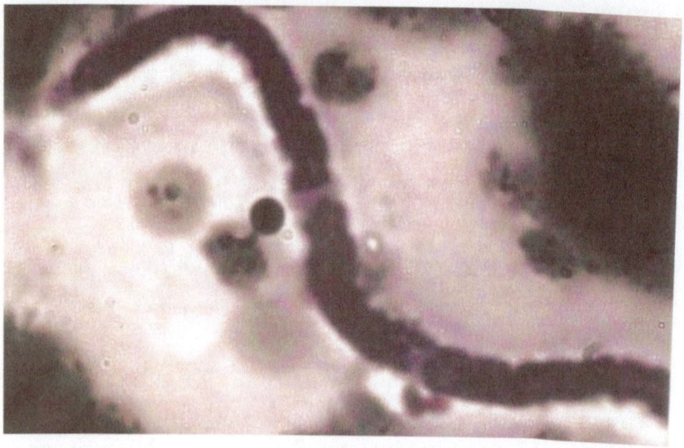

Fig. 3.2 Adult filarial worm in pleural fluid (Courtesy – Dr Miti Gupta) (magnified picture)

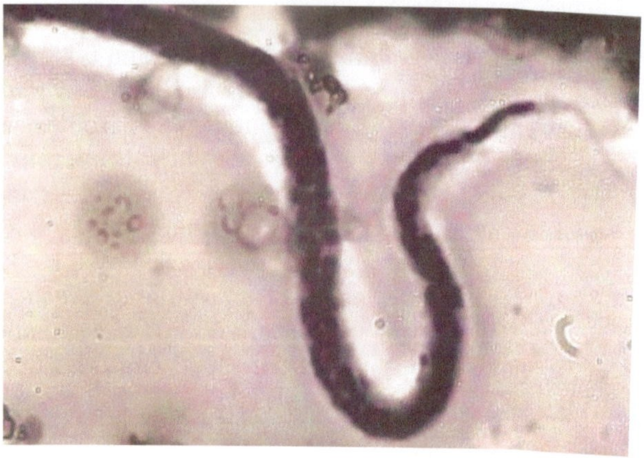

Fig. 3.3 Filarial worm in pleural fluid (Courtesy – Dr Miti Gupta) (magnified picture)

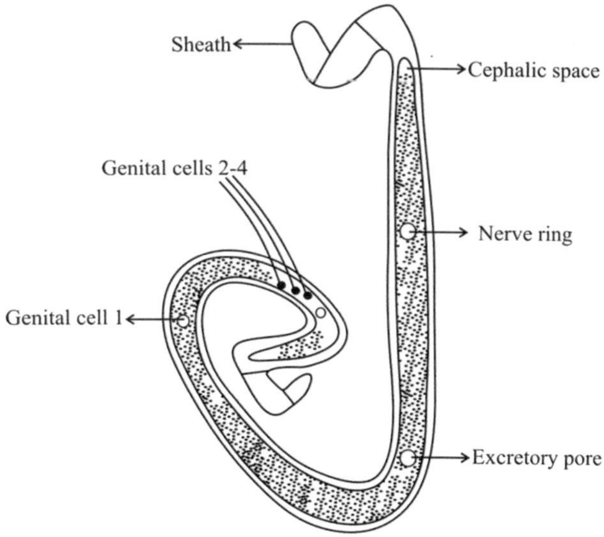

Fig 3.4 Microfilaria of *Wuchereria bancrofti*

3.2 *Brugia malayi*

- **Adult worm** – The adult worm looks like adult *W. bancrofti*, but it is smaller in size. A male brugian worm measures 13×23 mm×70–80 μm while the female measures 43–55 mm×130–170 μm.
- **Microfilariae** – They are smaller in size as compared to bancroftian microfilariae, measuring 177–230 μm×6 μm. The cephalic space is longer and the nuclear column appears blurred in Geimsa-stained films. The tail tip has two discrete nuclei, one at the extreme tip of the tail and other midway between the tip and the posterior column of the nuclei. It possesses secondary kinks and carries double stylets at the anterior end (Fig. 3.5).

3.2.1 Location of Adult Worms

Wuchereria bancrofti – The preferred site where the adult parasites live is the dilated scrotal lymphatics (Fig. 3.6a, b) in adult men or even in boys as seen by ultrasonography by the presence of "filarial dance sign" (Noroes et al. 1996; Dreyer et al. 1999a, b). Other common locations in women and children are breast and larger lymph vessels and lymph nodes draining the lower and upper extremities.

Kinmonth (1982) described a case of Bihari Indian aged 42 years who had filariasis of the scrotum and recurrent inguinal hernia. At time of surgery for hernia, it was found that the spermatic cord lymphatics were enormously dilated and undergoing spontaneous contractility at 10- to 20-s intervals. Through the walls of lymphatics lying in clear lymph were seen motile adult filarial worms.

Fig 3.5 Microfilaria of *Brugia malayi*

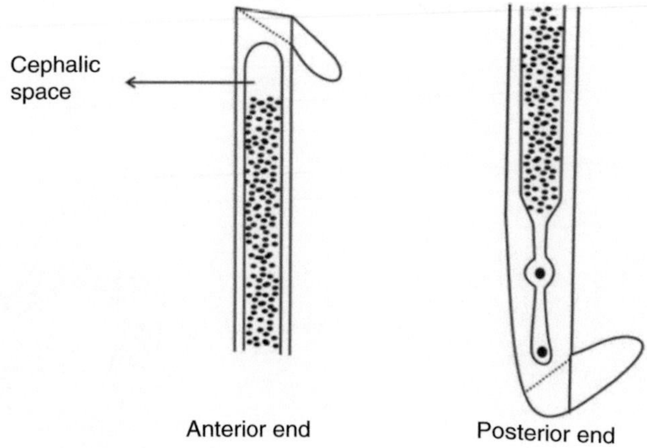

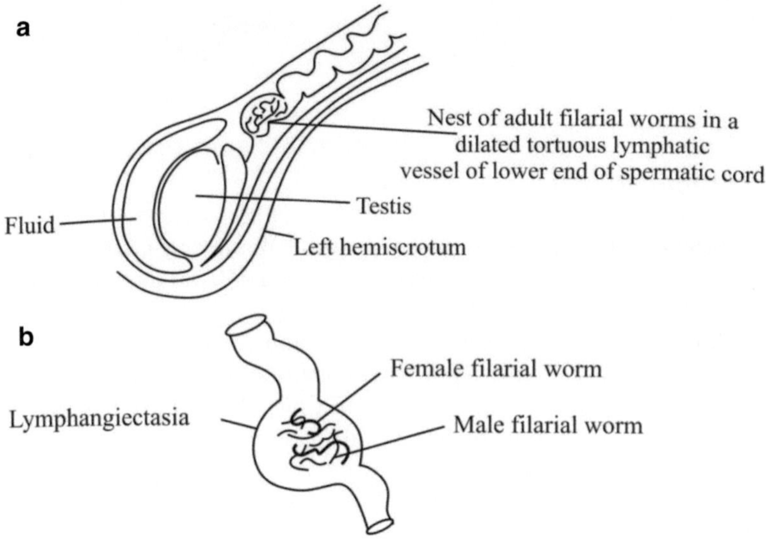

Fig. 3.6 (**a**) Adult filarial worms in a dilated lymphatic in the lower end of spermatic cord. (**b**) Nest of adult worms with female which is larger with many males which are smaller in a lymphangiectatic vessel of lower end of spermatic cord responsible for filarial dance sign seen in Doppler ultrasonography (location of microfilariae)

The dilating effect on lymphatics appears to be due to mechanical obstruction and to destruction of the valves rather than to any hypothetical paralyzing effect of toxins from the worms. The walls of vessels have healthy hypertrophied muscle and were contractile (Kinmonth 1982).

Brugia malayi – The adult worms as detected by ultrasonography live in the lymphatics of inguinal and axillary regions in children (Shenoy et al. 2007). They live in these sites for 6–8 years or more.

3.2.2 Location of Microfilariae

They live in blood most of the time but crowd the visceral capillaries during the day in nocturnal periodicity types.

3.2.3 Intermediate Host

W. bancrofti The female mosquitoes of genera Culex, Anopheles, and Aedes are the intermediate hosts of *W. bancrofti*. *Culex quinquefasciatus* is the most significant vector to transmit bancroftian infection in more than 50 % cases of filariasis. Anopheles species are the primary vectors of transmission in rural areas, which transmit malarial infection also.

B. malayi It is transmitted by Mansonia, Anopheles, and Aedes. In India, the intermediate hosts include *M. annulifera*, *M. indiana*, *M. uniformis*, and *Anopheles barbirostris*.

The differences between two main types of filarial parasites are given in the following Table 3.1

Table 3.1 Differences between two main types of filarial parasites

Features	*Wuchereria bancrofti*	*Brugia malayi*
Microfilaria		
Sheath	Sheathed	Sheathed
Appearance	Gracefully sweeping curves	Stiff with secondary multiple kinks
	Head and tail well separated	Folded with head close to tail
Measurement	245–295 μm × 7.5–10 μm	177–230 μm × 6 μm
Tail	Tapers to a point	Bulbous at the tip
	No terminal nuclei	Two terminal nuclei present
Cephalic space	As long as broad	Twice as long as broad
Body nuclei	Well-defined, spaced, and can be easily counted	Blurred, intermingled, and cannot be easily counted
Stylets	One	Two
Excretory cell	Small, near excretory pore	Large, far behind excretory pore
Periodicity	Usually nocturnal (10 pm – 2 am)	Nocturnal (partial), usually day time
Habitat	Blood	Blood
Adult worms		
Appearance	Long, thread-like, creamy white in color, closely intertwined	Long, thread-like, white in color, closely coiled together

(continued)

Table 3.1 (continued)

Features	*Wuchereria bancrofti*	*Brugia malayi*
Habitat	Adults in lymphatics and lymph nodes	Adults in lymphatics and lymph nodes
	Typically below the diaphragm	Typically above diaphragm
Male	2.5–4 cm × 0.1 mm	2–4 cm × 70–80 μm
Female	8–10 cm × 0.2–0.3 mm	7–10 cm × 130–170 μm
Intermediate host	*Culex quinquefasciatus*	Mansonia
	Anopheles	Anopheles
	Aedes	Aedes
Time taken for development in mosquito	10–11 days	6–8 days
Reservoir of infection	Human carriers only	Human carriers
		Cats, dogs, monkeys, and some birds, e.g., crows
Distribution	Widely distributed in tropics and subtropics of both hemispheres and on pacific islands	South India, Srilanka, Southeast Asia, South China, Northern coastal areas of China and South Korea
Urban/rural	Predominantly urban	Predominantly rural
Clinical features		
Elephantiasis		
Lower limb	+ + + may be total	+ + + below the knee
Upper limb	+ may be total	+ + below the elbow
Genitalia	+ +	Rare and not so gross
Hydrocele	+	–
Lymph scrotum	+	–
Chyluria	+	–
Pulmonary changes	Less common	Eosinophilia, pulmonary changes similar to those in bronchial asthma
Susceptibility to DEC	Susceptible	More susceptible, especially the adult worms

3.2.4 Life Cycle

The life cycle of the filarial worms is completed in two hosts – the man who is the definitive host and the mosquito who is the intermediate host (Fig. 3.7).

The adult worms live in the lymph nodes and afferent lymphatics of man, mate, and produce microfilariae. From the lymphatic system, they enter into blood circulation to produce microfilaremia. The female worms can release microfilariae for up to 5 years (Chandy et al. 2011).

The microfilariae in persons with microfilaremia are sucked up by a female mosquito when it has its blood meal. There should be at least 15 microfilariae in a drop

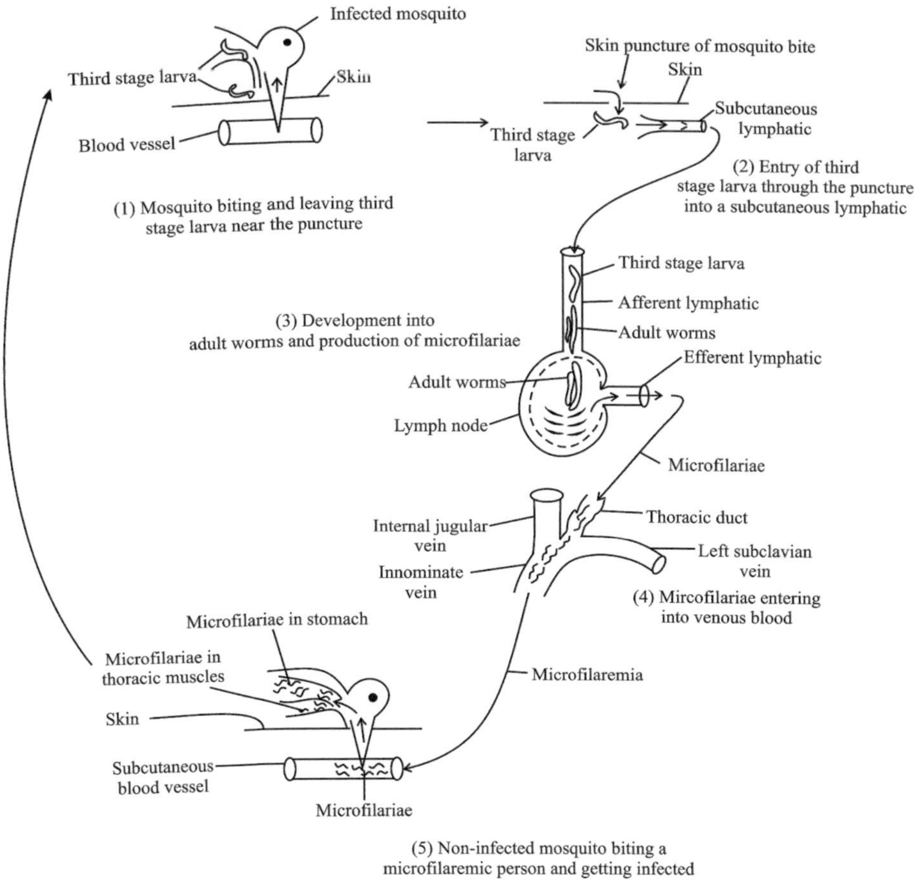

Fig. 3.7 Life cycle of filarial parasite

of blood in order to infect the mosquito. But if it is 100 or more, it kills the mosquito. The microfilariae complete their development in the mosquito to produce infective larvae.

Amaral et al. (1994) observed actively moving adult worms in dilated and tortuous lymphatic vessels by ultrasonography ("filarial dance sign").

3.2.4.1 Life Cycle in Mosquito

After entry with blood meal into the stomach of the mosquito, the microfilariae cast off their sheath in 2–6 h. They penetrate the stomach wall and reach the thoracic muscles in 4–17 h. Here they rest and grow in three stages.

First-stage larva – In the next 2 days, the slender snake-like organism changes to a thick, short, sausage-shaped (sausage larva) form with a short spiky "tail" measuring 124–250 μ × 10–7 μ.

Second-stage larva – In the next 3–7 days, the larva grows rapidly and moults (sheds its cuticle) once or twice. At the end of this stage, it measures 255–300 μ × 15–30 μ.

Third-stage larva – On 10–11th day, the metamorphosis is completed, i.e., the tail atrophies to a mere stump and the digestive system, body cavity, and the genital organs are fully developed. The larva now measures 140 × 200 μ × 18–23 μ. At this stage, it is infective to man and enters the proboscis sheath of mosquito on or about the 14th day. Due to their significant size, a mosquito carries only a limited number of infective larvae (Maizels et al. 1991). Hence, exposure to infective larvae must be intense and prolonged for the infection to occur (Ottesen 1993).

One microfilaria gives rise to one infective larva, as there is no multiplication in the vector. There may be several larvae remaining coiled up near the proboscis of the mosquito for an opportunity to infect man.

The larval development of *W. bancrofti* in mosquito is completed in 10–20 days (average 15 days) and of *B. malayi* in 6–8 days. This period is known as extrinsic incubation period. It depends upon the atmospheric temperature and the humidity and the species of mosquito.

3.2.4.2 Life Cycle in Man

When an infected mosquito bites a man, the third-stage larvae in its proboscis sheath are deposited near the puncture site. After the mosquito pulls out its proboscis, the larvae enter through the puncture or penetrate the skin on their own. The larvae are too big to pass through the proboscis. The minimum number of L3 (stage 3) larvae required to successfully transmit infection is not known. However, it is estimated that an average resident in an endemic area is exposed to 50–300 L3 larvae per year (Hati et al. 1989).

After entry into the tissues, they enter into the lymphatic system or are carried away by interstitial fluid to the ilio-inguinal lymphatics and nodes, as the lower extremity is the commonest site of mosquito bite. The third stage larvae prefer to reside in the lymphatics of spermatic cord where they form nests. Within lymphatics and lymph nodes, the L3 larvae undergo moulting to form L4 larvae. It takes about 7–10 days for both *W. bancrofti* and *B. malayi* to become L4 larvae. The L4 larvae have one more moulting to form adult worms. It occurs in about 4–6 weeks after L3 entry in *B. malayi*, and after several months in *W. bancrofti* (Cross et al. 1979; Ash and Schacher 1971), and then they become mature in 5–18 months. The adult worms take permanent residence in afferent lymphatics of the cortical sinuses of the lymph nodes. Male fertilizes the female who gives birth to as many as 50,000 microfilariae per day by viviparous reproduction, which enter the blood circulation through the thoracic duct. Thus the cycle is completed.

The time interval between the inoculation of L3 larvae and the first appearance of detectable microfilariae in the blood is known as "patent period" and the development of microfilariae from adult worms is known as patency. It varies from 8 to 15 days depending on species (Nutman 1991).

The life span of an adult worm is estimated to be about 5–10 years (Vanamail et al. 1989). The life span of bancroftian microfilariae is less than a week.

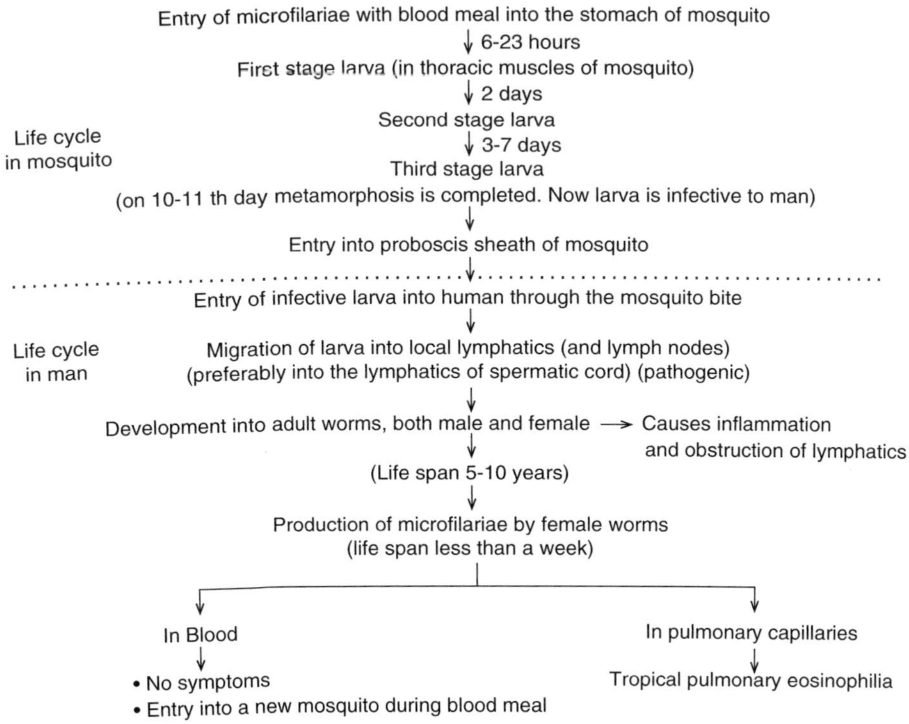

Flow Chart 3.1 Showing life cycle of a filarial parasite

Manson-Bahr (1960) described bancroftian filarial infection persisting as long as 12 years (Kinmonth 1982).

Life Cycle of *Brugia malayi* The life cycle of this parasite is same as that of *W. bancrofti*. The larval development is completed in 6–8 days, and it takes about 7 months for the larva to become adult after entry into man.

Summary of Life Cycle A microfilaria is born in man, grows in a mosquito into an infective larva, revisits another human host, matures, reproduces microfilariae, and dies. The life cycle of a filarial parasite is given in the following Flow Chart 3.1.

3.2.5 Endosymbiont – Wolbachia

Endosymbiont is a parasite that lives inside another parasite in symbiosis. Most of the filarial parasites infecting men are infected with a bacterial endosymbiont, Wolbachia which is an alfa-proteobacteria related to Rickettsia, Erlichia, and Anaplasma and is maternally inherited. The genome of filarial parasites is 1.1 Mb long. The brugian filarial endosymbiont has been fully sequenced (Ware et al. 2002).

Wolbachia is found in all life cycle stages of filarial parasite and is essential for adult worm viability and fertility, and larval development in men (Taylor and Hoerauf 1999). Hence, one of the modern method to treat filarial infection is to kill this bacteria by administering doxycycline.

3.2.6 Reservoirs of Infection

The man is the only source of infection of *W. bancrofti* and the periodic forms of *B. malayi*. The continuity of infection is maintained by interhuman transmission.

Cats, dogs, monkeys, and some birds, e.g., crows, may serve as a reservoir of infection of some forms of *B. malayi*.

3.2.7 Periodicity

The microfilariae are not present in the blood all the time. The periodicity refers to the time of the day when the microfilariae are most prevalent in the blood (Chandy et al. 2011). They appear in blood in good numbers depending upon the biting habits of transmitting mosquito. Accordingly, the filarial infection is of three types:

1. *Periodic infection* – In this type, there is a definite peak in the microfilarial count in the peripheral blood at the same time in 24 h while during the rest of the day the microfilariae are almost absent (or markedly reduced). The differences between the maximum and minimum count is often more than 100-fold. The periodic infection is of two types:
   (a) *Nocturnal periodicity* – Here the peak occurrence of microfilariae in peripheral blood occurs between 10 pm and 1.00 am at night (Dreyer et al. 1996c) and scarce during the day. It is most marked with bancroftian infection. The peak microfilaria rates are usually found in teenagers and young adults with the reduction of rates in older individuals which is likely to be correlated with acquisition of immunity (de Almeida and Freedman 1999).
   (b) *Diurnal periodicity* – It is the occurrence of maximum number of microfilaria in the blood during the day. The vectors of this parasite bite mainly during the day.

   When not in peripheral circulation, the microfilariae are found primarily in the capillaries and blood vessels of the lungs. The mechanism of filarial periodicity is not known. It may be adaptation to the biting habits of the transmitting vector as most of the mosquitoes bite at night. The other possible factors to which the periodicity is etiologically related include light and darkness, activity of the host, size of microfilariae, and vagal activity.

   The periodicity may be changed by reversing the sleeping and waking habits of the host. The reversal may take up to a week to complete.

2. *Subperiodic or nocturnally subperiodic infection* – In this type of periodicity, the microfilariae are present in the blood throughout the day but reach at maximal levels in the afternoon.
3. *Nonperiodic infection* – In this type, the microfilariae circulate at somewhat constant level during the day and night. In this infection, the mosquito bites mainly during the day.

It is interesting to note that microfilariae behave not as foreign material passively circulating in blood but as living organisms like fish in water which may in some measure actively choose its own favorable environment.

References

Amaral F, Dreyer G, Figueredo-Silva J, et al. Live adult worms detected by ultrasonography in human Bancroftian filariasis. Am J Trop Med Hyg. 1994;50(6):753–7.

Ash LR, Schacher JF. Early life cycle and larval morphogenesis of Wuchereria bancrofti in the jird, Mariones unguiculatus. J Parasitol. 1971;57:1043–51.

Chandy A, Thakur AS, Singh MP, Manigauha A. A review of neglected tropical diseases: filariasis. Asian Pac J Trop Med. 2011;4:581–6.

Cross JH, Partono F, et al. Experimental transmission of Wuchereria bancrofti to monkeys. Am J Trop Med Hyg. 1979;28:56–66.

de Almeida AB, Freedman DO. Epidemiology and immunopathology of bancroftian filariasis. Microbes Infect. 1999;1:1015–22.

Dreyer G, Noroes J, Addiss D, Santos A, Medeiros Z, Figueredo-Silva J. Bancroftian filariasis in a pediatric population: an ultrasonographic study. Trans Roy Soc Trop Med Hyg. 1999a;93: 633–6.

Dreyer G, Santos A, et al. Proposed panel of diagnostic criteria, including the use of ultrasound to refine the concept of 'endemic normals' in lymphatic filariasis. Trop Med Int Health. 1999b; 4:575–9.

Dreyer G, Pimentael A, Medeiros Z, Béliz F, Moura I, Coutinho A, de Andrade LD, Rocha A, da Silva LM, Piessens WF. Studies on the periodicity and intravascular distribution of Wuchereria bancrofti microfilariae in paired samples of capillary and venous blood from Recife Brazil. Trop Med Intl Health. 1996c;1:264–72.

Edesen JF. The epidemiology and treatment of infection due to Brugia malayi. Bull WHO. 1962;27(4–5):529–41.

Hati AK, Chandra G, Bhattacharya A, et al. Annual transmission potential of bancroftian filariasis in an urban and a rural area of West Bengal, India. Am J Trop Med Hyg. 1989; 40(4):365–7.

Kinmonth JB. The lymphatics. 2nd ed. London: Edward Arnold; 1982.

Maizels RM, Kurniawan A, Selkirk ME, Yazdanbakhsh M. Immune responses to filarial parasites. Immunol Lett. 1991;30:249–54.

Manson-Bahr P. Tropical diseases. 15th ed. London: Cassell; 1960.

Noroes J, Addiss D, Amaral F, Coutinho A, Medeiros Z, Dreyer D. Occurrence of adult Wuchereria bancrofti in the scrotal area of men with microfilaremia. Trans Roy Soc Trop Med Hyg. 1996;90:55–6.

Nutman TB. Experimental infection of humans with filariae. Rev Infect Dis. 1991;13: 1018–22.

Ottesen EA. Filarial infections. Infect Dis Clin North Am. 1993;7:619–33.

Shenoy RK, Suma TK, Kumaraswami V, Padma S, Rahmah N, Abhilash G, Ramesh C. Doppler ultrasonography detects adults worm nests in lymph vessels in children with brugian filariasis. Ann Trop Med Parasitol. 2007;101:173–80.

Taylor MJ, Hoerauf A. Wolbachia bacteria in filarial nematodes. Parasitol Today. 1999;15(11): 437–42.

Vanamail P, Subramaniam S, et al. Estimation of age-specific rates of acquisition and loss of Wuchereria bancrofti infection. Trans R Soc Trop Med Hyg. 1989;83:689–93.

Ware J, Moran L, et al. Sequencing and analysis of a 63 kb bacterial artificial chromosome insert from Wolbachia endosymbiont of human filarial parasite Brugia malayi. Int J Parasitol. 2002;32:159–66.

4 Lymphatic System

As filariasis is a disease of the lymphatic system, it is important to know its anatomy and physiology. The adult filarial worms live in the lymphatics and lymph nodes and produce all its clinical manifestations residing in them.

4.1 History

Erasistratus in Alexandria, more than 2000 years ago, described the lymphatic system for the first time. In the late eighteenth century, William Hunter described the physiology of lymphatic system. Henry Starling studied the hydrostatic and hemodynamic forces regulating the movement of fluid across the capillaries (Homer-Vanniasinkam and Russell 2013).

4.2 Embryology

The lymphatic system develops from lymphatic endothelial cells which are derived from embryonic veins in the jugular and perimesonephric areas from where they migrate to form the primary lymph sacs and plexus. The transcription, e.g., Prox 1 and growth factors, e.g., vascular endothelial growth factors (VEGFs) are required for their development.

During embryonic life four lymph sacs develop at 6–7 weeks gestation as cystic spaces one on each side of neck and one in each groin. These sacs enlarge and develop communications with the loco-regional lymphatics. The groin lymph sacs drain the lymph of lower limbs and abdomen into cisterna chyli from where it drains via the thoracic duct into the left internal jugular vein at its confluence with the left subclavian vein. The lymph from right half of head and neck, right upper extremity and right hemithorax is drained by right lymphatic duct into the confluence of right internal jugular and right subclavian veins. In addition there are additional lympho-venous shunts at the level of lymph nodes and around major veins, e.g., jugular, subclavian and iliac veins.

T.C. Goel, A. Goel, *Lymphatic Filariasis*, DOI 10.1007/978-981-10-2257-9_4

4.3 Anatomy

The lympahtics are present all over the body and accompany the veins except in cortical bone, central nervous system, and eyeball although the latter two systems possess cerebrospinal fluid and aqueous humor, respectively. Other structures where the lymphatics are not found include epidermis, cornea, cartilage, tendon, and muscle (Pipinos and Baxter 2012).

The dermis is very rich in lymphatics that it is not possible to puncture the dermis without puncturing a dermal lymphatic (McMaster 1937). This fact is important to understand the mechanism of entry of third-stage larvae in the lymphatics following mosquito bite.

The lymphatic system consists of lymphatic channels and lymph nodes which are being described here.

4.4 Lymphatic Capillaries

They develop in the interstitial fluid space from specialized endothelialized capillaries (initial lymphatics) or nonendothelialized channals, e.g., space of Disse in the liver. The initial lymphatics are much larger (50 μm) and blind-ended. They permit the entry of molecules up to 1000 kDa size (even cells and microbes) as the basement membrane is fenestrated, tenuous, or even absent and the endothelium has intracellular and intercellular pores. They are attached to interstitial matrix by filaments (4–6 nm) tethering the interstitial matrix to the endothelial cells. In the resting state, the initial lymphatics are collapsed. When the interstitial fluid volume and pressure rise, the initial lymphatics and their pores are kept open by these filaments to facilitate interstitial fluid (ISF) drainage.

4.5 Terminal (Collecting) Lymphatics

Many initial lymphatics drain into terminal lymphatics which have bicuspid valves and endothelial cells having actin, a contractile protein. Larger terminal lymphatics are surrounded by smooth muscle fibers and have valves that divide the lymphatics into segments (lymphangions) which contract sequentially to propel lymph into the lymph trunks (Fig. 4.1).

4.6 Lymph Trunks

Many terminal lymphatics join to form lymph trunks which are of two types – superficial trunks that form lymph bundles of various sizes that are located within strips of fatty tissue along with major superficial veins, and deep trunks accompanying the main neurovascular bundles. The deep lymphatics transport only about 10 % of lymph of the extremities. There are only a few communications among the

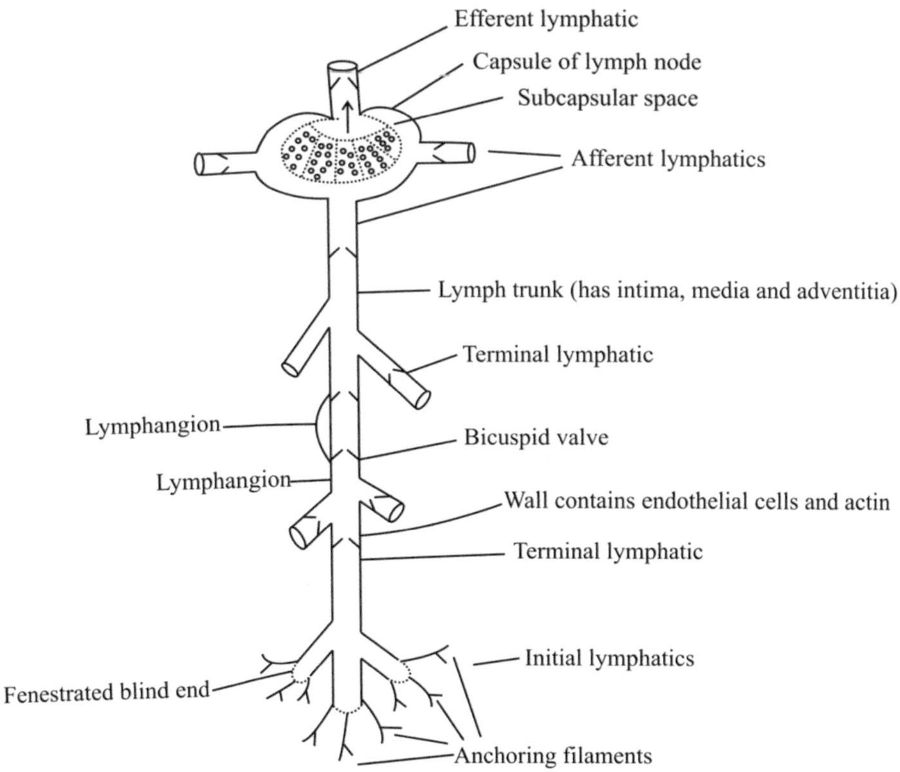

Fig. 4.1 Anatomy of lymphatics

superficial and deep lymphatics with direction of flow from superficial to deep lymphatics (Handley 1908; Manokaran 2005).

The lymph trunks have a structure similar to that of veins, i.e., a single layer of endothelial cells lying on a basement membrane. External to this layer, there is media consisting of smooth muscle cells which has sympathetic, parasympathetic, and sensory nerve endings. Then there is a layer of adventetia of fibrous connective tissue.

4.7 Cisterna Chyli

It is a 5–7-cm-long saccular dilatation of the beginning of thoracic duct situated in front of first and second lumbar vertebral body immediately to the right of back of abdominal aorta (Fig. 4.2). It is joined by right and left lumbar trunks and intestinal lymphatic trunks (Williams and Warwick 1980).

The lumbar trunks are formed from the efferent lymphatics from lumbar lymph nodes that receive the lymph from the liver, extremities, the walls and viscera of the

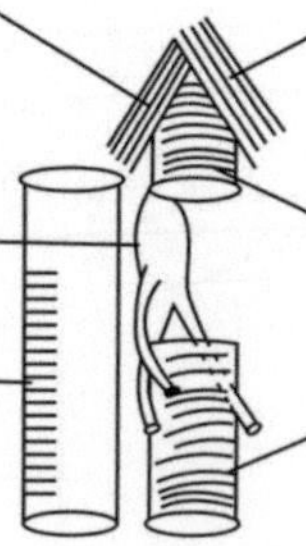

Fig. 4.2 Cisterna chyli

pelvis, the kidneys and adrenals, testes or ovaries, and the deep lymphatics of most of the abdominal wall.

The intestinal lymph trunks comprise the large lymph vessels that receive the lymph from stomach, intestine, pancreas, and spleen and lower and anterior part of liver.

4.8 Thoracic Duct

It is the main lymphatic channel that drains most of the lymph of the body, i.e., the lymph of lower half of body and left half of body above diaphragm. It is a muscular tube (Moncure 1994) of about 18 in. (45 cm) in length and starts from the upper end of cisterna chyli, i.e., lower border of body of 12th thoracic vertebra and enters the thorax through the aortic orifice of diaphragm (Fig. 4.2). It ascends up through the posterior mediastinum between thoracic aorta on the left, azygos vein on the right, and esophagus anteriorly. At the level of fifth thoracic vertebra, it inclines to the left, ascends up by left side of esophagus, and enters the neck where it travels behind the left common carotid artery, left internal jugular vein and left vagus nerve, and anterior to left vertebral vessels, sympathetic trunk, and thyrocervical trunk, and opens in the junction of left internal jugular vein with left subclavian vein at the level of seventh cervical vertebra. Here there is a one-way bicuspid valve (Fig. 4.3). This duct can be visualized by radio-opaque contrast study (Fig. 4.4).

It is segmented by the provision of one-way valves in it. It has multiple connections with the lymphatics of chest and abdomen; hence a single block does not cause chylothorax or chylous ascites.

The normal thoracic duct has intrinsic rhythmic contractility which can be seen at operations in the neck (Kinmonth and Taylor 1956). Later, Kinmonth and Sharpey-Schafer (1959) recorded pressure waves in the normal human thoracic ducts occurring about 4/mt and with amplitudes of 10 mmHg or more. Further, they found that the pressure in the thoracic duct may build up to 50 mmHg if it is obstructed. The high pressures thus obtained have a bearing of the possible opening of lympho-venous shunts under abnormal obstructive situations (Kinmonth 1982). These shunts are not visible in normal persons (Edwards and Kinmonth 1969).

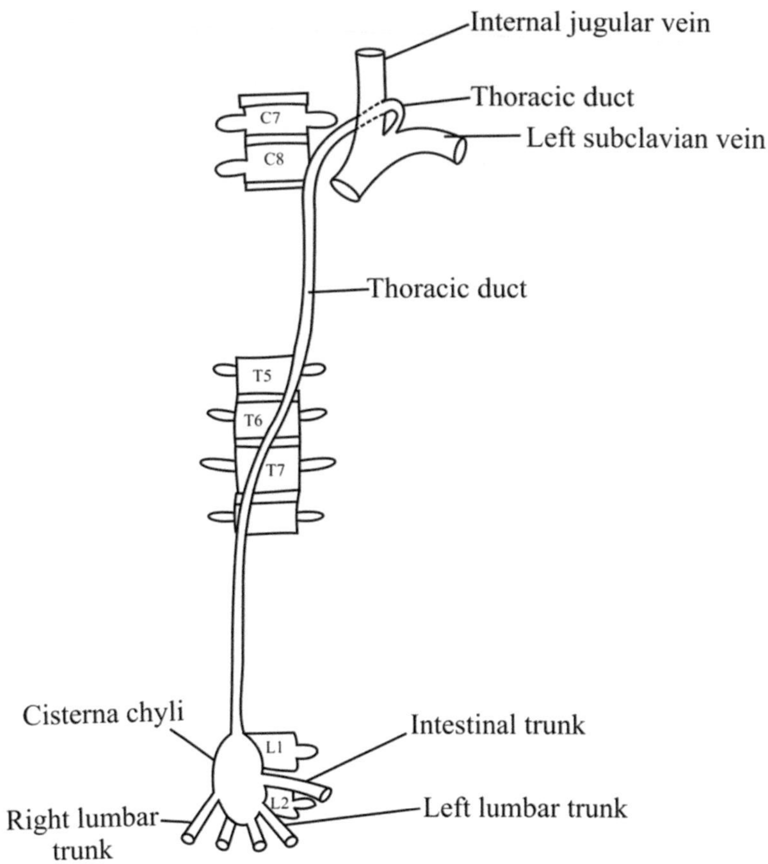

Fig. 4.3 Thoracic duct

4.9 Right Lymphatic Duct

It is present in the root of the neck on the right side and is about 1 cm in length. It receives lymph from right half of head and neck through right jugular trunk, right upper extremity through right subclavian trunk and from right half of thorax and its contents through right bronchomediastinal trunk. It runs along the medial border of scalenus anterior in the root of neck and opens into the junction of right subclavian with right internal jujular vein where there is a bicuspid valve which prevents reflux of blood into the duct (Fig. 4.5).

The anatomy of the lymphatic vascular system is described in the following Flow Chart 4.1:

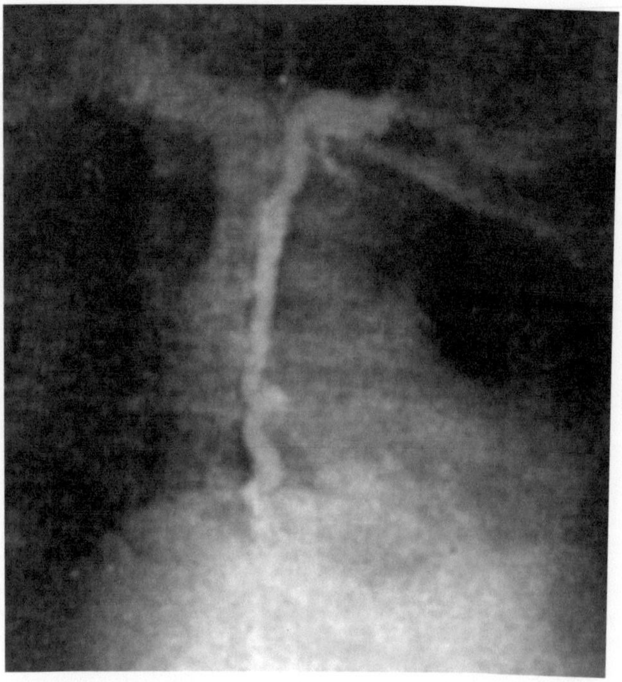

Fig. 4.4 Right oblique view of chest showing opacified thoracic duct

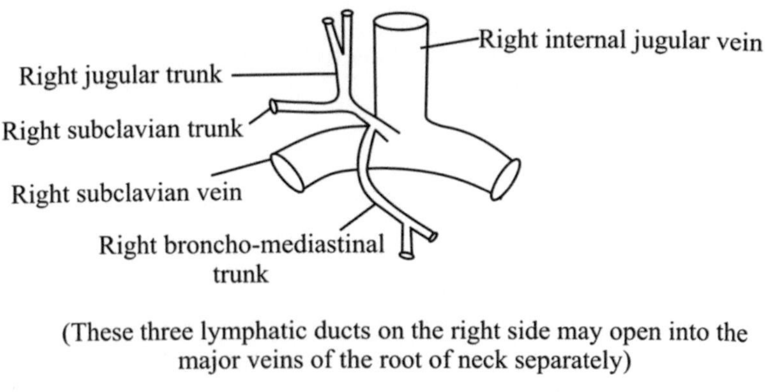

Fig. 4.5 Right lymphatic duct

4.10 Lymph Nodes

The lymph nodes are flattened, ovoid, or reniform structures that vary in size from a pinhead to 2.5 cm or more in diameter. They are situated in the course of lymph vessels so that the lymph passes through them on its way to drain into the

Initial lymphatics at periphery
(blind ended, a little larger than 50 μm)
↓
Terminal lymphatics
(thin wall made of endothelial cells and contractile protein actin,
have bicuspid valves inside to direct the lymph flow)
↓
Lymph trunks along the main vessels
(wall structure similar to that of a vein but thinner than that of vein)

↓ Thoracic duct
(lymph of subdiaphragmatic half of body and left supradiaphragmatic half)
↓
Left jugulo-subclavian venous junction in left side of neck
↘ Systemic blood circulation

↓ Right lymphatic duct
(lymph of right half of head and neck, right upper extremity and right hemithorax
↓
Right jugulo-subclavian venous junction on right side of neck
↙ Systemic blood circulation

Flow Chart 4.1 The lymphatic vascular system

venous circulation (Williams and Warwick 1980). Most of them are located in axilla, inguinal region (groin) and along large vessels of neck, thorax, and abdomen.

The cross-section of a lymph node shows its capsule and a framework of trabeculae and reticular fibers and lymphocytes entangled in it. For descriptive purposes, it can be divided into subcapsular space, cortex, paracortex, and medulla. The capsule is made of connective tissue and attached to the surface only at the hilum. In the subcapsular space, the afferent lymphatics are open from all the directions. They have unidirectional valves which open towards the lymph nodes.

There is a depression on one side called hilum through which enters the supplying artery and comes out the draining vein and efferent lymphatic (Fig. 4.6).

Cortex It occupies the whole of the convexity of the surface except the hilum, and consists of several layers of lymphoid follicles each having a pale germinal center (Last 1963). Each lymphoid follicle has a large collection of lymphocytes. It has a pale center because the lymphocytes here are loosely packed and their nuclei are less dense. The majority of cells are B- and T-lymphocytes (bone and thymus derived), though macrophages are also frequent. The cortex is penetrated by fibrous trabeculae from the capsule which are surrounded by a space continued from subcapsular lymph space.

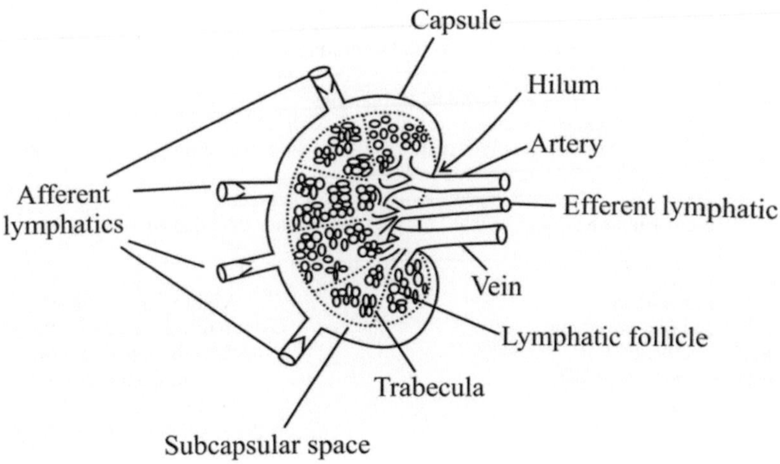

Fig. 4.6 Microanatomy of a lymph node

Medula It consists of a meshwork of trabeculae which reaches the surface at the hilum where the cortex is missing. The artery and vein enter the lymph node through it and ramify along the trabeculae. The lymph of subcapsular space passes through the follicles of cortex and the interstices of medulla to emerge at the hilum by fewer but larger efferent lymphatics (Last 1963). Thus, the lymph from any tissue or organ traverses one or more lymph nodes before it eventually drains into venous blood stream (Williams and Warwick 1980). An efferent lymphatic of one lymph node may become afferent lymphatic of a proximal lymph node.

Paracortex It is an ill-defined zone located between cortex and medulla. It contains T-lymphocytes (Sriram Bhat 2013). It is related to cell-mediated immunity, hence expands when cell-mediated immunity enhancement is needed.

Both cortex and medulla are associated with humoral immunity.

Functions The functions of lymph nodes are production of lymphocytes and antibodies, filteration of tissue fluid of particulate material including bacteria, and reduction of volume of tissue fluid by half.

4.11 Interstitial Fluid (ISF)

The tissues and cells of the body need oxygen, water, and nutrition for their metabolic needs and survival, and they reach them through the arteries into the capillary network (Fig. 4.7). At the arterial end of the capillary, the blood pressure is 32 mmHg and the oncotic pressure of plasma is 25 mmHg. Hence the nutrition-rich (O_2+) fluid comes into the interstitial space due to this pressure difference of 7 mmHg. At the venous end of capillary, the blood pressure is 16 mmHg (and the oncotic pressure of plasma is 25 mmHg). Hence, the interstitial fluid returns into the capillary at

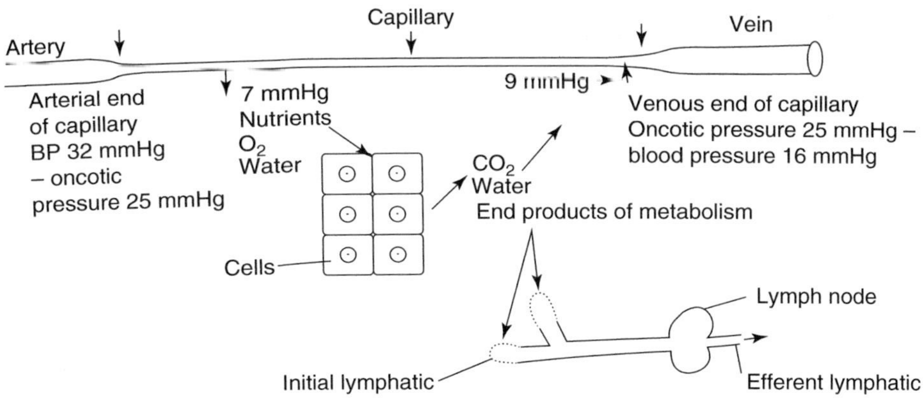

Fig. 4.7 Tissue circulation

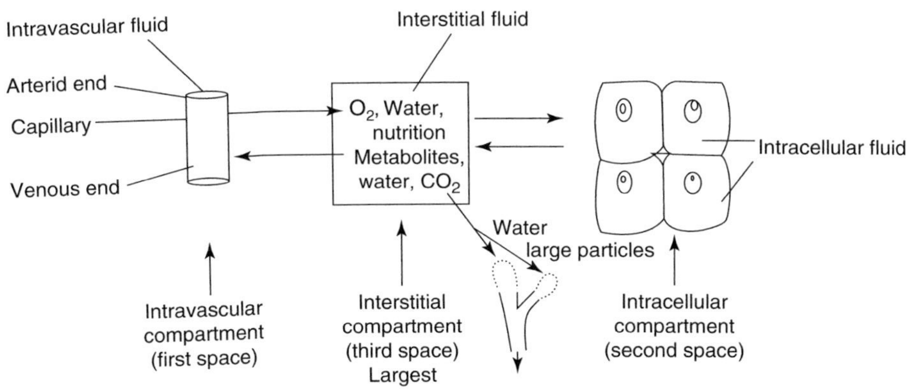

Fig. 4.8 Fluid compartments and tissue perfusion

9 mmHg pressure difference (intracapillary blood pressures pushes the fluid out while the intracapillary oncotic pressure pulls the fluid inside).

There are two sources of water in the interstitial fluid – one is arterial end of capillaries and second is endogenous production from oxidation of glucose. A part of water and large particles which cannot enter the blood capillaries are removed by lymphatics (initial lymphatics) which have large pores (Fig. 4.8).

4.12 Lymph

The term lymph is derived from Latin word lympha which means clear water as it is a clear watery fluid which may be faintly yellow or slightly opalescent. It is collected by the lymphatic capillaries from the interstitial fluid contained in the extracellular extravascular space of various organs and tissues. It has the same constituents as present in the plasma, i.e., electrolytes, protein, and many lymphocytes (Moore 1992).

Chyle It is the lymph draining from the small bowel 2–3 h after a fat-rich meal. It contains emulsified fat, fatty acids, glycerol, aminoacids, and glucose and may be milky. It is drained by lacteals of mesentery into cisterna chyli.

4.13 Physiology (Functions of Lymphatic System)

Although the lymphatic system is not an integral component of the cardiovascular system, it provides a functional and anatomical link between the interstitial fluid compartment and the intravascular compartment, i.e., blood circulation (Fig. 4.8) (Cuschieri and Giles 1995). The lymphatic system has the following functions:

- *Transport of protein-rich interstitial or tissue fluid into the blood circulation through the lymphatico-venous junctions in the neck* – It is the main function of the lymphatic system. The items returned in this manner include water, electrolytes, low-molecular-weight moieties (polypeptides, cytokines, and growth factors), and macromolecules (fibrinogen, albumin, globulins, and coagulation and fibrinolytic factors). Every day 50–100 % of intravascular proteins are filtered into interstitial space and returned to blood.
- *Return of interstitial fluid into the lymphatics* – The source of interstitial fluid (ISF) is arterial blood from where its formation depends upon the balance of the hydrostatic and oncotic pressures between the two compartments (Starling's forces) along with the relative impermeability of blood capillary membrane to molecules above 70 kDa which are removed by lymphatics. In healthy persons, there is a balance between the capillary filtration and drainage of ISF by the lymphatics and venous end of capillaries.
- *Transport of particles* – The large particles in ISF enter the initial lymphatics through the interendothelial openings and intra-endothelial pores such as bacteria, parasites, and even malignant cells. The macrophages actively phagocytose the large particles and transport them.
- In the small intestine, the absorbed resynthesized triglycerides, lipoproteins (chylomicrons), cholesterol, long-chain fatty acids, and fat-soluble vitamins (A. E, D, and K) are carried in the intestinal lymphatics as chyle by the intestinal lymph trunks to cisterna chyli bypassing the liver. The chylomicrons are large particles, hence cannot enter into the capillaries of intestinal villi but can negotiate the lymphatic vessels as the latter do not possess a basement membrane.
- *Transport of lymph* – The resting interstitial pressure is –2 to –6 mm of water and the intralymphatic pressures are positive, even then the prograde lymphatic flow occurs because of the following reasons:
  1. The main driving force in the extremities is the compression of local lymphatics by the contraction of adjacent skeletal muscles pushing the lymph upwards similar to the mechanism of venous return (Cuschieri and Giles 1995).
  2. Contraction and relaxation of lymphangions in a sequence from below up without reflux because of competent valves in the lymphatics – the contraction of lymphangions is enhanced by noradrenaline, serotonin, some prosta-

glandins, and thromboxanes and endothelin 1. The pressures up to 30–50 mmHg have been found in normal lymph trunks. The lymphatics may modify their contractility by producing nitric oxide and other modulators.
3. The negative intra-thoracic pressure together with a positive intra-abdominal pressure pulls/pushes the lymph from abdomen (lower half of body) to thorax. This movement synchronizes with the movements of diaphragm.
4. Negative pressure in neck veins – The venous pressure in the neck veins is always negative. Hence the lymph is sucked into neck veins during diastole of right atrium.
5. Arterial pulsation – The pulsation of arteries in the vicinity of lymphatic trunks may help in the movements of lymph.

- *The other important function of the lymphatic system* is the trafficking of the lymphocytes and monocytes between blood and lymph nodes. This function is crucial to both cellular and humoral immune responses.

4.14 Lymphatics of Inferior Extremity

The commonest or the main target of filarial infection is the lymphatic system of lower extremity; hence, it is being described here.

The lower limb is drained by extensive subcutaneous network of lymphatics into the inguinal and popliteal lymph nodes which are described below.

4.14.1 Inguinal Lymph Nodes

They are situated at the root of thigh below the inguinal ligament (Fig. 4.9). They are classified as described below.

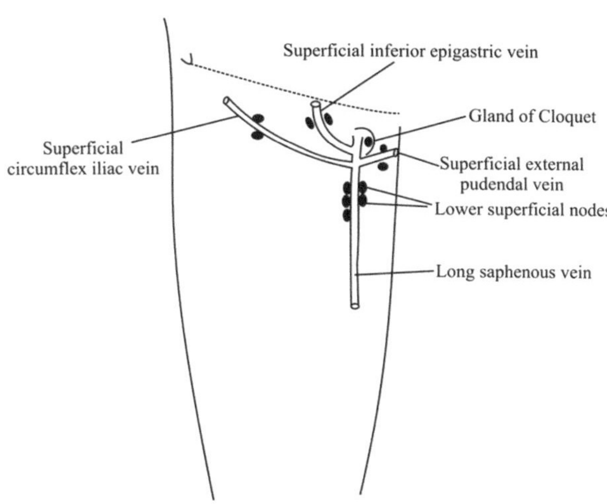

Fig. 4.9 Inguinal lymph nodes

1. Superficial inguinal lymph nodes
   (a) Upper (transverse) group
   (b) Lower (longitudinal) group
2. Deep inguinal lymph nodes

Superficial inguinal lymph nodes They are present in the subcutaneous tissue of the root of thigh superficial to fascia lata (deep fascia). They are arranged in two sets – upper and lower. The lymph nodes of upper group are five to six in number and are situated below and parallel to inguinal ligament. They are located along the superficial circumflex iliac, superficial inferior epigastric, and superficial external pudendal veins from lateral to medial side and named accordingly.

The lower group of superficial lymph nodes are four to five in number and are situated along the terminal part of long saphenous vein.

All the superficial lymph nodes send the lymph to external iliac lymph nodes, some traversing the femoral canal and others passing in front of or lateral to femoral vessels.

Deep inguinal lymph nodes They are usually one to three in number and situated deep to fascia lata of thigh. One is present just below the angle formed by the union of long saphenous vein with the femoral vein, one in the femoral canal (gland of Cloquet), and one lateral to femoral ring. The third one may be absent.

4.14.2 Popliteal Lymph Nodes

They are embedded in the popliteal pad of fat and are six to seven in number. One lymph node is constantly present in the angle formed by the junction of short saphenous vein with the popliteal vein, another is present between the posterior surface of knee joint and popliteal artery. Other lymph nodes are present along the popliteal vessels. They drain along the popliteal vessels to deep inguinal nodes but a few lymphatics may go along the long saphenous vein and drain into superficial inguinal lymph nodes.

The inguinal lymph nodes drain the lower extremity, external genitalia in male (except testis), and external genitalia in female below hymen, lower quadrant of abdomen below the level of umbilicus, gluteal region, perineum, and anus.

The popliteal lymph nodes drain the lateral aspect of leg and foot, especially the heel.

The details of the lymphatics of lower extremity are given below in Table 4.1.

4.15 Lymphatics of Abdomen and Pelvis

After the lymphatics of lower extremity, the lymphatics and lymph nodes of the abdomen and pelvis are next involved in lymphatic filarial infection.

Table 4.1 Lymph nodes of inferior extremity

Name of lymph node group	Number	Drained area
Superficial circumflex iliac nodes (along the vein of same name)	2	Gluteal region, lower lateral half of back
Superficial inferior epigastric (along the vein of same name)	1–2	Lower lateral abdominal quadrant
Superficial external pudendal (along the vein of same name)	1–2	External genitalia except testis in male and ipsilateral half of perineum
Lower (longitudinal) group (along terminal part of long saphenous vein)	4–5	Thigh and leg
Deep inguinal lymph nodes (along the femoral vein)	1–3	Deep tissues of lower extremity, deep to deep fascia
Popliteal lymph nodes (in popliteal fossa along popliteal vessels)	6–7	Leg and foot, especially posterolateral part

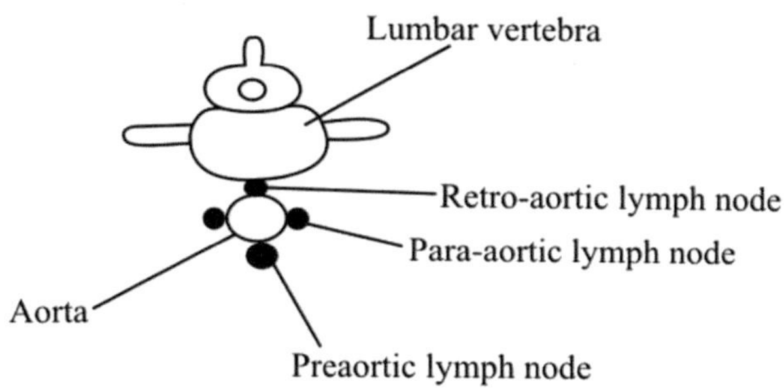

Fig. 4.10 Lymph nodes of abdomen

There are about 800 lymph nodes in the body, out of these about 200 are present in the abdomen and pelvis. They drain all the organs and tissues of these cavities which are drained into the veins of the neck via the thoracic duct. These lymph nodes are described in relation to aorta and its branches; hence they are of three types – preaortic, para-aortic, and retro-aortic (Fig. 4.10).

1. *Preaortic lymph nodes* – They are situated directly anterior to abdominal aorta and drain the subdiaphragmatic part of alimentary canal, hepatobiliary tract including pancreas and spleen. Their efferents form the intestinal trunks which enter the cisterna chyli. They are divided into celiac, superior mesenteric, and inferior mesenteric groups intimately related to the origins of these arteries.
2. *Para-aortic lymph nodes* – The para-aortic or lateral lymph nodes lie on each side of aorta up to its bifurcation in front of medial margin of psoas major, crus of diaphragm and sympathetic trunk, and also by the side of its main divisions in the abdomen and pelvis. They drain these organs – kidneys, suprarenals, testes, ovaries, abdominal ureters, fallopian tubes, and upper part of uterus. The lymphatics from these structures form a lumbar trunk on each side which drains into cisterna chyli.

In the pelvis, these lymph nodes lie by the sides of common iliac, internal iliac, and external iliac vessels and include common iliac, internal iliac, external iliac, and sacral lymph nodes. They drain most of the pelvic viscera and deep pelvic parietes.

3. *Retroaortic lymph nodes* – They are placed behind the aorta and are closely related to para-aortic lymph nodes. They drain the deeper layer of abdominal wall especially the posterior wall. The details of lymphatics of abdomen and pelvis are given in the Flow Chart 4.2 and Table 4.2.

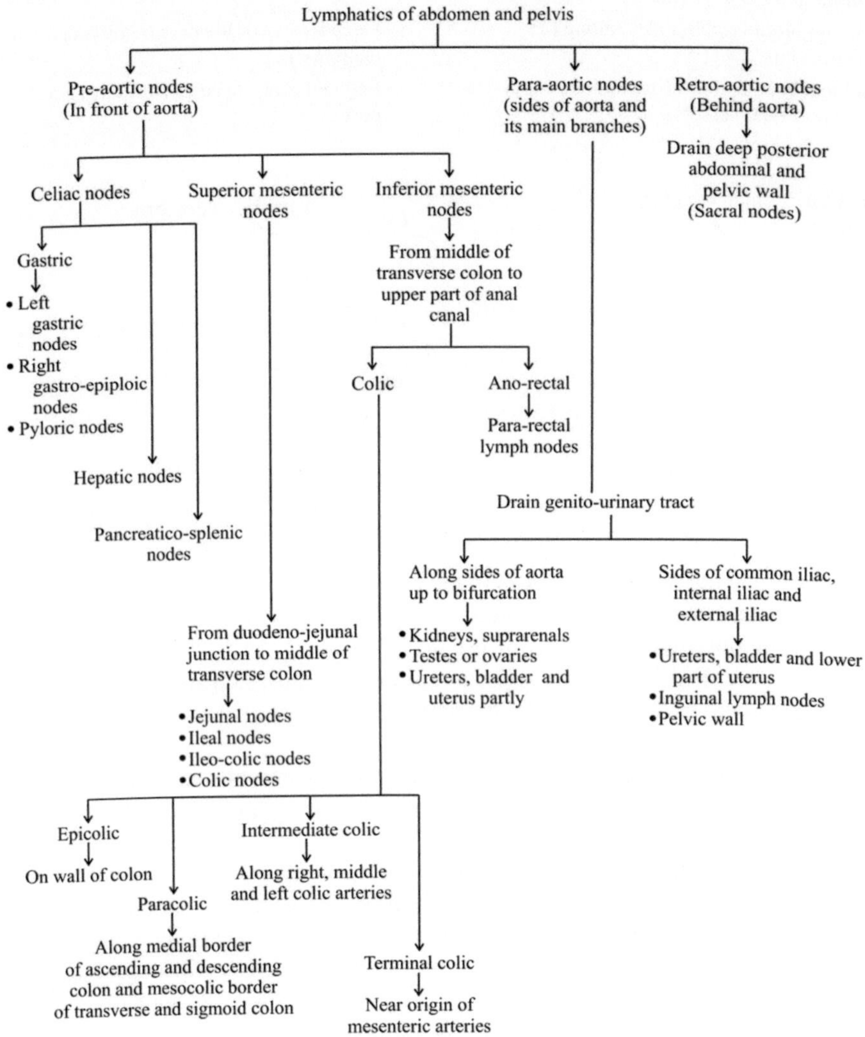

Flow Chart 4.2 Lymphatics of abdomen and pelvis

Table 4.2 Lymph nodes of abdomen and pelvis

Lymph node group	Site	Drained structures	Efferent
Preaortic	In front of aorta, including lymph nodes of mesentery	Subdiaphragmatic part of alimentary canal, hepatobiliary tract including pancreas	Intestinal trunks
Para-aortic	By the side of aorta and its main pelvic branches	Genitourinary tract and suprarenals including kidneys, ureters, testes, ovaries, uterus, and urinary bladder	Lumbar trunks
Retroaortic	Behind the aorta	Deeper abdominal wall, especially deep posterior parietes	Lumbar trunks

4.16 Lymphatics of Upper Extremity Including Breast

The lymphatics of the upper extremity are less commonly involved than those of lower extremity in lymphatic filariasis. All the lymphatics of the upper extremity drain into a terminal group of lymph nodes in the axilla. They are of two types – superficial and deep. The superficial lymphatic vessels lie in the subcutaneous plane along with the superficial veins. The deep vessels are below the deep fascia and accompany the principal vascular and neurovascular bundles of axilla.

4.16.1 Axillary Lymph Nodes

They vary from 20 to 30 in number, are of a relatively large size, and are divided into five groups depending upon their anatomical location.

1. *Anterior or pectoral group* – They are four to five in number and situated along the lower border of pectoralis minor in relation to lateral thoracic vessels. They drain the skin and muscles of anterior and lateral walls of the body above the level of umbilicus, and the central and lateral parts of breast. The efferents of these nodes drain into central and apical group of lymph nodes.
2. *Posterior or subscapular group* – They are six to seven in number and placed on the lower border of posterior axillary fold in relation to subscapular vessels. They drain the skin and muscles of lower part of back of neck and back of trunk up to iliac crest. Their efferents pass to the apical and central axillary nodes.
3. *Lateral group* – They are four to six in number and lie medial and behind the axillary vein. They drain the whole upper extremity except for the part whose lymph vessels accompany the cephalic vein. Their efferents drain partly to central and apical groups and partly to lower deep cervical lymph nodes.

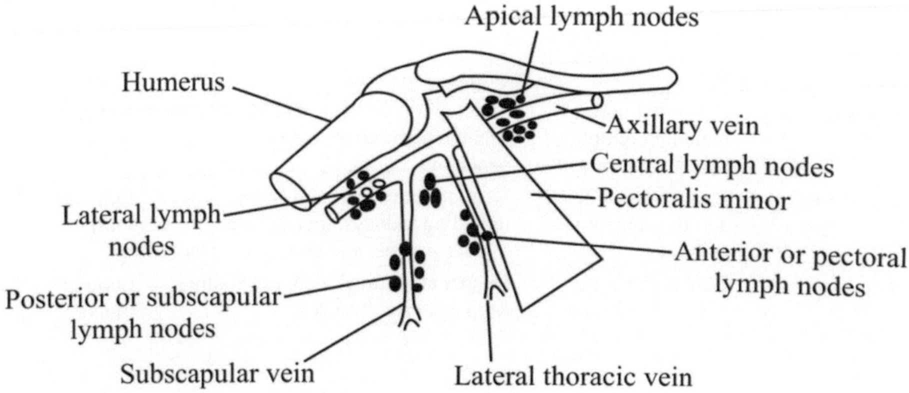

Fig. 4.11 Lymph nodes of right axilla

4. *Central group* – They are three to four large lymph nodes which are embedded in the axillary fat. This group receives afferent from all the three groups described above. Its efferents drain into the apical group.
5. *Apical group* – It consists of 6–12 lymph nodes situated partly posterior to upper part of pectoralis minor and partly above its upper border and extends upwards into the apex of axilla along the medial side of axillary vein. It receives the afferents which accompany the cephalic vein, and also from upper and peripheral part of breast. It drains all other axillary lymph nodes (Fig. 4.11).

The efferents of this group join to form the subclavian trunk which drains directly into the junction of subclavian and internal jugular veins or into the jugular trunk on the right side. On the left side, it opens into the thoracic duct.
A few efferents from this group of lymph nodes go directly to lower deep cervical lymph nodes.

4.16.2 Other Lymph Nodes

1. *Supratrochlear lymph nodes* – They are one to two in number, and are situated on medial side of upper arm above medial epicondyle along the basilic vein. They drain the medial border of forearm and hand. Their efferents pass along the basilic vein to join the deep lymph vessels of axilla.
2. *Infraclavicular lymph nodes* – They are one to two in number situated along cephalic vein in the deltopectoral groove below the clavicle. They drain the upper part of chest wall including the breast. Their efferents penetrate the clavipectoral fascia and drain into apical lymph nodes. Some efferents may pass anterior to clavicle to drain into lower deep cervical (supra-clavicular) nodes.

Lymphatic drainage of breast More than 75 % of lymph of the breast drains into axillary lymph nodes. The superficial parts of breast drain into subareolar plexus of

Sappey and the deep parts drain into the submammary plexus, and both communicate freely through the breast tissue. The submammary plexus lies on the deep fascia of chest wall.

From these two plexuses, the lymph of lateral half of breast drains into the pectoral group of axillary nodes. The upper convexity of breast drains into infraclavicular nodes. The medial convexity communicates across the midline with the submammary plexus of opposite breast and drains through the intercostal spaces (mainly the second, third, and fourth) into the glands along the internal mammary vessels and thence to the mediastinal glands. The inferior convexity communicates through the abdominal parietes with the lymphatics of extraperitoneal areolar tissue.

The lymphatics of upper extremity and breast are summarized in Table 4.3.

Table 4.3 Lymph nodes of upper extremity

Lymph node group	Site	Number	Drained area (afferents)	Drain into (efferents)
Anterior or pectoral group	Lower border of pectoralis minor along lateral thoracic vessels	4–5	Anterior chest wall including breast	Central and apical group of axillary lymph nodes
Posterior or subscapular group	Lower border of posterior axillary fold along subscapular vessels	6–7	Parietes of lower part of back of neck and trunk up to iliac crest	Central and apical group of axillary lymph nodes
Lateral group	Lateral part of axilla medial and behind the axillary vein	4–6	Nearly whole of upper extremity	Central and apical groups and partly to lower deep cervical nodes
Central group	Embedded in axillary fat	3–4 large lymph nodes	All three groups of axillary nodes described above	Apical group
Apical group	Apex of axilla behind upper part of pectoralis minor and above along medial side of axillary vein	6–12	Afferents that accompany cephalic vein, upper and peripheral breast and all axillary nodes	Subclavian trunk or jugular trunk on right side, and thoracic duct on left side A few efferents to lower deep cervical nodes
Supra or epitrochlear nodes	Medial side of upper arm above medial epicondyle along basilic vein	1–2	Medial border of forearm and hand	Efferents along basilic vein to lateral group of lymph nodes of axilla
Infraclavicular group	Along cephalic vein in deltopectoral groove below clavicle	1–2	Upper chest wall and upper part of breast	Apical nodes, a few to lower deep cervical nodes

4.17 Lymphatics of Thorax

4.17.1 Superficial Parietal Lymphatics

The lymph of superficial tissues of the chest wall is drained in axillary (lateral thoracic) lymph nodes.

4.17.2 Deep Parietal Lymphatics

They drain the deeper tissues of thoracic wall. They include three sets of lymph nodes as described below:

1. *Parasternal or internal thoracic lymph nodes* – They are four to five in number and are situated by the side of sternum in the intercostal spaces in relation to internal thoracic vessels. They receive the afferents from breast, deep part of anterior thoracic wall, deep part of anterior abdominal wall above umbilicus, and from retro-xiphoid lymph nodes. Their efferents usually join with those of tracheobronchial and brachiocephalic nodes to form bronchomediastinal trunk which may end directly into the junction of internal jugular and subclavian veins. On the right side, it may join the right subclavian trunk and on the left the thoracic duct.
2. *Intercostal lymph nodes* – These lymph nodes are situated in the posterior part of intercostal spaces in relation to the neck of ribs. They receive afferents from posterolateral part of chest wall and breast. The efferents of lower four to five intercostal spaces descend to drain into cisterna chyli or commencement of thoracic duct. The efferents of upper left lymph nodes drain into thoracic duct and right upper nodes into the right lymphatic duct.
3. *Diaphragmatic lymph nodes* – They are situated on the superior surface of diaphragm and are arranged in four sets – anterior, right lateral, posterior, and left lateral.

Anterior group consists of two to three small nodes situated behind the base of xiphoid which receive the efferents from convex surface of liver, and one to two lymph nodes on each side near the costochondral junction of seventh rib which receive the lymph from anterior part of diaphragm. The efferents from this group drain into parasternal nodes.

The lateral group consists of two to three lymph nodes situated close to the site where the phrenic nerve enters the diaphragm. They drain the middle part of diaphragm. Their efferents drain into posterior mediastinal, parasternal, and brachiocephalic nodes.

Posterior group of nodes are situated on the back of crus of diaphragm. They are connected on one side with lateral aortic nodes and on the other with posterior mediastinal nodes.

4.17.3 Visceral Lymphatics (Mediastinal Nodes)

They drain the thoracic viscera and are situated in the mediastinum. They are classified into the following groups:

1. *Superior mediastinal (brachiocephalic) nodes* – They are 20–35 in number and are situated in superior mediastinum in front of brachiocephalic veins and large aortic branches. They receive efferents from thymus, thyroid, pericardium, and lateral diaphragmatic lymph nodes. Their efferents join with those of tracheobronchial nodes to from right and left bronchomediastinal trunks.
2. *Posterior mediastinal lymph nodes* – These lymph nodes are present behind the pericardium around esophagus and descending thoracic aorta. They drain the esophagus, posterior part of pericardium, diaphragm, lateral and posterior diaphragmatic nodes, and sometimes left lobe of liver. Their efferents mostly drain into the thoracic duct and a few into tracheobronchial nodes.
3. *Tracheobronchial lymph nodes* – They include some of the largest lymph nodes of the body and consist of five groups:
   (a) *Paratracheal lymph nodes* – They are situated on the sides of trachea and in the tracheoesophageal groove.
   (b) *Superior tracheobronchial lymph nodes* – They are situated in the angles between the trachea and bronchi.
   (c) *Inferior tracheobronchial lymph nodes* – They are situated in the angle between the two bronchi where the keel-shaped cartilage is situated. Hence they are often called carinate nodes.
   (d) *Bronchopulmonary nodes* – They are present in the hilum of each lung (hilar nodes).
   (e) *Pulmonary nodes* – They are present in lung parenchyma around larger bronchi.

   The afferents of tracheobronchial nodes drain the lungs and bronchi and heart. Their efferents unite with efferents of parasternal and brachiocephalic nodes to make the right and left bronchomediastinal trunks. They drain into the lymphatic trunks of root of neck (Williams and Warwick 1980; Pani 2013).

4.18 Lymphatics of Head and Neck

There are about 800 lymph nodes in the body of which about 300 lymph nodes are present in the neck. Hence, the neck is the part of the body that has maximum number of lymph nodes. It is probably due to the presence of air and food passages in the neck through which various micro-organisms enter the body. Depending upon the site, these lymph nodes are classified into two broad groups – superficial lymph nodes and deep lymph nodes.

4.18.1 Superficial Lymph Nodes

These lymph nodes are present in the subcutaneous tissue of the neck superficial to deep fascia (fascia colli). According to their anatomical arrangement, they are classified into two types:

A. Transverse group (external Waldeyer ring)
   1. Submental nodes
   2. Submandibular nodes
   3. Preauricular nodes
   4. Postauricular (mastoid) nodes
   5. Superficial parotid nodes
   6. Buccal (facial) nodes
   7. Occipital nodes

B. Longitudinal group
   - Anterior midline nodes
     1. Submental nodes
     2. Suprahyoid nodes
     3. Infrahyoid nodes
     4. Suprasternal nodes (in space of Burns)
   - Lateral cervical nodes along the external jugular vein

4.18.2 Deep Lymph Nodes

They are situated deep to fascia of neck (fascia colli) and are arranged anterior or posterior to sternocleidomastoid muscle. They are classified as described below.

A. Anterior deep cervical group
   - Upper set
     1. Submandibular nodes
     2. Jugulodigastric nodes
     3. Sublingual nodes
   - Lower set
     1. Retropharyngeal nodes
     2. Retrotracheal nodes
     3. Paratracheal nodes

B. Posterior deep cervical group
   - Upper set
     1. Suboccipital nodes
     2. Jugular nodes (in vicinity of internal jugular vein)
     3. Deep occipital nodes
   - Lower set
     1. Juguloomohyoid nodes
     2. Supraclavicular nodes (including Virchow's lymph node on left side)
     3. Subclavian nodes

All the lymphatics of head and neck region drain into deep cervical lymph nodes along the carotid sheath either directly or indirectly after draining into the nodes in the vicinity. The efferents of deep cervical nodes form a jugular trunk of either side. On the right side, it may end in the junction of internal jugular vein and subclavian vein (Fig. 4.5) or may join the right lymphatic duct. On the left side, it usually enters the thoracic duct (Fig. 4.3), although it may join either the left internal jugular or left subclavian vein (Williams and Warwick 1980).

The cervical lymph modes are very rarely involved in the lymphatic filariasis. Hence, the details of these lymph nodes are not described here (Pani 2013).

References

Cuschieri A, Giles GR. Blood flow, the microcirculation, lymphatic system, fluid and electrolyte disorders, pH balance and blood transfusion. In: Cuschieri A, Giles GR, Moosa AR, editors. Essential surgical practice. 3rd ed. Oxford: Butterworth Heinemann; 1995. p. 63.

Edwards JM, Kinmonth JB. Lymphovenous shunts in man. Br Med J. 1969;4(5683):579–81.

Handley WS. Lymphangioplasty: a new method for the relief of the brawny edema of breast cancer and for similar conditions of lymphatic oedema – preliminary note. Lancet. 1908;1:783.

Homer-Vanniasinkam S, Russell DA. Lymphatic disorders. In: Williams NS, Bulstrode CJK, O'Connell PR, editors. Bailey & Love's short practice of surgery. 26th ed. London: CRC Press; 2013. p. 923–40.

Kinmonth JB. The lymphatics. 2nd ed. London: Edward Arnold; 1982.

Kinmonth JB, Sharpey-Schafer EP. Manometry of human thoracic duct. J Physiol (Lond). 1959;145:3.

Kinmonth JB, Taylor GW. Spontaneous rhythmic contractility in human lymphatics. J Physiol (Lond). 1956;133:3.

Last RJ. Lymphoid tissue. In: Anatomy, regional and applied. 3rd ed. London: J & A Churchill Ltd; 1963. p. 25–7.

Manokaran G. Management of genital manifestations of lymphatic filariasis. Indian J Urol. 2005;21:39–43.

McMaster PD. The lymphatics and lymph flow in the edematous skin of human beings with cardiac and renal disease. J Exp Med. 1937;65(3):373–92.

Moncure AC. Chylothorax. In: Morris PJ, Malt RA, editors. Oxford textbook of surgery, vol. I. New York: Oxford University Press; 1994. p. 1933–5.

Moore KL. Lymphatics and the lymphatic system. In: Clinically oriented anatomy. 3rd ed. Baltimore: Williams & Wilkins; 1992. p. 26.

Pani S. Pani's filariasis. 3rd ed. New Delhi: Jaypee Brothers; 2013.

Pipinos II, Baxter BT. The lymphatics. In: Townsend Jr CM, Beauchamp RD, Evers BM, Mattox KL, editors. Sabiston textbook of surgery, vol. II. 19th ed. Philadelphia: Elsevier Saunders; 2012. p. 1819.

Sriram Bhat M. SRB's manual of surgery. 4th ed. New Delhi: Jaypee; 2013. p. 271.

Williams PL, Warwick R. Angiology: reticulo-endothelial and lymphatic system. In: Gray's anatomy. 36th ed. Edinburgh: Churchill Livingstone; 1980. p. 767–73.

Pathology of Lymphatic Filariasis

5

The lymphatic filarial infection is present in the body in three developmental forms:

1. Third-stage larvae entering into the local lymphatics at the site of mosquito bite.
2. Adult worms in afferent lymphatics and lymph nodes, i.e., ilio-inguinal and retroperitoneal lymphatics as the lower extremity is the commonest site bitten by the mosquitoes.
3. Microfilariae present in the blood, i.e., microfilaremia.

5.1 Third-Stage Larvae

The third-stage larvae are deposited or left on the skin of the host by the site of puncture. They enter into the body through the skin puncture produced by the mosquito and carry with them local bacteria, e.g., streptococci and staphylococci into the local tissues and lymphatics to produce cellulitis, lymphangitis, and lymphadenitis (adenolymphangitis and acute dermatolymphangioadenitis).

Repeated mosquito bites at different–different times at different–different sites in the lower extremity affect most or all of the lymphatics and lymph nodes of the extremity.

5.2 Adult Worms

The mature male and female worms reside in the lymphatics of the lower extremity, inguinal canal, scrotum, upper limb and thorax (i.e., breast in a female) (Olds 1994). They are resistant to the host's immune attack.

As the adult worms reside in the lymphatic system, there is hardly any reaction as long as the worms are alive except for lymphatic dilatation and thickening of the vessel wall due to their activity and secretory metabolic products ("toxins").

T.C. Goel, A. Goel, *Lymphatic Filariasis*, DOI 10.1007/978-981-10-2257-9_5

Contrary to this view, the dilatation appears to be due to mechanical obstruction and to the destruction of valves rather than to any hypothetical paralyzing effect to toxins from the worms, as the walls of vessels have healthy hypertrophied muscle that is contractile (Kinmonth 1982).

When the worm dies, it becomes highly antigenic and causes a sudden severe inflammatory reaction at the local site with infiltration of plasma cells, eosinophils, and macrophages in and around the infected lymphatic containing often fragmented dead worms along with endothelial and connective tissue proliferation. An abscess may form around a dead worm. The other changes include formation of new lymphatics, damaged lymph valves, and tortuosity of lymphatics (Figueredo-Silva et al. 2002).

It is postulated that as long as the adult worms are alive, the lymphatic vessels, though damaged, still remain patent (Babu and Nutman 2005). The death of the worm, however, results in progressive fibrosis, lymphatic obstruction by granuloma and thrombi formation, and extensive perilymphangitis. The final result is irreversible lymphatic damage.

The overall result of lymphatic filarial pathology is adenolymphatic obstruction, which causes hydrocele, chronic lymphedema, elephantiasis, and chylous manifestations.

With passage of time, the filarial parasitic granulomas containing segments of dead worms may calcify.

Role of Endosymbiont Wolbachia Many studies have revealed that the potent inflammatory response shown by the filarial worms is due to endotoxin-like activity of Wolbachia. It involves the pattern recognition receptors, CD14 and TLR4 (Taylor et al. 2000; Taylor et al. 2001; Taylor & Hoeranf, 2001).

Thus, the whole filarial disease occurs in two phases with considerable overlap, i.e., inflammatory phase and fibrous obstructive phase with their different clinical manifestations.

Basically, the filariasis is a parasitic infection of lymphatics and lymph nodes, the tissues and organs containing these structures or drained by them are affected secondarily. The pathological changes, i.e., the site, nature, and extent in filariasis, depend upon the following factors:

1. Number of infected mosquito bites
2. Number of entering third-stage larvae
3. The time period between the infected bites, i.e., short or long spread-out over many years
4. The site of bite and localization of adult worm, e.g., when the mosquito bites the lower extremity, the worms are localized in the inguinal or inguino-scrotal lymphatics resulting in filarial manifestations in lower limb and external genitalia (external genitalia in bancroftian filariasis only).
5. The severity of immunologic reaction
6. Presence of secondary infection and other complicating diseases, e.g., varicose veins of lower extremity
7. The age at which the patient was first infected

The changes in the lymphatic structure and function can be seen by Doppler ultrasonography, lymphography, lymphoscintigraphy, and MRI.

Summarizing the pathology of lymphatic filariasis, it includes damage to the lymphatics due to tissue alterations related to live adult parasites, tissue alterations related to dead adult worms, host inflammatory response to living and dead parasite, the host inflammatory response to the endosymbiont Wolbachia, and tissue alterations due to secondary bacterial and fungal infection (Babu and Nutman 2005).

5.3 Microfilariae

The living microfilariae generally do not produce any lesion except some pulmonary changes in tropical pulmonary eosinophilia which may be due to concentration of microfilariae in the lungs (Olds 1994). It occurs in some patients infected with *W. bancrofti* and *B. malayi* (Ottesen and Nutman 1992). These patients are immunologically hyper-responsive to filarial antigens (Ottesen and Nutman 1992) and reveal high levels of filaria-specific IgG and IgE. The lung biopsy may show inflammatory foci around degenerating microfilariae. These findings suggest that TPE is antibody-mediated microfilarial destruction in the lungs. The lungs may be normal or may show increased bronchovascular markings, diffuse miliary lesions, or mottled opacities (Khoo and Danaraj 1960).

In this syndrome, the rapid clearance of microfilariae and parasite antigens from the blood by the lungs results in symptoms (O'Bryan et al. 2003).

Further trapping of microfilariae in the reticuloendothelial elements in many organs and tissues may cause their enlargement, i.e., hepatomegaly, splenomegaly, or lymphadenopathy (Neva and Ottesen 1978).

The dead microfilariae do not have any effect on the body except when microfilariae die rapidly in large numbers following diethylcarbamazine therapy.

Asymptomatic microfilaremic persons if examined by Doppler ultrasonography show dilatation of lymphatics and contained live adult worms (filiarial dance sign), and other lymphatic structural abnormalities.

5.4 Immunity in Lymphatic Filariasis

The immune system of the body is very much likely to be affected as the adult filarial worms live in the lymphatics and lymph nodes for many years, mate, and produce microfilariae that remain alive for days and weeks in the blood (Grove and Forbes 1979). These two are the main sites of defense establishment of the body (cantonment areas). This cannot happen without modifying or suppressing the immune status of the body.

A normal host does not show any reaction to living adult worms and microfilariae. However, there is marked immunity to both adult worms and microfilariae that have died naturally or after administration of antifilarial drugs (Manson-Bahr and Apted 1982).

The immune response in filariasis is both humoral and cellular and is mainly directed against the microfilariae. The humoral antibodies thus produced include complement fixing, hemagglutinating, and fluorescent. Both IgG and IgE are increased in patients with microfilaremia (Moreau et al. 1972) and tropical pulmonary eosinophilia. A humoral response to dead microfilariae of immediate sensitivity type occurs following diethylcarbamazine therapy.

Some of the other findings in lymphatic filariasis include impairment of specific antibody production and suppression of delayed hypersensitivity skin reactions in patients with asymptomatic mircofilaremia and in those with obstructive filarial disease. The antibody response to tetanus toxoid is significantly impaired in patients with filariasis (D'Alesandro and Klei 1976).

Therefore, the patients with bancroftian filariasis are particularly prone to develop cutaneous infection. Other factors such as lymph stasis contribute to infection. Ottesen et al. (1977) have demonstrated a specific cellular immune unresponsiveness in filariasis. They observed that the lymphocyte transformation in response to stimulation with filarial antigens was grossly reduced in chronic filariasis especially in children with persistent microfilaremia.

The mechanism by which the specific and nonspecific immunity is suppressed is not clear, but it may include the activity of suppressor lymphocytes, serum inhibitors of cell-mediated immunity, interference with macrophage function, presence of immune complexes, disruption of lymphocyte traffic, and production of lymphotoxins by the parasite (Ogilvie and Wilson 1976). The pathogenetic significance of immune suppression is not clear, but it may be a means by which the filarial worms can evade the host's immune response.

5.5 Protective Immunity

Protective immunity has never been found in this disease as the epidemiological analysis of age-infection patterns in endemic areas have not shown reduction of infection prevalence with advancement of age which is expected as an effect of acquired immunity (Michael et al. 2001; Stolk et al. 2004).

References

Babu S, Nutman TB. Lymphatic filariasis. In: Cox FEG, Wakelin D, Gillespie SH, Despommier DD, editors. Topley & Wilson's microbiology & microbial infections, Parasitology. 10th ed. London: Hodder Arnold; 2005. p. 769–80.

D'Alesandro DA, Klei TR. Evidence of immunodepression in Syrian hamsters and Mongolian jirds by Dipetalonema viteae infection. Trans R Soc Trop Med Hyg. 1976;70:534–5.

Figueredo-Silva J, Noroes J, et al. The histopathology of bancroftian filariasis revisited the role of the adult worm in the lymphatic vessel disease. Ann Trop Med Parasitol. 2002;96:531–41.

Grove DI, Forbes IJ. Immunosuppression in bancroftian filariasis. Trans R Soc Trop Med Hyg. 1979;73:23–6.

Khoo FY, Danaraj TJ. The roentgenographic appearance of eosinophilic lung (tropical eosinophilia). Am J Roentgenol Radium Ther Nucl Med. 1960;83:251–9.

Kinmonth JB. The lymphatics. 2nd ed. London: Edward Arnold; 1982.

Manson-Bahr PEC, Apted FIC. Filariases. In: Manson's tropical diseases. 18th ed. London: Bailliere Tindal; 1982. p. 148–80.

Michael E, Simonsen PE, Malecela M, et al. Transmission intensity and the immuno epidemiology of bancroftian filariasis in East Africa. Parasite Immunol. 2001;23:373–88.

Moreau JP, Cuzon G, Pichon G, Outin-Fabre D, Lagraulet J. Serum proteins in lymphatic filariasis due to Wuchereria bancrofti var. pacifica. Electrophoretic study and immunochemical assay of A, M, G, and E immunoglobulins. Bull Soc Pathol Exot Filiales. 1972;65(3):456–63.

Neva FA, Ottesen EA. Tropical (filarial) eosinophilia. N Engl J Med. 1978;298:1129–31.

O'Bryan L, Pinkston P, et al. Localized eosinophil degranulationmediates disease in tropical pulmonary eosinophilia. Infect Immun. 2003;71:1337–42.

Ogilvie BM, Wilson RJ. Evasion of immune response by parasites. Br Med Bull. 1976;32:177–81.

Olds GR. Infections caused by Helminths. In: Stein JH, Sande MA, editors. Internal medicine. 4th ed. St. Louis: Mosby; 1994. p. 2274–89.

Ottesen EA, Nutman TB. Tropical pulmonary eosinophilia. Annu Rev Med. 1992;43:417–24.

Ottesen EA, Weller PF, Heck L. Specific cellular immune unresponsiveness in human filariasis. Immunology. 1977;33:413–21.

Stolk WA, Ramaiah KD, Van Oortmarssen GI, et al. Meta analysis of age prevalence patterns in lymphatic filariasis: no decline in microfilaraemia prevalence in older age groups as predicted by models with acquired immunity. Parasitology. 2004;129:605–12.

Taylor MJ, Cross HF, Bilo K. Inflammatory responses induced by the filarial nematode Brugia malayi is mediated by lipopolysaccharide-like activity from endosymbiont Wolbachia bacteria. J Exp Med. 2000;191:1429–36.

Taylor MJ, Cross HF, et al. Wolbachia bacteria in filarial immunity and disease. Parasite Immunol. 2001;23:401–9.

Taylor MJ, Hoerauf A. A new approach to the treatment of filariasis. Curr Opin Infect Dis. 2001;14:727–31.

6 Clinical Features

Lymphatic filariasis is the one among the most important parasitic diseases of man (Rosenthal 2015).

Prepatent Period It is the time from the entry of third-stage infective larvae to the first appearance of microfilariae in the peripheral blood. It varies from 80 to 150 days depending on species (Nutman 1991).

Incubation Period It is the time of entry of infection into the body to the appearance of symptoms. It is generally 8–26 months in expatriates but may be longer in endemic areas.

The filarial infection is characterized by a wide range of clinical presentations which vary from asymptomatic infection to symptomatic disease.

6.1 Asymptomatic Group or Subclinical Microfilaremia

This group includes:

1. The people who have not been sufficiently exposed to infection
2. The people with prepatent infection or adult worm infection without microfilaremia
3. The people who have cleared the infection
4. The people who have microfilaremia without obvious clinical manifestations. Some of these people remain microfilariaemic and asymptomatic for years or even for the rest of their life. Nearly all of these patients have microscopic hematuria and/or proteinuria (Nutman and Weller 2012). These individuals are carriers of infection and the reservoir for ongoing transmission.

Recent studies employing ultrasonography and lymphoscintigraphy have shown subclinical lymphatic abnormalities, especially dilatation of lymphatic vessels

T.C. Goel, A. Goel, *Lymphatic Filariasis*, DOI 10.1007/978-981-10-2257-9_6

(lymphangiectasia) in infected but apparently asymptomatic people with or without microfilaremia (Dreyer et al. 2002; Friedman et al. 1994).

It is important because about 30 % of children in certain endemic communities acquire filarial infection by the age of 4 years as shown either by presence of microfilariae or W bancrofti antigen in blood (Addiss et al. 1997).

6.2 Symptomatic Group

Age The filarial infection is mostly acquired during childhood and its incidence increases up to about 20–30 years of age after which it reaches a plateau (Dondero et al. 1976; Day et al. 1991). In endemic areas, all the patients tend to acquire infection by third decade of life. Hence, it commonly manifests clinically in middle ages.

Many children in endemic areas suffer with ADLA[1] attacks, hydrocele, and lymphedema of extremities (Ramaiah and Kumar 2000). It has also been confirmed by prevalence studies of microfilaremia and filarial antigenemia in children (Wilt and Ottesen 2001; Lammie et al. 1998). Ultrasonography and lymphoscintigraphy have shown live adult worms in lymphatics and lymphatic abnormalities, respectively, in children 3–15 years of age. The earliest age of detection of bancroftian microfilariae in blood of children is 7–10 months and that of brugian microfilariae 3.5 months (Babu and Nutman 2005). Thus, in endemic areas, nearly one third of children are infected before 5 years of age (Lammie et al. 1994; Simonsen et al. 1996; Steel et al. 2001).

Sex The gender of the individual appears to have an important influence on the incidence of chronic manifestations of filariasis, i.e., the males are more susceptible than females (Brabin 1990).

The acute disease is not significantly different between males and females but the chronic disease is more in males than females. The cause of this gender difference may be both environmental, i.e., men are more exposed to mosquito bite than women, and genetic, i.e., sex hormonal influence on innate and adoptive immunity.

Clinical filariasis is characterized by many symptoms and signs that are principally due to inflammatory or overexuberant response to developing, mature, and dying worms as described below (Babu and Nutman 2005):

Fever with Rigor It appears a few months to many years after patency. The patient suffers with recurrent attacks of fever with rigor lasting for 3–15 days. It may be associated with headache, bodyache, and malaise. It may or may not be accompanied by any of the clinical manifestations of filariasis.

Pain It occurs at the site of inflammation and present in all inflammatory manifestations of filariasis, e.g., lymphadenitis, lymphangitis, epididymoorchitis, funiculitis,

[1] It is acute inflammation of skin, subcutaneous tissue, lymphatics and lymph nodes (acute dermatolympangioadenitis).

cellulitis, and abscess. The pain is constant and severe in acute filariasis. It is increased by making the affected part dependent. In chronic disease, it is variable in severity.

Lymphatic filariasis is one of the commonest causes of pain in the inguino-scrotal region.

Swelling In inflammatory manifestations like adenolymphangitis, funiculitis, epididymoorchitis, etc., the patient has a tender local swelling.

In obstructive phase of disease, the swelling is distal to the site of adenolymphatic obstruction, e.g., hydrocele, lymphedema, elephantiasis, and lymph varix (Figs. 6.1, 6.2, and 6.3).

The initial manifestation of filarial infection is often acute lymphangitis with fever, painful lymph nodes, edema, and inflammation spreading peripherally from involved lymph nodes.

Discharge Discharge is an uncommon symptom. The lymphatic leak (lymphorrhea) from the skin of scrotum and lower limb is the most common discharge. It is due to ilioinguinal adenolymphatic obstruction.

Sometimes, the adenolymphatic obstruction affects the chyle-bearing lymphatics which may manifest as chyluria (milky urine), chylous diarrhea, and chylorrhea.

Filariasis may sometimes present as hematuria and hematochyluria.

Depending upon the mode of onset, duration, and clinical presentation, filarial disease is of three types – acute, chronic, and occult.

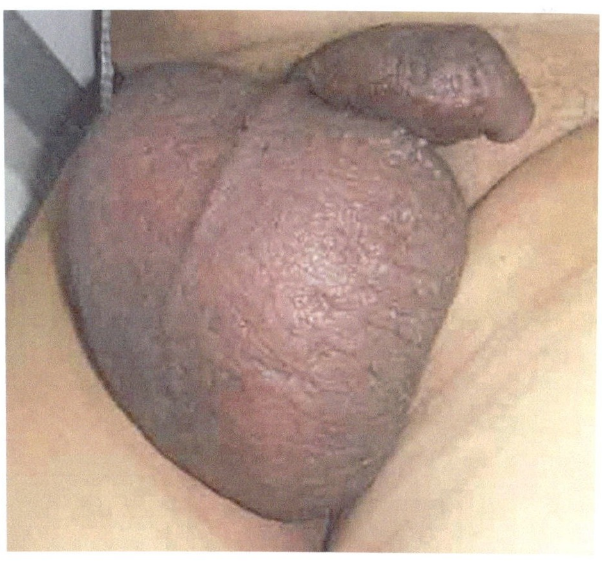

Fig. 6.1 Bilateral filarial hydrocele. The left is bigger than the right. On the left hemiscrotum, a few lymph vesicles are seen in the skin associated with elephantoid changes

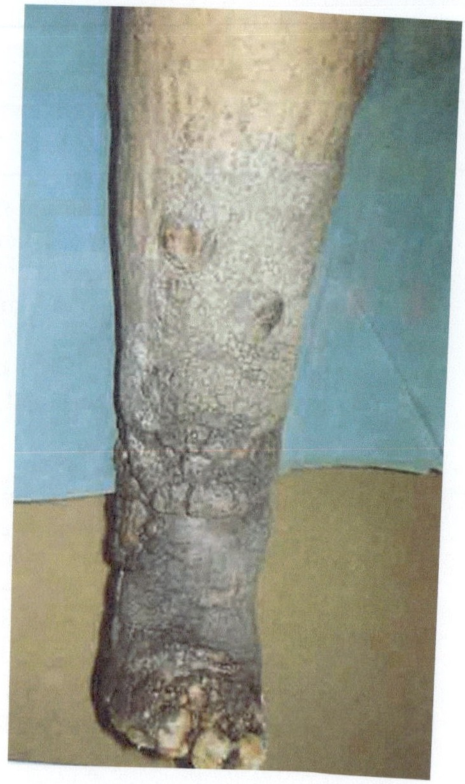

Fig. 6.2 Swelling, pigmentation, and nodularity of skin due to filarial elephantiasis of leg and foot (Courtesy – Dr Surajit Bhattacharya)

Acute Filariasis It is characterized by acute attacks of fever with rigor with or without inflammation of lymphatics and lymph nodes that occur at irregular intervals and last for several days.

In inflammation of lymphatics and lymph nodes (adenolymphangitis), the lymph nodes are affected first and then the infection spreads to local lymphatics in retrograde manner unlike the bacterial infection of these structures. The lymphangitis and lymphadenitis commonly affects the extremities, mostly the lower extremity.

As the disease progresses, epididymitis, orchitis, and funiculitis as well as the involvement of ilioinguinal and retroperitoneal lymph nodes may occur.

Chronic Filariasis It is characterized by the manifestations of adenolymphatic obstruction, e.g., scrotal hydrocele, elephantiasis, lymph varix, chyluria, chylous ascites, chylocele, etc.

Some patients present with lymphadenopathy.

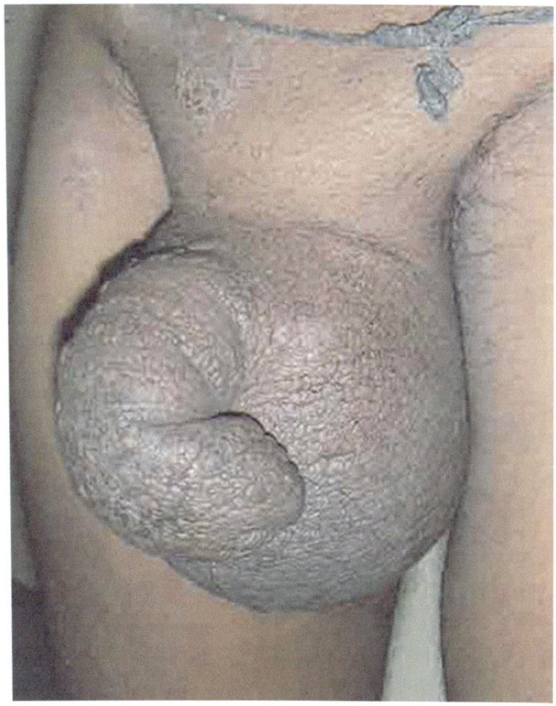

Fig. 6.3 Filarial elephantiasis of penis (ram-horn penis) and scrotum

Occult Filariasis Some infected persons have occult disease in which there are no classic symptoms and signs of filariasis and no microfilariae in the blood. These patients have microfilariae in tissues as seen in lungs in tropical pulmonary eosinophilia.

6.3 Differences Between the Clinical Types of Lymphatic Filariasis

The bancroftian filariasis involves the entire affected extremity, the genitals, or the breasts producing both acute and chronic clinical manifestations including chyluria.

The *Brugia malayi* infection differs in that the lymphedema involves only the leg below the knee and forearm below the elbow, without any genital or breast involvement. ADLA attacks occur in both infections (World Health Organization 1992). The clinical manifestations of *Brugia timori* are like that of *Brugia malayi* except that the scrotal lesions are almost absent (Supali et al. 2002) (see the table given below).

Features	Bancroftian filariasis	Brugian filariasis
Incidence	Very common (90 %)	Less common (10 %)
Hydrocele and other genital manifestations	Common	Rare
Chronic lymphedema–elephantiasis	Entire extremity	Legs below the knee and forearms below elbow
Breasts	May be involved	Not involved
Chyluria	Occur	Not seen or rare

6.4 Travelers and Transmigrants into Endemic Region

Following sufficient number of bites by infected mosquitoes, usually over 3–6 months period, the patient may develop acute lymphatic or scrotal inflammation with or without urticaria and localized angioedema. Epitrochlear, axillary, femoral, or inguinal lymphadenitis is often followed by retrogradely evolving lymphangitis. Acute attacks are of short duration and are not usually accompanied by fever. With prolonged exposure to infection and no treatment, the disease may become more severe with permanent lymphatic damage.

References

Addiss DG, Beach MI, Streit TG, et al. Randomised placebo-controlled comparison of ivermectin and albendazole alone and in combination for Wuchereria bancrofti microfilaremia in Haitian children. Lancet. 1997;350:480–4.

Babu S, Nutman TB. Lymphatic filariasis. In: Cox FEG, Wakelin D, Gillespie SH, Despommier DD, editors. Topley & Wilson's microbiology & microbial infections, Parasitology. 10th ed. London: Hodder Arnold; 2005. p. 769–80.

Brabin L. Sex differentials in susceptibility to lymphatic filariasis and implications for maternal child immunity. Epidemiol Infect. 1990;105:335–53.

Day KP, Gregory WF, Maizels RM. Age-specific acquisition of immunity to infective larvae in a bancroftian filariasis endemic area of Papua New Guinea. Parasite Immunol. 1991;13: 277–90.

Dondero Jr TJ, Bhattacharya NC, et al. Clinical manifestations of Bancroftian filariasis in a suburb of Calcutta, India. Am J Trop Med Hyg. 1976;25:64–73.

Dreyer G, Addiss G, Roberts J, et al. Progression of lymphatic vessel dilatation in the presence of living adult Wuchereria brancrofti. Trans R Soc Trop Med Hyg. 2002;96:157–61.

Friedman DO, Filho PJA, Besh S, et al. Lymphoscintigraphic analysis of lymphatic abnormalities in symptomatic and asymptomatic human filariasis. J Infect Dis. 1994;70:927–33.

Lammie PJ, Hightower AW, Eberhard ML. Age-specific prevalence of antigen in a Wuchereria bancrofti exposed population. Am J Trop Med Hyg. 1994;51:348–55.

Lammie PJ, Reiss MD, Dimock KA, Streit TG, Roberts JM, Eberhard ML. Longitudinal analysis of the development of filarial infection and antifilarial immunity in a cohort of Haitian children. Am J Trop Med Hyg. 1998;59:217–21.

Nutman TB. Experimental infection of humans with filariae. Rev Infect Dis. 1991;13: 1018–22.

Nutman TB, Weller PF. Filarial and related infections. In: Longo DL, Fauci AS, Kasper DL, Hauser SL, Jameson JL, Loscalzo J, editors. Harrison's internal medicine. 18th ed. New York: McGraw Hill; 2012. p. 1745–8.

Ramaiah KD, Kumar KN. Effect of lymphatic filariasis on school children. Acta Trop. 2000;76:197–9.

Rosenthal PJ. Lymphatic filariasis. In: Papadakis MA, McPhee SJ, editors. Current medical diagnosis & treatment. 54th ed. New York: McGraw Hill; 2015. p. 1513–4.

Simonsen PE, Lemnge MM, et al. Bancroftian filariasis, the patterns of filarial-specific immunoglobulin G1 (IgG1), IgG4 and circulating antigens in an endemic community of Northeastern Tanzania. Am J Trop Med Hyg. 1996;55:69–75.

Steel C, Ottesen EA, et al. Worm burden and host responsiveness in Wuchereria bancrofti infection: use of antigen detection to refine earlier assessment from the South Pacific. Am J Trop Med Hyg. 2001;65:498–503.

Supali T, Wibowo H, Ruckert P, et al. High prevalence of Brugia timori infection in the highland of Alor Island, Indonesia. Am J Trop Med Hyg. 2002;66:560–5.

Wilt C, Ottesen EA. Lymphatic filariasis: an infection of childhood. Trop Med Int Health. 2001;6:582–606.

World Health Organization. Lymphatic filariasis: the disease and its control. Fifth report of the WHO Expert Committee on Filariasis. World Health Organ Tech Rep Ser. 1992; 821:1–71.

7 Investigations

7.1 Blood

The blood counts are usually raised, especially the eosinophils. Their count may be as high as 80 % (Chambers 1994). In chyluria patients, hypoproteinemia and lymphocytopenia may be found and the albumin–globulin ratio is reversed (Tanagho and Kane 2013).

7.2 Parasitological

7.2.1 Microfilariae

- *Microfilariae in blood* – The most common method of diagnosing lymphatic filariasis is by finding microfilariae in blood (and other tissues and fluids) (Fig. 7.1). In the indigenous persons, they are uncommon in the first 2–3 years, abundant as the disease advances, and again uncommon in the obstructive phase. Hence, the absence of microfilariae does not exclude the presence of infection. Further, there is no correlation between microfilarial density and the severity of disease.

The peripheral blood is collected during the night (10 pm to 2 am) in areas of nocturnal periodicity, and during the day (10 am to 2 pm) in areas of subperiodic lymphatic filariasis, and anticoagulated, and stored at ambient temperature till examination is done, as early as possible.

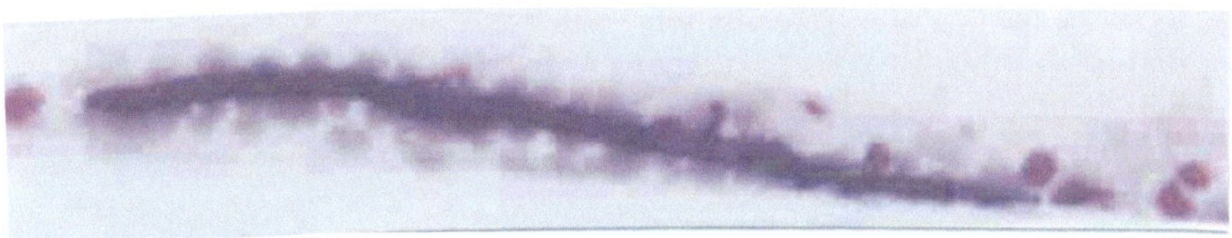

Fig. 7.1 Blood smear showing a microfilaria (Courtesy – Dr Vineeta Dwivedi)

T.C. Goel, A. Goel, *Lymphatic Filariasis*, DOI 10.1007/978-981-10-2257-9_7

Many methods are available for detecting the microfilariae in blood:

1. *Counting chamber technique* – This method of examination is fast, quantitative, and cheap (McMahon et al. 1979a). An aliquot of 1.00 mL of finger-prick blood is added to a tube containing 0.9 mL of 3 % acetic acid. It is put in a counting chamber under the low power of a compound microscope and microfilariae are identified and counted. If only one species of filarial infection is present in that geographical area, this method is ideal for routine diagnosis and also for field surveys. Species identification is difficult with this method.
2. *Blood film technique* – The simplest method is microscopic examination of a wet film of blood for motile larvae having undulating motion displacing the red blood cells from side to side as they move.

Identification of the Type of Microfilariae It is done by examining the blood film after staining it with Giemsa and Delafield's hematoxylin. The Giemsa will stain the nuclei and hematoxylin the sheath, if present. The morphologic differences between two main microfilariae are given below.

Microfilariae	Size	Sheath stain	Cephalic space	Tail	Stylet	Nuclei	Other feature
W. bancrofti	245–295 × 7.5–10 μm Average 260 × 8 μm	Pink	Long and broad	Pointed	One	Small discrete stop short of tail	Lies in gentle or smooth curves
B. malayi	177–230 × 6 μm	Deep pink	Short and broad	Blunt	Two	Large two nuclei in tail	Lies in sharp angles or multiple kinks

The blood film techniques are simple to perform but the sensitivity is rather low owing to small volume of blood examined and some loss of microfilariae during staining (Simonsen 2009).

If the results are negative, the blood specimen is concentrated for the parasite by Knott's method or filtration technique or by DEC provocation.

3. *Knott's concentration method* – 20 mL of whole blood is added to 20 mL of 2 % formalin and centrifuged for 20 min at 2000 rpm and the sediment is examined for microfilariae. Here the microfilariae will not be seen moving as the formalin kills them.

   If instead of formalin equal volumes of 1 % saponin in saline is used, actively motile microfilariae can be seen.
4. *Filtration method* – 20 mL of blood is taken into sodium citrate (anticoagulant) and drawn into a syringe which is connected to a Swinnex holder having 5 μm

pore size Nucleopore membrane. The blood is gently pushed through the membrane. Now 10 mL of normal saline taken in a syringe is also pushed through the membrane. Next step is to push some air taken in a syringe through the membrane to clear it. The membrane is removed from the holder and put on a slide. A drop of normal saline is put on it followed by a cover slip, and it is examined with a 10× objective for motile microfilariae. The film is examined again after putting a drop of methylene blue at the edge of cover slip to make it run under the cover slip due to capillary action using a 40× objective.

5. *Diethylcarbamazine (DEC) provocative day test* – If the microfilariae are at a low level, the nocturnally periodic microfilariae of *W. bancrofti* and *B. malayi* may be provoked by giving a dose of 2 mg/kg of DEC to enter in the peripheral blood during day time. Usually, 100 mg DEC is given to adults and 50 mg to children below 12 years of age (McMahon et al. 1979b). The blood is taken after 30–60 min. The peak levels are usually reached within 15–20 min after administration of the drug. In hospitalized patients and those in whom the sleep rhythm is changed, this test has hardly any value.

This test should not be done in onchocerciasis-endemic regions because of the risk of severe Mazzotti reaction. Daytime administration of ivermectin or albendazole does not have any provocative effect on microfilariae (Dunyo et al. 1999).

One must remember that amicrofilaremia does not rule out filarial disease and nor does microfilaremia denote it. The investigative findings must be correlated with the clinical picture.

- Microfilariae in urine and hydrocele fluid – These fluids are centrifuged at 2000 rpm for 5 min, the supernatant is thrown away, and the deposit is put on a slide, covered with a cover slip and examined microscopically (Fig. 7.2).
- Another method is filtration technique in which these fluids are filtered and the deposit on the membrane is examined microscopically.

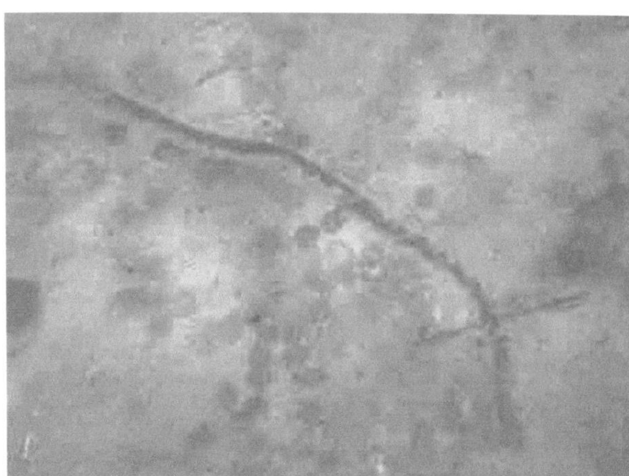

Fig. 7.2 Smear of urinary sediment of a patient with hematuria showing a microfilaria and red blood cells

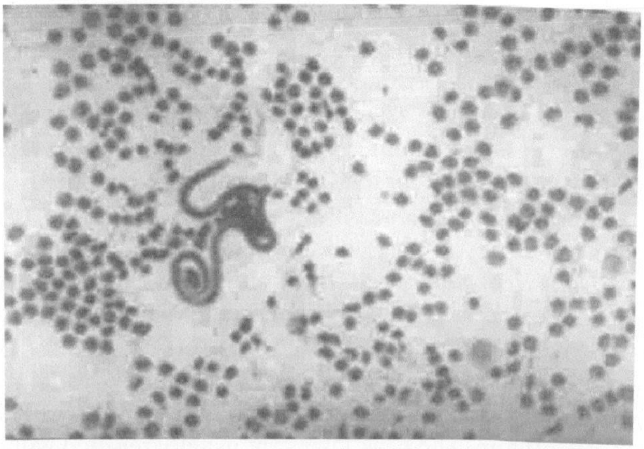

Fig. 7.3 Microphotograph showing microfilariae in the aspirate of a lymph node

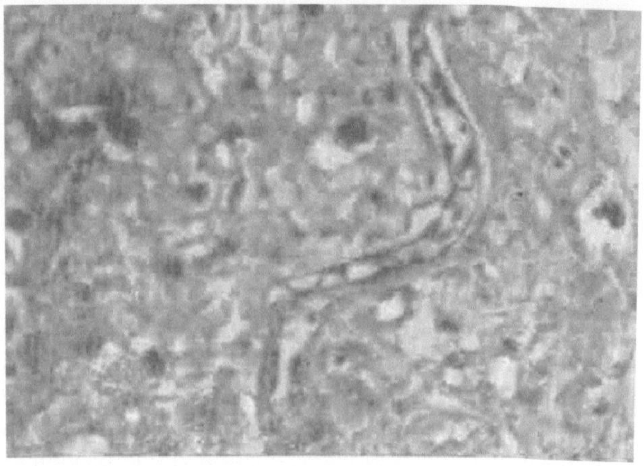

Fig. 7.4 Microphotograph showing a microfilaria in a nodule removed from spermatic cord

- The microfilariae may be present in other tissue fluids and body aspirates. Apart from blood, urine, and hydrocele fluid, the microfilariae have been detected in aspirate of lymph nodes, subcutaneous nodules of breast, bone marrow, and pus from filarial ulcers (Kar et al. 2013) (Figs. 7.3, 7.4, and 7.5). Apart from these, they may be present in nipple secretion (Lahiri 1975).
- *Microfilarial culture* – Efforts are being made to do microfilarial culture (Pani 2013). For this purpose, special culture media are required (Sneller and Weinstein 1982).

7.2.2 Adult Worms

- *In lymphatics* – The live motile adult worms can be seen within the lymphatics of scrotum, breast (Dreyer et al. 1996), and spermatic cord in infected areas using ultrasonography in conjunction with pulse wave Doppler using a 7.5- or 10-MHz probe (Chandy et al. 2011). The live worms wriggle continuously inside dilated lymphatics. It is called "filarial dance sign." Adult *W. bancrofti* are found

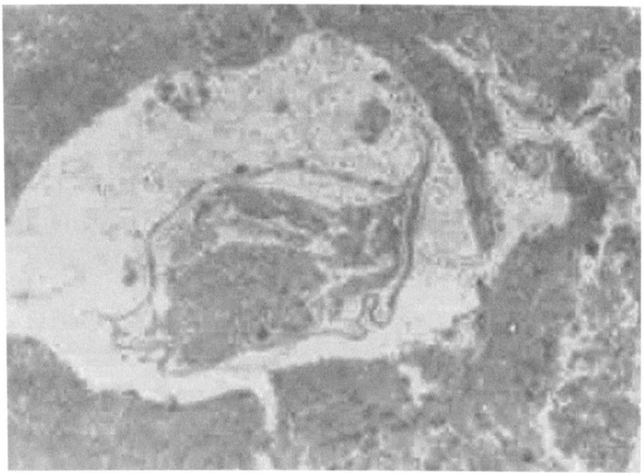

Fig. 7.5 Microphotograph showing microfilariae in a dilated lymphatic vessel

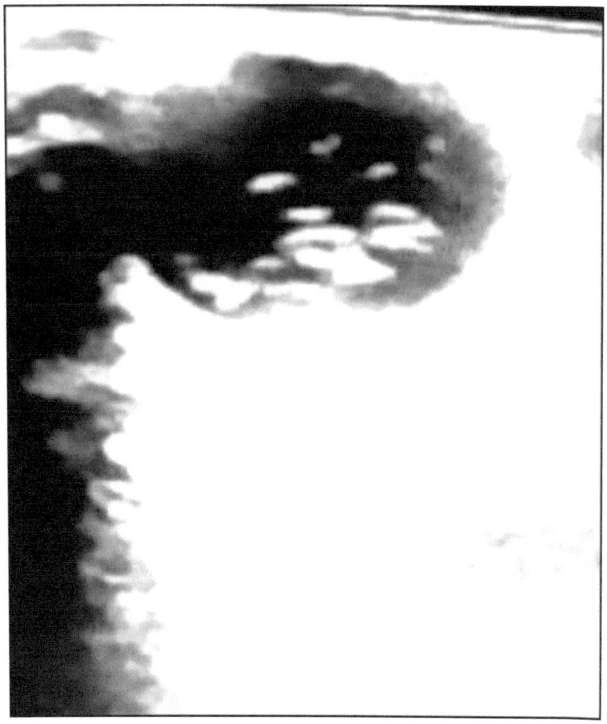

Fig. 7.6 The filarial dance sign in a varicose lymphatic of upper arm (Courtesy – Dr Ravi Mishra)

in the lymphatics in up to 80 % of infected persons (Fig. 7.6). Frequently, there are several worms clumped together and that show a remarkable long-term stability in location (Amaral et al. 1994). They are more difficult to detect in the lymphatics of infected females (Mand et al. 2004).

Adult *B. malayi* are not found in scrotal lymphatics but are detected in the breast, thigh, and calf lymphatics and in inguinal lymph nodes of infected persons (Mand et al. 2006).

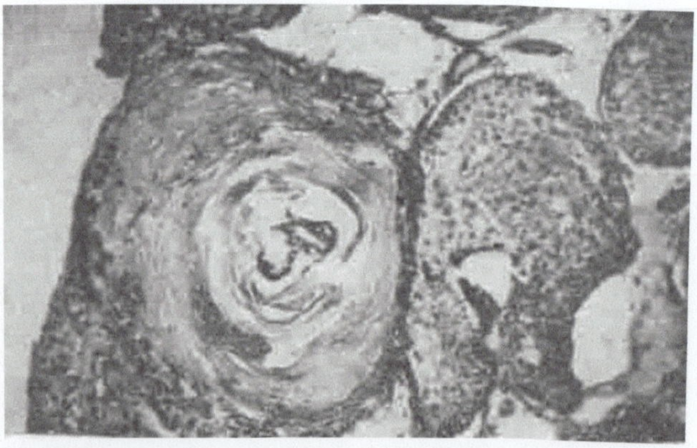

Fig. 7.7 Microphotograph showing a filarial worm in testis

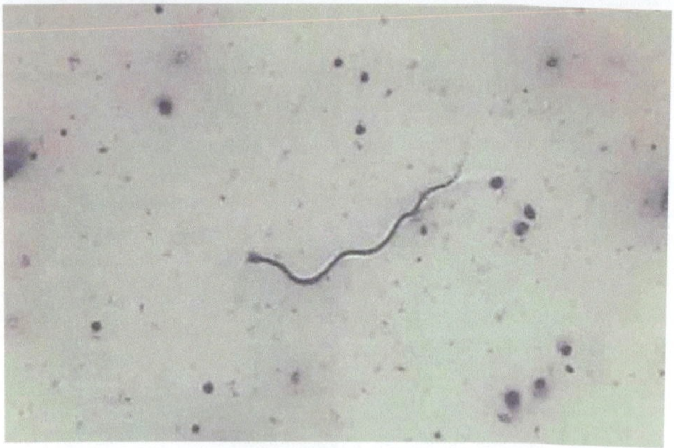

Fig. 7.8 Microfilarial worm found in testicular aspirate in a case of infertility (Courtesy – Dr Miti Gupta)

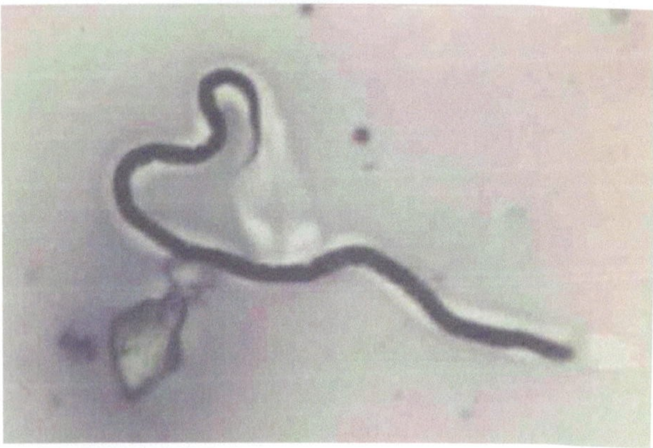

Fig. 7.9 Adult filarial worm in pleural fluid (Courtesy – Dr Miti Gupta)

- *In lymph nodes and other structures* – They may be detected in the biopsied lymph nodes during histopathological examination and at other places (Figs. 7.7, 7.8, and 7.9).

7.3 Immunological Tests

(a) *Antigen assays* – Specific circulating filarial antigens (CFAs) of bancroftian filariasis can be detected in the serum, plasma, or blood with the use of specific monoclonal antibodies. The CFA-based tests diagnose the adult worm infection and not just microfilaremia. The sensitivity and specificity of these tests is nearly 100 %. These tests are not dependent on microfilarial periodicity. Hence, the blood sample can be taken and tested for infection anytime of the day. Two tests are commercially available in the antigen assays (Simonsen and Dunyo 1999; Walther and Muller 2003).

- *Tropo-Bio Og4C3 Test (TropoBio, Australia)* – It is a semiquantitative sandwich ELISA for detection of CFA in serum or plasma of the patient. A subversion of this test is used on finger-prick blood collected on filter paper disks. It is based on one of two well-characterized monoclonal antibodies, Og4C3 or AD12 (Weil et al. 1997). It has a sensitivity approaching 100 % and specificity of 90–100 %.
- *NOW Filariasis Test (Binax Inc. USA)* – It is an immunochromatographic card test (ICT) done with serum or fresh finger-prick blood specimens which gives the results within a few minutes. It has a sensitivity of 96–100 % and specificity of 95–100 %.

An immune chromatographic test is a rapid screening tool that may be used to find the prevalence and distribution of *W. bancrofti* infection. It may be used in the global program to eliminate lymphatic filariasis. It is used to assess the residual antigen levels following antifilarial treatment. Schuetz et al. (2000) found that antigens persist in microfilaria negative persons for up to 3 years following treatment.

(b) *Antibody assays* – Specific IgG4 antibodies can be detected in blood. It is a good marker of active infection particularly of *B. malayi*. A rapid format dip stick test (Brugia Rapid) in the whole blood is under field trial studies (Ismail et al. 2005). Specific IgG4 can also be detected in urine of patients infected with *W. bancrofti* (Weerasooriya et al. 2003).

(c) *Polymerase chain reaction (PCR)* – PCR-based assays of DNA of both types of filarial parasites in blood are also available (Williams et al. 2002; Fischer et al. 2003). They have a specificity and sensitivity equal or greater than parasitological methods. This test needs at least one microfilaria in the volume of blood employed for DNA extraction.

The immunological tests have a limited value in endemic areas as most of the people there are positive for filarial antibodies due to continued long-term exposure. Further they cannot differentiate the past and present infection and they have cross-reactions with other nematode infections. They may be of some value in diagnosing this disease in visitors to endemic areas who develop symptomatic disease without microfilaremia.

7.4 Visualization of Lymphatics

7.4.1 Lymphoscintigraphy (Isotope Lymphography)

It is radioisotopic visualization of lymphatics after injection of radioiodinated human albumin or 99 m-Tc-labeled sulfur colloid into the first interdigital space of foot or hand and the use of a whole body gamma camera.

Lymphoscintigraphy has emerged as the investigation of choice in patients with suspected lymphedema (Barrett et al. 2006; Szuba et al. 2003).

A small amount of radiopharmaceutical, i.e., 2–3 mCi in 0.2 mL of saline is injected intradermally in first and second web spaces of each foot in equal divided doses and the migration of the radiopharmaceutical within the lymphatics is monitored after a brisk walk. Whole body anterior and posterior images are taken immediately and 2 h later (Subramanyam and Palaniswamy 2012) with a whole body gamma camera.

It shows the major lymphatic channels of the extremity and the degree of radioactivity in the inguinal (or axillary) lymph nodes 30–60 min after injection.

Some signs of filarial lymphatic disease are dermal backflow, obstruction, and abnormal tracer collection.

An uptake value less than 0.3 % of the total injected dose at 30 min is diagnostic of lymphedema, the normal value being 0.6–1.6 %. In edema secondary to venous disease (phlebedema) the isotope clearance is very rapid with more than 2 % ilio-inguinal uptake. (Pipinos and Baxter 2012). Further, it shows the site of lymphatic obstruction and leaks.

It has a sensitivity of 70–90 % and a specificity of almost 100 % in differentiating lymphedema from other causes of swollen extremity.

It is a simple, safe, nontraumatic, quick, and reproducible method with low exposure of radioactivity, but it requires a nuclear lab.

7.4.2 Lymphography

It is radiographic visualization of lymphatics after injection of a contrast medium, i.e., ultrafluid lipiodol or ethiodized oil. It provides the finest details of lymphatic anatomy (Weissleder and Weissleder 1989).

A peripheral lymphatic of the first intermetatarsal space of dorsum of foot is identified by injection of patent blue violet or isosulfan blue, carefully dissected under local anesthesia and cannulated. It often necessitates the use of magnification optics (an operating microscope). After lymphatic cannulation, the contrast material is slowly injected, and serial radiography is done. Usually, 7–10 mL of contrast is ideal for lower extremity and 4–5 mL for upper extremity (Pipinos and Baxter 2012).

It may be a unipedal or bipedal procedure to visualize the whole lymphatic system of lower body, but usually unipedal procedure is done as it identifies the crossover lymphatics.

It is a difficult, time-consuming, technically demanding procedure and potentially damaging to lymphatics. Hence, it is usually not done. Other complications include allergic reactions and pulmonary embolism if the oil-based contrast enters the venous side through lymphovenous anastomosis. Hence, it is reserved for preoperative evaluation of patients considered for direct surgery on lymphatic vessels. It has 90 % sensitivity and 100 % specificity.

The differences between the two methods of visualization of lymphatics are given in the following table (Dalela 2005; Sriram Bhat 2013):

Features	Lymphography	Lymphoscintigraphy
Definition	Radiographic visualization of lymphatics	Radioisotopic visualization of lymphatics
Medium used	Lipiodol	Tc99m serum albumin sulfur colloid
Ease of doing	Technically more demanding	Simple, less demanding, and safe
Time taken	Takes more time	Takes less time
Invasion	More invasive; extravasation of dye can occur	Less invasive
Image resolution	Very good	Poor
Effects on lymphatics	Damages the lymphatics	Does not damage the lymphatics
Recommendation	Not recommended for routine use	Recommended for routine use

Contrast Magnetic Resonance Lymphangiography

It is a most promising new test to image the lymphatics (Liu et al. 2009). It is performed after the intracutaneous injection of gadobenate dimeglumine into the interdigital webs on the dorsum of the foot. This investigation is capable of visualizing the anatomy and functional status of lymph flow of lymphatics and lymph nodes of lymphedematous extremities. The lymphatics can also be imaged by contrast CT scan (Figs. 7.10, 7.11, and 7.12), but the images of MRI are better than those of CT scan.

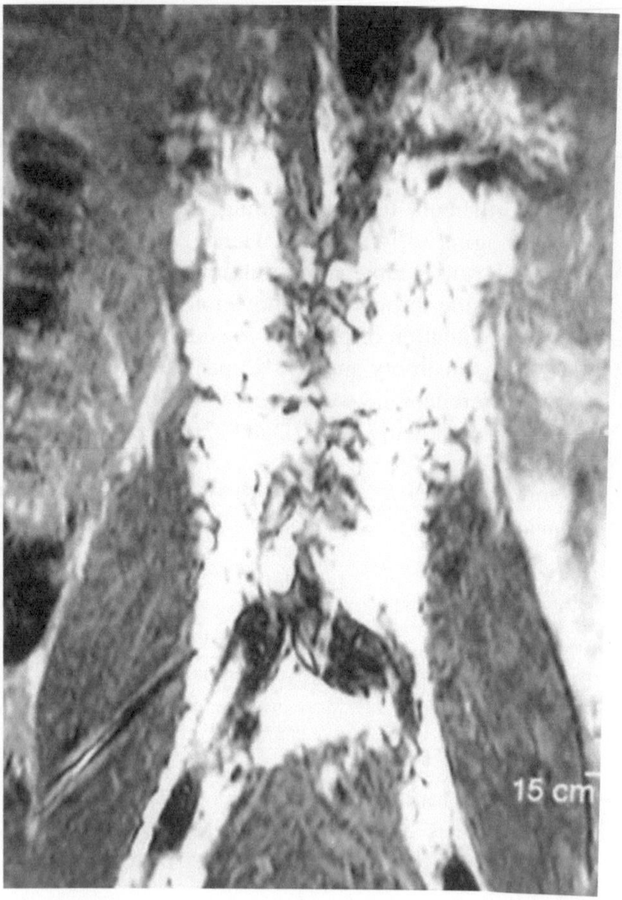

Fig. 7.10 Coronal CT scan of abdomen showing varicose retroperitoneal lymphatics

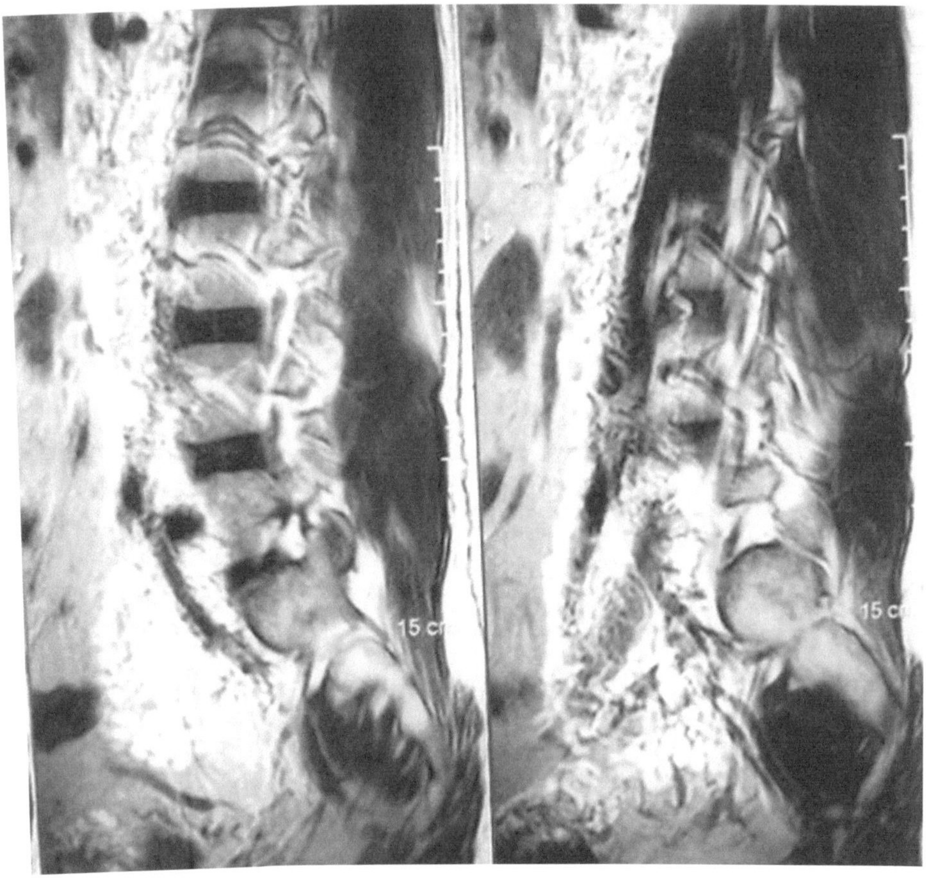

Fig. 7.11 Sagittal CT scan of lumbosacral region of retroperitoneum showing varicose retroperitoneal lymphatics

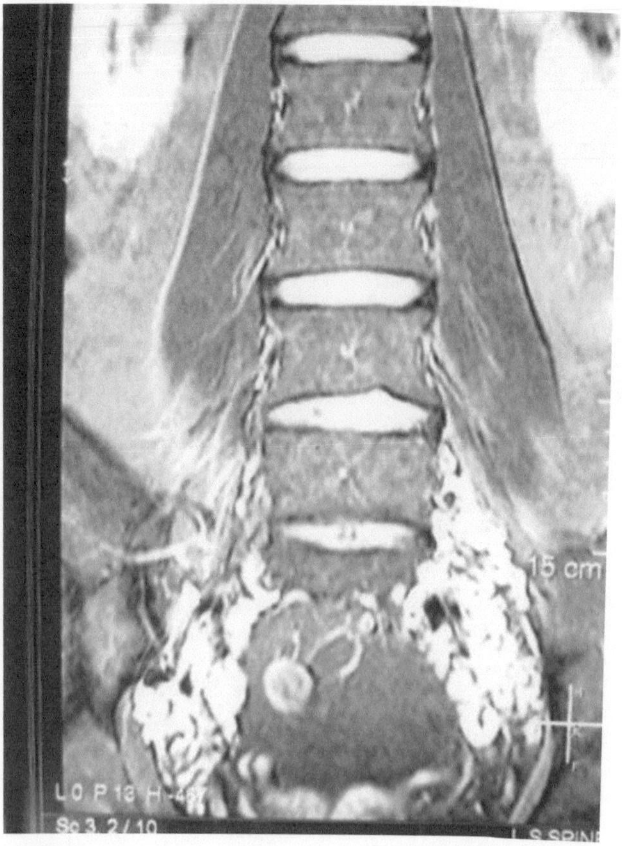

Fig. 7.12 Coronal CT scan of abdomen and upper part of pelvis showing varicose pelvic lymphatics

7.4.3 Retrograde Pyelography

It is done to visualize the pyelolymphatic fistulae in patients of chyluria (Figs. 7.13, 7.14, and 7.15). A retrograde ureteral catheter is passed into renal pelvis and the contrast is instilled in the renal pelvis without pressure or force (gravity propelled filling) and radiographs are taken. Normally, no lymphatics are visualized, but if there are pyelolymphatic fistulae, the communicating lymphatics are opacified.

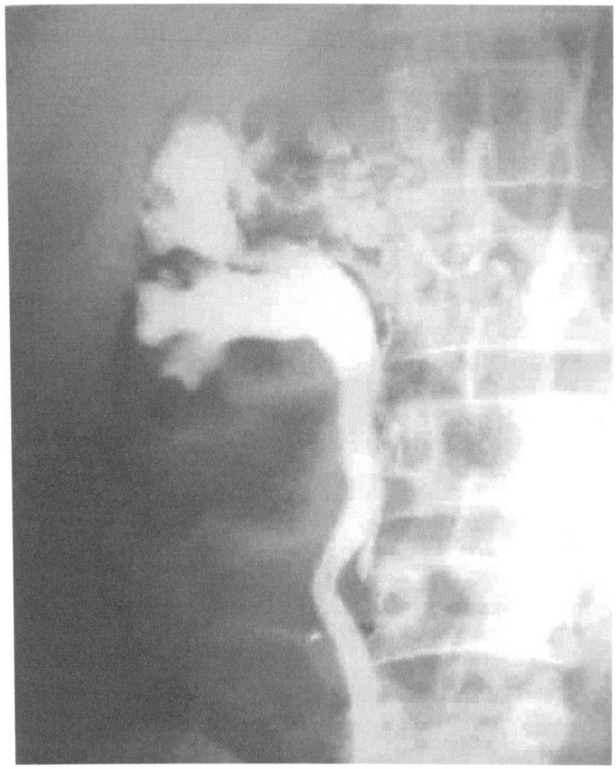

Fig. 7.13 Right retrograde pyelogram (RGP) showing pyelolymphatic backflow (Courtesy – Professor D Dalela)

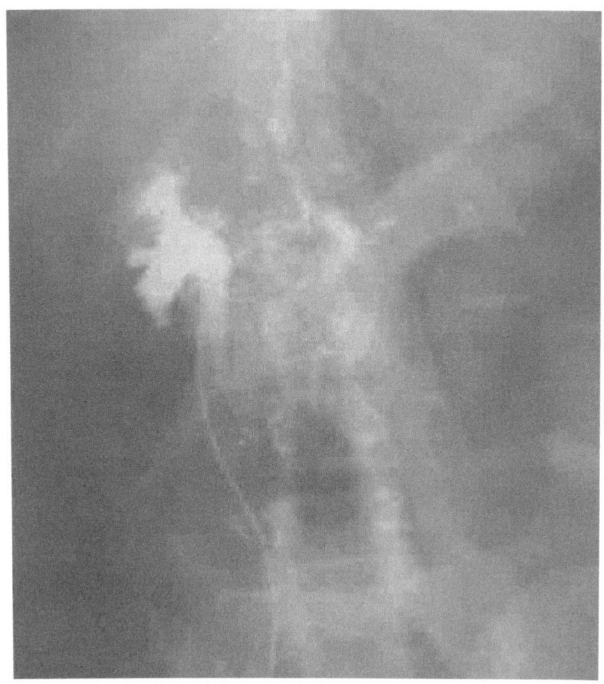

Fig. 7.14 Right-sided retrograde pyelography showing pyelolymphatic backflow and fistulae

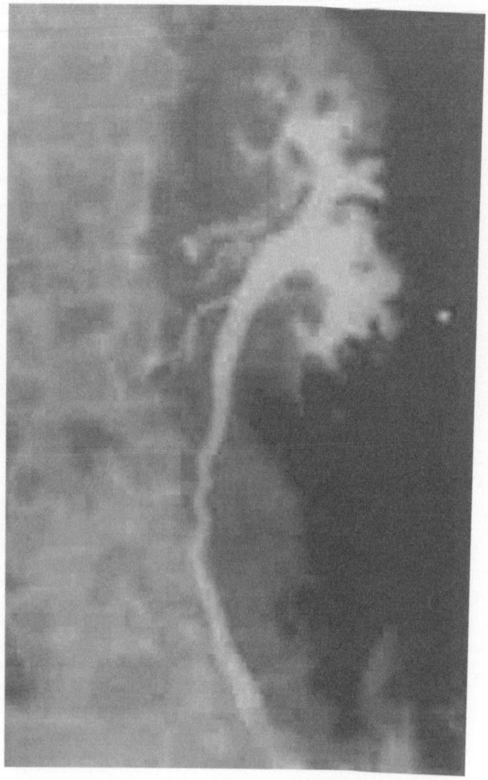

Fig. 7.15 Retrograde pyelography showing pyelo-lymphatic fistulae on left side

7.5 Clinico-Investigative Correlation

Many workers have reported about their experience of clinico-investigative correlation in lymphatic filariasis. The findings of two such studies are described below.

Simonsen et al. (2002) did clinico-investigative correlation after studying the clinical filarial disease, infection, and specific antibody response pattern in a high- and low-endemicity community in East Africa and found microfilaremia and filarial antigenemia in 24.9 and 52.2 % in the high, and 2.7 and 16.5 % in the low-endemicity communities, respectively. A positive history of attacks of acute adenolymphangitis (ADL) was present in 12.2 and 7.1 % of the people, 4.0 and 0.9 % of adults presented with lymphedema, and 25.3 and 5.3 % of adult males had scrotal hydrocele in the high- and low-endemicity communities, respectively. Both infection and disease occurred earlier and reached higher levels in the high-endemicity community.

The overall levels of filarial-specific IgG1, IgG2, IgG4, and IgE were significantly higher in the high-endemicity than in the low-endemicity people. Contrary to these findings opposite pattern was found for IgG3.

IgG4 has been claimed to be a marker of infection in lymphatic filariasis (Kurniawan et al. 1993).

Ebenezer et al. (2011) studied the relationship between the microfilarial density, antigenemia, and the clinical presentation of Bancroftian filariasis in Epie Creek communities in Nigeria in 1803 individuals and found microfilaremia and circulating filarial antigen (CFA) in 7 and 11.3 %, respectively. The infection rate was higher in males as compared with females, i.e., microfilaremia in 7.5 % and circulating filarial antigen in 11.5 % males, and microfilaremia in 6.5 %, and circulating filaria antigen in 11 % females. These two figures decreased with age.

Higher microfilarial density was seen in age bracket of 10–19 years while higher circulating filarial antigen was found in the age bracket of 20–29 years. The clinical signs of filariasis decreased with age with more clinical signs among 40–60 year olds. The commonly observed clinical manifestations were febrile attacks, chyluria, hydrocele, and elephantiasis of leg and breast. 7.5 % of subjects who were microfilaremic and 4.2 % amicrofilaremic subjects were found positive for circulating filarial antigen.

References

Amaral F, Dreyer G, Figueredo-Silva J, et al. Live adult worms detected by ultrasonography in human Bancroftian filariasis. Am J Trop Med Hyg. 1994;50(6):753.

Barrett T, Choyke PL, Kabayashi H. Imaging of the lymphatic system: new horizons. Contrast Media Mol Imaging. 2006;1:230–45.

Chambers III HF. Fever and infections in travelers. In: Stein JH, Sande MA, editors. Internal medicine. 4th ed. Mosby: St. Louis; 1994. p. p. 1966.

Chandy A, Thakur AS, Singh MP, Manigauha A. A review of neglected tropical diseases: filariasis. Asian Pac J Trop Med. 2011;4:581–6.

Dalela D. Issues in etiology and diagnosis making of chyluria. Indian J Urol. 2005;21:18–23.

Dunyo SK, Nkrumah FK, Simonsen PE. A study on the provocative day test effect of ivermectin and albendazoleon nocturnal periodic Wuchereria bancrofti microfilaremia. Trans R Soc Trop Med Hyg. 1999;93:608–10.

Dreyer G, et al. Studies on the periodicity and intravascular distribution of Wuchereria bancrofti microfilariae in paired samples of capillary and venous blood from Recife, Brazil. Trop Med Int Health. 1996;1:264–72.

Ebenezer A, Amadi EC, Agi PI. Studies on the microfilaria, antigenermia and clinical signs of bancroftian filariasis in Epie creek communities, Niger delta. Nigeria Inter Res J Microbiol. 2011;2(9):370–4.

Fischer P, Broakye D, Hamberger J. Polymerase chain reaction-based detection of lymphatic filariasis. Med Microbiol Immunol. 2003;192:3–7.

Ismail MM, Andrew K, Junaidi D, et al. Field validation of sensitivity and specificity of rapid test for detection of Brugia malayi infection. Trop Med Int Health. 2005;10:99–104.

Kar H, Singh G, Urhekar AD, et al. Microfilariae in pus sample of an ulcer over elephantiasis leg: an unusual case presentation. Int J Curr Microbiol App Sci. 2013;2(7):147–50.

Kurniawan A, Yazdanbakhsh M, Van-Ree R, et al. Differential expression of IgE and IgG4 specific antibody responses in asymptomatic and chronic human filariasis. J Immunol. 1993;150: 3941–50.

Lahiri VL. Microfilariae in nipple secretion. Acta Cytol. 1975;19:154–5.

Liu NF, Lu Q, Jaing JH, et al. Anatomic and functional evaluation of the lymphatics and lymph nodes in diagnosis of lymphatic circulation disorders with contrast magnetic resonance lymphangiography. J Vasc Surg. 2009;49:980–7.

Mand S, Debrah A, Batsa L, et al. Reliable and frequent detection of adult Wuchereria bancrofti in Ghanaian women by ultrasonography. Trop Med Int Health. 2004;9:1111–4.

Mand S, Supali T, Djuardi J, et al. Detection of adult Brugia malayi filaria by ultrasonography in humans in India and Indonesia. Trop Med Int Health. 2006;11:1375–81.

McMahon JE, Marshall TFC, Vaughan JP, et al. Bancroftian filariasis: a comparison of microfilaria counting techniques using counting chamber, standard slide and membrane (nucleopore) filtration. Ann Trop Med Parasitol. 1979a;73:457–64.

McMahon JE, Marshall TFC, Vaughan JP, et al. Tanzania filariasis project: a provocative day test with diethylcarbamazine for the detection of microfilariae of nocturnally periodic Wuchereria bancrofti in the blood. Bull World Health Organ. 1979b;57:759–65.

Pani S. Pani's filariasis. 3rd ed. Jaypee Brothers: New Delhi; 2013.

Pipinos II, Baxter BT. The lymphatics. In: Townsend Jr CM, Beauchamp RD, Evers BM, Mattox KL, editors. Sabiston textbook of surgery, vol. II. 19th ed. Philadelphia: Elsevier Saunders; 2012. p. 1819.

Schuetz A, Addiss DG, Eberhard ML, Lammie PJ. Evaluation of the whole blood filariasis ICT test for short-term monitoring after antifilarial treatment. Am J Trop Med Hyg. 2000;62(4):502–3.

Simonsen PE, Dunyo SK. Comparative evaluation of three new tools for diagnosis of bancroftian filariasis based on detection of specific circulating antigens. Trans R Soc Trop Med Hyg. 1999;93:278–82.

Simonsen PE, Meyrowitsch DW, Jaoko WG, et al. Bancroftian filariasis infection, disease, and specific antibody response patterns in a high and a low endemicity community in East Africa. Am J Trop Med Hyg. 2002;66(5):550–9.

Simonsen PE. Filariases. In: Cook GC, Zumla AI, editors. Manson's tropical diseases. 22nd ed. Philadelphia: Saunders Elsevier; 2009. p. p. 1–15.

Sneller V, Weinstein PP. In vitro development of Dirofilaria immitis microfilariae: selection of culture media and serum levels. Int J Parasitol. 1982;12:233–8.

Subramanyam P, Palaniswamy SS. Images in clinical tropical medicine. Lymphoscintigrapy in unilateral lower limb and scrotal lymphedema caused by filariasis. Am J Trop Med Hyg. 2012;87(6):963–4.

Sriram Bhat M. SRB's manual of surgery. 4th ed. New Delhi: Jaypee; 2013. p. 271.

Szuba A, Shin WS, Strauss HW, et al. The third circulation: radionuclide lymphoscintigraphy in the evaluation of lymphedema. J Nucl Med. 2003;44:43–57.

Tanagho EA, Kane CJ. Specific infections of the genitourinary tract. In: McAninch JW, Lue TF, editors. Smith & Tanagho's general urology. 18th ed. New York: McGraw Hill Medical; 2013. p. 234–5.

Walther M, Muller R. Diagnosis of human filariasis (except onchocerciasis). Adv Parasitol. 2003;53:149–93.

Weerasooriya MV, Itoh M, Islam MZ, et al. Prevalence and levels of filaria-specific urinary IgG4 among children less than five years of age and the association of antibody positivity between children and their mothers. Am J Trop Med Hyg. 2003;68:465–8.

Weil GJ, Lammie PJ, Weiss N. The ICT filariasis test: a rapid-format antigen test for diagnosis of bancroftian filariasis. Parasitol Today. 1997;13:401–4.

Weissleder H, Weissleder R. Interstitial lymphangiography: initial clinical experience with a dimeric nonionic contrast agent. Radiology. 1989;170:371–4.

Williams SA, Laney SJ, Bierwert LA, et al. Development and standardization of rapid PCR based method for the detection of Wuchereria bancrofti in mosquitoes for xenomonitoring the human prevalence of bancroftian filariasis. Ann Trop Med Parasitol. 2002;96:541–6.

Treatment and Prognosis

8

The prompt removal of a recently infected patient from the endemic area almost always results in relief in symptoms and signs in early disease (Tanagho and Kane 2013).

The World Health Organization (WHO) has identified lymphatic filariasis as the second leading cause of permanent and long-term disability in the world after leprosy. Hence it should be given early and prompt treatment to control it and to prevent further attacks.

8.1 Antifilarial Drugs

- Diethylcarbamazine (DEC) is the drug of choice as it is a microfilaricidal agent which is also capable of killing a proportion of adult *W. bancrofti*, *B. malayi*, and *B. timori*. It is given 2 mg/kg orally three times daily for 10–14 days (average 12 days). It rapidly kills circulating microfilariae (microfilaricidal) but kills the adult worms (macrofilaricidal) slowly and incompletely (20 %). The drug is well-tolerated and the side effects are rare, but the immunological reactions may occur due to dying parasites. They are more commonly seen in bancroftian filariasis than in *Brugia malayi* infection. These reactions are frequent, rapid, and sometimes severe and include fever, headache, malaise, hypotension, dizziness, and bronchospasm. Hence the treatment may begin with a lower dose (50–100 mg first day) with escalation over the first 4 days of treatment.

  A single dose of DEC of 6 mg/kg may be equally efficacious (Kimura et al. 1992; Dreyer et al. 1995; Kazura et al. 1993).
- Ivermectin – It is the drug of choice in the areas where onchocerciasis coexists with filariasis. It is given in 400 μg/kg as a single dose. In these areas, DEC is contraindicated because of the possibility of severe reaction to dying microfilariae of both parasites.

T.C. Goel, A. Goel, *Lymphatic Filariasis*, DOI 10.1007/978-981-10-2257-9_8

- Combination treatment – A combination of a single dose of albendazole 400 mg with DEC 6 mg/kg body weight or ivermectin 400 μg/kg have been demonstrated to have a sustained microfilaricidal effect (Horton et al. 2000).
- Doxycycline – It may be given 100–200 mg daily orally for 4–6 weeks to kill obligate intracellular (endosymbiont) bacteria, Wolbachia leading to death of adult filarial worms (Rosenthal 2015).

This treatment may prevent the development of lymphatic damage by eliminating the adult worms. It has no effect on already filaria-induced lymphatic damage or on chronic obstructive disease.

8.2 Treatment of Clinical Manifestations

- Acute manifestations, e.g., filarial fever, lymphangitis, lymphadenitis, funiculitis, epididymitis, and epididymo-orchitis are given bed rest, antipyretic analgesics, and antibiotics for secondary infection. In acute epididymo-orchitis, the scrotum is supported by a suspensory bandage. Diethylcarbamazine is not given during the acute attack, but given after the subsidence of acute symptoms, usually after 3–4 days.
- Acute dermatolymphangioadenitis (ADLA) attacks are controlled with foot care combined with administration of antibiotics, and local application of antifungal drugs to foot lesions.
- Scrotal hydrocele is treated by eversion or excision of sac depending upon the condition of tunica vaginalis, but WHO has recommended complete excision of sac with electrocautery to prevent the postoperative complications of lymph scrotum and elephantiasis.
- Chronic lymphedema–elephantiasis of lower extremity is treated with postural drainage, centripetal massage, and pressure bandage or garment. Advanced disease is treated with lympho-venous shunt or excision of elephantoid tissue.
- Chronic lymphedema–elephantiasis of scrotum, penis, vulva, and breast is treated by excision and repair or reconstruction.
- Lymphangiovarix and lymphadenovarix are excised.
- Chyluria – Majority of patients are relieved by conservative treatment including DEC, removal of precipitating factor, if any, and restriction of dietary fats and substitution with medium-chain triglycerides (MCTs). If this treatment does not give relief, the leaking renal pelvis is treated by instillation of sclerosing agents like diluted betadine or 1 % silver nitrate. If sclerotherapy fails excision of varicose lymphatics of renal hilum and around the kidney and may be around the ureter (Patna operation) may be required. Management of lymphatic filariasis is summarized in the following two flow charts: (Flow Charts 8.1 and 8.2.

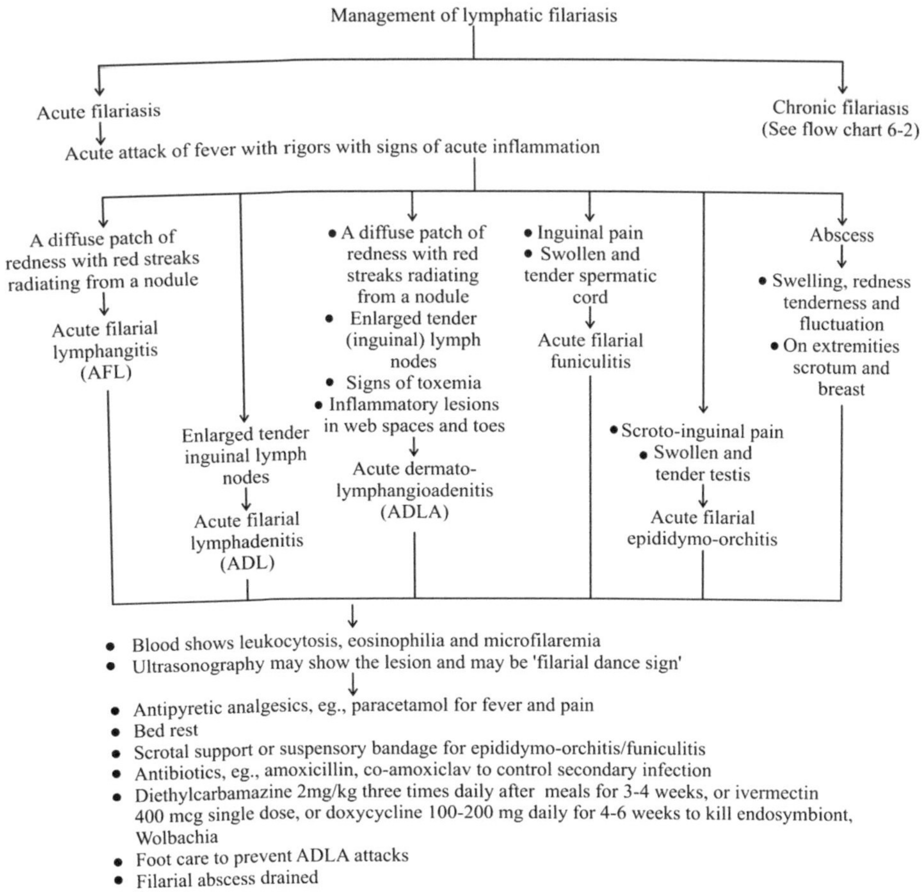

Flow Chart 8.1 The management of acute manifestations of lymphatic filariasis

8.3 Prognosis

- The prognosis is good in early and mild disease if it is properly and promptly treated and further attacks are prevented. The damaged lymphatics never return to normal in spite of treatment, but the further damage is prevented by early and prompt treatment.
- The chronic or advanced disease has significant morbidity. The total Disability Adjusted Life Years (DALYs) lost in India is around 2.06 million resulting in a wage loss of US$840 million to 1.5 billion per annum (Pani et al. 2005).
- It rarely kills its victim, e.g., a patient of severe uncontrolled chyluria may die of nutritional deficiency, but such cases are rare.

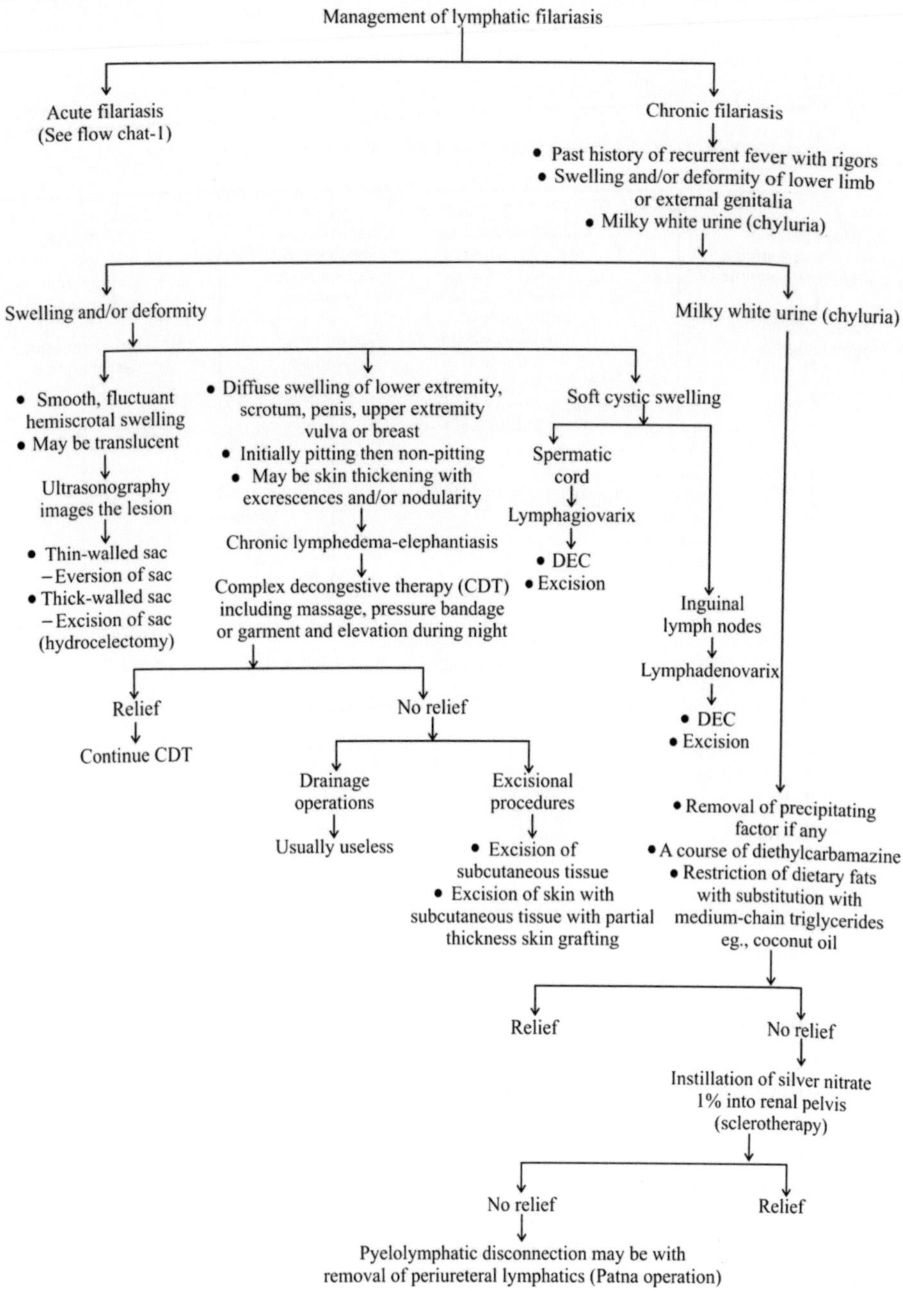

Flow Chart 8.2 Management of chronic manifestations of lymphatic filariasis

References

Dreyer G, Coutinho A, et al. Treatment of bancroftian filariasis in Recife, Brazil: a two year comparative study of the efficacy of single treatments with ivermectin or diethylcarbamazine. Trans R Soc Trop Med Hyg. 1995;89:98–102.

Horton J, Witt C, et al. An analysis of the safety of the single dose, two drug regimens used in programmes to eliminate lymphatic filariasis. Parasitology. 2000;Suppl:S147–60.

Kazura JW, Greenberg J, et al. Comparison of single dose diethylcarbamazine and ivermectin for treatment of bancroftian filariasis in Papua New Guinea. Am J Trop Med Hyg. 1993;49:804–11.

Kimura E, Spears GF, et al. Long-term efficacy of single dose mass treatment with diethylcarbamazine citrate against diurnally subperiodic Wuchereria bancrofti: eight year's experience in Samoa. Bull World Health Organ. 1992;70:769–76.

Pani SP, Kumaraswami V, Das LK. Epidemiology of lymphatic filariasis with special reference to urogenital manifestations. Indian J Urol. 2005;21:44–9.

Rosenthal PJ. Lymphatic filariasis. In: Papadakis MA, McPhee SJ, editors. Current medical diagnosis & treatment. 54th ed. New York: McGraw Hill; 2015. p. 1513–4.

Tanagho EA, Kane CJ. Specific infections of the genitourinary tract. In: McAninch JW, Lue TF, editors. Smith & Tanagho's General Urology. 18th ed. New York: McGraw Hill Medical; 2013. p. 234–5.

9 Prevention and Control

Lymphatic filariasis has many disfiguring and debilitating clinical manifestations resulting in much suffering and severe socioeconomic consequences. But it is a preventable disease as the cause and mechanism of this problem are now well known.

The National Filaria Control Program (NFCP) was launched in our country in 1955 which was based on prevention of mosquito bite, but it failed and filariasis increased with increase in population and urbanization manifold during last four decades. Currently, there may be up to 27 million microfilaremics, 21 million symptomatic patients, and about 554 million individuals potentially at risk of infection (Sebasan et al. 2000). Bihar has the highest endemicity and Goa the lowest.

9.1 Prevention at Mosquito Level

9.1.1 Mosquito Control

Effective mosquito control rapidly reduces transmission of infection, but it is slow to reduce the prevalence of filariasis, and it is difficult to attain effective mosquito control.

The main antivector measures include environmental control of breeding sites, larviciding, and use of insecticides against adult mosquitoes. Environmental control varies from filling in of temporary pools, clearing of refuse that collects dirty water, and construction of closed drainage system.

Culex Quinquefasciatus It breeds in highly polluted water and plays a major role in the transmission of *W. bancrofti* in urban and semiurban areas. A new method of its control in stagnant water utilizes a layer of expanded polystyrene beads that float on the water surface and prevent the mosquito larvae from breathing. This method has proven long-lasting and has been used successfully in Zanzibar. Another method is the use of *Bacillus sphaericus*, a toxin-producing bacteria which is being further studied.

T.C. Goel, A. Goel, *Lymphatic Filariasis*, DOI 10.1007/978-981-10-2257-9_9

Anopheles Vectors They are responsible for transmission of much of rural filariasis. In areas where malaria and filaria are transmitted by the same Anopheles species, malaria vector control program may help in filariasis control also as happened in Solomon Islands.

Mansonia Its larvae are best controlled by the destruction of host plants.

Aedes vectors have scattered and inaccessible sites, hence their control is not easy.

Even though the vector control is ideal, it is difficult to achieve in practice. The disadvantages of use of chemical insecticides include high cost and environmental damage. In spite of these problems, the use of insecticides is a major weapon of vector control.

9.1.2 Prevention of Mosquito Bite

It is done by use of mosquito nets, especially pyrethrin-impregnated bed nets, mosquito repellants, and proper clothing to cover most of the parts of body during sleep (e.g., use of longer trousers than the lower limb length, and shirt with longer sleeves with a rubber band tied at the end, and a light cover for head, forehead, and pinnae).

9.1.3 Vaccines

So far, there is no antifilarial vaccine available which can be used to prevent filariasis in endemic areas.

Unfortunately, the complex multiple stage life cycle of filarial parasite along with its ability to downgrade the immune system suggests that development of a vaccine is improbable, if not impossible (de Almeida and Freedman 1999).

9.2 Global and National Lymphatic Filariasis Control Program

Lymphatic filariasis is considered one of the six potentially eradicable diseases by the World Health Organization (WHO).

Hence now for many years, Global (WHO) and National Filariasis Control Program (NFCP) are being run to eliminate this disease. The control of lymphatic filariasis is possible because of:

1. Availability of better tools of diagnosis
2. Availability of safe and effective antifilarial drugs which can be used for chemoprophylaxis – The cost of diethylcarbamazine is not much, but albendazole and

ivermectin are relatively costly. Hence the filarial control program is supported by large-scale donation of albendazole by Glaxo SmithKline and the expansion of Mectizan (ivermectin) Donation Program for onchocerciasis to include free ivermectin for elimination of lymphatic filariasis (and onchocerciasis) in Africa where two infections often co-exist.

3. Almost exclusive human reservoir as there is no evidence of any animal being infected with *Wuchereria bancrofti* that causes 90 % of clinical lymphatic filariasis. The nocturnally periodic forms of *Brugia malayi* occur only in men, but the subperiodic form is found in a large variety of domestic and wild animals, e.g., monkeys, cats, etc. But it is a small number that does not have much epidemiological importance. There is no animal reservoir for *Brugia timori*.

Hence, in the year 2000 under the leadership of World Health Organization (WHO) emerged the Global Alliance for the Elimination of Lymphatic Filariasis (GAELF). The goals of this alliance were set to eliminate lymphatic filariasis as a public health menace by 2020. It has two arms consisting of:

(a) Interruption of transmission of infection by mass drug administration (MDA) to the local people to eliminate filarial infection in the communities
(b) Alleviation of disability in those who already have the disease (Seim et al. 1999)

9.3 Mass Drug Administration (MDA, Prevention at Human Reservoir)

It is the main method of prevention which is based on the administration of antifilarial drugs to the total population of the area at risk without doing any parasitological or other tests, thus reducing the cost of program. It reduces the load of microfilariae in a given community to such a low level that the mosquitoes will not be able to effectively transmit the infection. The drugs used are diethylcarbamazine, ivermectin, and albendazole. In India, it consists of a single annual dose of two-drug regimen, including diethylcarbamazine 6 mg/kg and albendazole 400 mg for a period of 4–6 years. Children under 2 years of age, pregnant women, and severely ill persons are excluded from MDA. The estimated fecundity life of the adult worms is 4–6 years, which is the basis for continuing the MDA program for the duration mentioned (Ottesen 2000).

DEC-fortified salt Another attractive alternative is the use of 0.1–0.4 % DEC-fortified salt. Hawking and Marques (1967) introduced this idea in Brazil when they found that this drug was stable after cooking. Subsequently, it has been used successfully in various parts of China, Taiwan, and India. After 6 months of use of 7.2 g of DEC, the microfilaremia rate decreased from 9 % to less than 1 % (Gelband 1994).

Ivermectin It is a drug which is used for the treatment of onchocerciasis. It is also a potent microfilaricidal for bancroftian and brugian infections. Hence it is used in areas where onchocerciasis or loiasis coexists with lymphatic filariasis, therefore diethylcarbamazine is contraindicated (Boussinesq and Gardon 1997). It is given in the dose of 400 μg/kg in a single dose annually.

Combination Therapy Recently, albendazole, a broad spectrum anthelmintic used in the treatment of a variety of intestinal worms, has been found to be an efficient microfilaricidal drug especially when used in combination with ivermectin or DEC (Ismail et al. 1998).

Bockarie et al. (1998) found that in the communities where a single-dose combination of DEC and ivermectin was used, the microfilarial density reduced over 90 % after 1 year of treatment, but if single-dose DEC treatment was given, the microfilarial density reduced by 70 %. In another study, combination of albendazole with ivermectin was found to be significantly more efficacious than either drug alone with no increase in adverse effects (Addiss et al. 1997).

The modern recommended combination regime is DEC 6 mg/kg and albendazole 400 mg single annual dose in non-onchocerciasis areas and ivermectin 400 μg/kg with albendazole 400 mg in onchocerciasis areas.

The annual single-dose co-administration of two drugs reduces microfilaremia by 99 % at 1 year, while annual single dose of one drug either ivermectin or DEC results in 90 % reduction.

The mass drug administration (MDA) to eliminate lymphatic filariasis is already in action in 51 out of 83 endemic countries. In India, MDA with single dose of DEC was taken up as a pilot project in 13 districts of 7 states covering 41 million populations in 1996–1997. It was extended to cover 77 million people by 2002 and 468 million people in 202 districts during 2004. From 2007, the entire population at risk of 590 million people in 250 districts was the target for MDA. Very high treatment coverage, probably more than 85 % is required to achieve interruption of transmission and elimination.

The benefits of global MDA (2000–2007) have been remarkable. In treated communities, an estimated 6.6 million newborns who would otherwise have acquired this infection, about 1.4 million cases of scrotal hydrocele, 800,000 cases of lymphedemas, and 4.4 million cases of subclinical disease have been averted in their lifetime. Further, MDA has protected 9.5 million asymptomatic people from developing overt disease, i.e., hydrocele six million and lymphedema 3.5 million.

9.4 Alleviation of Disability

It is an important arm of GAELF as it will be really effective if it is combined to address the suffering and the disability caused by this disease especially acute attacks (ADLA), hydrocele, and lymphedema.

9.4.1 Acute Attacks (ADLA)

The most important aspect of disability of lymphatic filariasis is acute attacks of dermato-lymphangio-adenitis (ADLA) which are characterized by pain, fever, and swollen limb that confine the patient to bed and prevent him to do his job for several days.

- An attack can be easily treated with bedrest, relief of pain and fever by paracetamol, maintenance of local hygiene, local antibiotic or antifungal ointment application on digital or web space lesions of foot, and/or administration of oral or parenteral antibiotics depending upon local and general condition of the patient. Commonly used antibiotics include penicillin, tetracycline, amoxicillin, ampicillin, and cotrimoxazole depending upon the culture and sensitivity report of swabs of entry lesions. Systemic use of antifungal drugs is usually not required as the fungal infection is confined to toes or web spaces and does not cause ADLA (Olszewski et al. 1999). These attacks are responsible for progressive damage to the lymphatics resulting in chronic lymphedema–elephantiasis.
- Ideally, these attacks (ADLA) should be prevented which can be done by very simple and cheap measures as described below (Shenoy et al. 1999; Suma et al. 2002):

1. Washing and cleaning the affected part, especially the grooves and folds, and webs of the toes with soap and water once or twice daily and wiping dry with a clean cloth. A hair-dryer set on low temperature may be used, if available. An emollient may be applied to keep the skin soft.
2. The nail should be kept clean and clipped at regular intervals.
3. Prevention of injuries and infections of foot by regular use of a comfortable and proper footwear, and promptly treating them if they occur by antibiotic ointments.
4. Fungal infections are treated by applying antifungal ointment to webs of toes, skin folds, and sides of feet.
5. Keeping the affected limb elevated at night by using 6-in. blocks (to elevate the foot end of bed above heart level)

Diethylcarbamazine has no role in the prevention and treatment of acute attacks. Proper foot care should be taught to children in the endemic areas as the filarial infection is usually acquired during childhood as indicated by irreversible lymphatic damage.

9.4.2 Lymphedema

In early stages, it may respond to treatment with diethylcarbamazine, elevation of limb, and prevention of attacks of ADLA (Addiss 2010). Once elephantiasis occurs, it cannot be cured but can be kept under control by the following measures:

1. Keeping the limb elevated at night by putting 6-in. blocks under the foot end of the bed after removing the bandage or compression garment
2. Elastic crepe bandaging or compression garment during the day when the patient is moving about
3. Regularly exercising the affected extremity
4. Centripetal massage to stimulate lymph flow from below up towards the larger patent vessels
5. Intermittent pneumatic compression of the swollen limb using single or multi-cell jackets
6. Heat therapy using either wet heat or hot oven – In China the lymphedema is treated with alternate local hot and cold fomentation.
7. Surgical procedures to drain the static lymph by nodo-venous shunt or omental transposition, or to debulk the limb by excision of elephantoid tissue

The lymphedema of external genitalia and other organs or parts can be treated successfully by surgery.

9.4.3 Hydrocele

It may have a silent onset or may be preceded by one or more attacks of funiculitis or epididymo-orchitis. In early stages, it may disappear completely following treatment of filariasis, but over the years, it appears gradually and may progress with thickening of tunica vaginalis. Simple hydrocele can be managed in a small peripheral hospital (level I facility) but a large hydrocele may require referral to a bigger city hospital (level II facility).

Mass Surgery Weeks (MSW) for Treatment of Hydrocele Mass Surgery Weeks program may be held in areas where the filarial hydrocele is very common, majority of people are poor, and the treatment facilities are scarce. It may be held as a part of lymphatic filariasis disability alleviation programs (WHO 2005). Thomas et al. (2009) have reported their experience of holding a pilot program of MSW in Central Nigeria in which 425 surgical repairs of hydrocele were done in 301 men in 5 Mass Surgical Weeks in 3 rural Nigerian community hospitals between 2002 and 2005. The most common (94 %) operation done was eversion of sac which was most familiar to local doctors. Excision of sac was done in 19 patients (6.3 %) where the tunica was too thick for eversion. Orchiectomy was required in 17 patients when the testis was found to be necrotic or infected. No chylocele was encountered in this series.

The overall results were good. Postoperative complications included hematoma (3.7 %) and wound infection (3 %) and one death due to uncontrolled infection due to unrecognized diabetes mellitus. One hundred and fifteen patients could be followed for 1–3 years with 7 % recurrence. The redundant skin of the scrotum may shrink and return to normal or may persist. No case of lymph scrotum was seen.

In such camps, strict attention must be paid to preoperative screening of the patient and asepsis.

WHO in 2002 published a guideline manual for doing hydrocelectomy in Mass Surgical Weeks. Some of these recommendations are:

1. Facility of pulse oximetry and electrocautery should be available – both these facilities were not available in LGA level hospitals where Thomas et al. (2009) held MSW, and they could manage these patients well without them.
2. Hydrocelectomy should involve "complete excision of sac" and not eversion (WHO 2004), but in the Nigerian MSW, only 19 excision operations were done because of the following reasons:
   (a) Excision operation requires more meticulous hemostasis which is best obtained with the use of electrocautery (DeVries 2002). Though it is possible to do excision without the use of electrocautery, but then it will take some additional time to obtain hemostasis.
   (b) In spite of the use of electrocautery, the incidence of postoperative scrotal hematoma is higher after excision of sac than after eversion.
   (c) Local doctors who performed the surgery were not aware of "another technique" that would have given better results.
   (d) They did not encounter a single case of lymph scrotum or "uncomfortable scrotal swelling" in their series of 115 followed up patients for 1–3 years after operation.

Hence, in a subsequent WHO publication (2006), a contradictory recommendation (to the previous one) was given, i.e., "because there are different recommended methods of hydrocelectomy, the choice of method will largely depend on the practice adopted by the surgical service of the district."

The success of this program depends on strict attention to the details of use of familiar techniques, commitment to patient's safety, maximal attention to sterility, and close coordination of all involved personnel. There is some difficulty in suture removal which can be improved by providing prepacked sterile disposable suture removal kits to patients at the time of discharge to ensure sterility during suture removal.

9.4.4 Benefits of Elimination of Lymphatic Filariasis

Apart from stoppages of transmission of lymphatic filariasis, the benefits of elimination of lymphatic filariasis are the following (Molyneux 2003):

1. The intestinal parasitic burden in reduced.
2. The anemia caused by ankylostomiasis in alleviated.
3. The nutritional status of community improves.
4. School attendance improves.
5. The health systems are strengthened.

References

Addiss DG, Beach MI, Streit TG, et al. Randomised placebo-controlled comparison of ivermectin and albendazole alone and in combination for Wuchereria bancrofti microfilaremia in Haitian children. Lancet. 1997;350:480–4.

Addiss DG. Global elimination of lymphatic filariasis: addressing the public health problem. PLoS Negl Trop Dis. 2010;4(6):e741.

Bockarie MJ, Alexander ND, Hyun P, Dimber Z, Bockarie F, Ibam E, Alpers MP, Kazura JW. Randomized community-based trial of annual single-dose diethylcarbamazine with or without ivermectin against Wuchereria bancrofti in human beings and mosquitoes. Lancet. 1998;351:162–8.

Boussinesq M, Gardon J. Prevalences of Loa loa microfilaremia throughout the area endemic for infection. Ann Trop Med Parasitol. 1997;91:573–89.

de Almeida A, Freedman DO. Epidemiology and immunopathology of bancroftian filariasis. Microbes Infection. 1999;1:1015–22.

DeVries CR. The role of the urologist in the treatment and elimination of lymphatic filariasis worldwide. BJU Int. 2002;89 Suppl 1:37–43.

Gelband H. Diethylcarbamazine salt in the control of lymphatic filariasis. Am J Trop Med Hyg. 1994;50:655–62.

Hawking F, Marques RJ. Control of bancroftian filariasis by cooking salt medicated with diethylcarbamazine. Bull WHO. 1967;37:405–14.

Ismail MM, Jayakody RL, Well GJ, et al. Efficacy of single dose combination of albendazole, ivermectin and diethylcarbamazine for the prevention and treatment of bancroftian filariasis. Trans R Soc Trop Med Hyg. 1998;92:94–7.

Molyneux D. Lymphatic filariasis (elephantiasis) elimination: a public health success and development opportunity. Filaria J. 2003;2:13.

Olszewski WL, Tripathi FN, Manokaran G et al. Mycotic flora of legs with filarial lymphedema. Progress in lymphology XVII: Proceedings of the 17th International Congress of Lymphology, Chennai, 1999. p. 141–3.

Ottesen EA. The global programme to eliminate lymphatic filariasis. Trop Med Int Health. 2000;5(9):591–4.

Sebasan S, Palaniyandi M, Das PK, Michael E. Mapping of lymphatic filariasis in India. Ann Trop Med Parasitol. 2000;94:591–606.

Seim AR, Dreyer G, Addiss DG. Controlling morbidity and interrupting transmission; twin pillars of lymphatic filariasis elimination. Rev Soc Brazil Med Trop. 1999;32:325–8.

Shenoy RK, Kumaraswami V, Suma TK, et al. A double-blind placebo controlled study of the efficacy of oral penicillin, diethylcarbamazine or local treatment of the affected limb in preventing acute adenolymphangitis in lymphedema caused by brugian filariasis. Ann Trop Med Parasitol. 1999;93(4):367–77.

Suma TK, Shenoy RK, Kumaraswami V. Efficacy and sustainability of foot-care programme in preventing acute attacks of adenolymphangitis in brugian filariasis. Trop Med Int Health. 2002;7(9):763–6.

Thomas G, Richards Jr FO, Eigege A, Dakum NK, Azzuwut MP, Sarki J, Gontor I, et al. A pilot program of mass surgery weeks for treatment of hydrocele due to lymphatic filariasis in Central Nigeria. Am J Trop Med Hyg. 2009;80(3):447–51.

World Health Organization. Surgical approaches to the urogenital manifestations of lymphatic filariasis. Geneva: World Health Organization; 2002. p. 1–29.

World Health Organization. Lymphatic filariasis progress in disability prevention activities. Wkly Epidemiol Rec. 2004;79:417–24.

World Health Organization. Global program to eliminate lymphatic filariasis: progress report for 2004. Wkly Epidemiol Rec. 2005;80:202–12.

World Health Organization. Informal consultation on preventing disability from lymphatic filariasis. Wkly Epidemiol Rec. 2006;81:373–83.

10 Antifilarial Drugs

These drugs kill the filarial worms or their larvae, i.e., microfilariae, and used in the treatment of lymphatic filariasis. Their classification is given below:

- Most commonly used drugs
  1. Microfilaricidal and macrofilaricidal drug – Diethylcarbamazine
  2. Microfilaricidal drug – Ivermectin
  3. Macrofilaricidal drug – Benzimidazole derivative – Albendazole
- Not commonly used but effective macrofilaricidal drug – Doxycycline
- Drugs having antifilarial activity but not used clinically to treat lymphatic filariasis
  1. Microfilaricidal drugs
     - Metrifonate
     - Levamisole
  2. Macrofilaricidal drugs
     - Suramin
     - Benzimidazole derivative – Mebendazole
     - Amodiaquine

10.1 Diethylcarbamazine (DEC)

During the Second World War, there were about 1500 cases of filariasis among the American military personnel (Wartman 1947). Hence there was an acute search for effective filaricides. It resulted in the discovery of the piperazine derivatives of which the diethylcarbamazine is most important member (Hawking 1979; Mackenzie and Kron 1985).

Chemistry Diethylcarbamazine is chemically NN diethyl, 4-methyl–1–piperazine carboxamide (synthetic piperazine derivative) with following chemical structure:

T.C. Goel, A. Goel, *Lymphatic Filariasis*, DOI 10.1007/978-981-10-2257-9_10

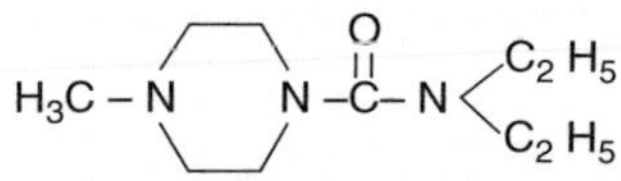

The drug is commonly available as a water-soluble citrate salt. It is tasteless, odorless, water soluble and stable to heat.

10.1.1 Pharmacological Actions

The exact mechanism of action of diethylcarbamazine is not known, but it appears to exert a direct action on *W. bancrofti* microfilariae by causing organelle damage and apoptosis. The mechanism of action against the adult worms is also not understood. Some studies suggest that DEC compromises intracellular processing and transport of certain macromolecules to the plasma membrane. It may also affect some specific immune and inflammatory responses of the host by undefined mechanisms which may sensitize the adult worms as well as the microfilariae to the phagocytic action of reticuloendothelial system.

Microfilariae Diethylcarbamazine causes rapid disappearance of microfilariae of *W. bancrofti*, *B. malayi*, and *Loa loa* from blood within 48–72 h of administration. The microfilariae of *Onchocerca volvulus* disappear from skin but form nodules that contain adult (female) worms. It has little action on microfilariae in vitro. It may act by changing the parasite so that it becomes susceptible to host's normal immune response (Rang et al. 2007a). It has no effect on the bancroftian microfilariae in a hydrocele despite penetration into the fluid. It has two types of action:

1. It decreases the muscular activity to immobilize the worm due to hyperpolarizing effect of piperazine moiety.
2. It produces alterations in the microfilarial surface membranes rendering them more susceptible to destruction by host defense mechanism (Mackenzie and Kron 1985).

Adult Worms Diethylcarbamazine kills the adult worms of *Loa loa* and probably also of *W. bancrofti* and *B. malayi*. But it has little action on adult *Onchocerca volvulus*. However, the mechanism of action is not known (Hawking 1979). It may compromise intracellular processes and transport of certain macromolecules through the plasma membrane (Spiro and Parsons 1986).

Diethylcarbamazine kills the microfilariae rapidly and nearly completely but the adult worms incompletely and slowly after administration.

10.1.2 Absorption, Fate, and Excretion

Diethylcarbamazine is rapidly and almost completely absorbed after oral administration and is widely distributed in non-fatty tissue. Peak plasma levels occur within 1–2 h after a single oral dose, and the plasma half-life varies from 2 to 10 h depending on the urinary pH.

It is rapidly metabolized in the body (Faulkner and Smith 1972) and excreted by both urinary and extra-urinary routes. More than half of oral dose is excreted in acidic urine as the unchanged drug, but this level is decreased if the urine is alkaline (Edwards et al. 1981). Hence, alkalinizing of urine may raise the plasma levels, prolong the plasma half-life, and increase both the therapeutic effect and toxicity of the drug (Awadzi et al. 1986). Hence, the dose may have to be reduced in patients with renal dysfunction or sustained alkaline urine. There is little tendency for accumulation.

10.1.3 Therapeutic Uses

Diethylcarbamazine is used for individual and community treatment of systemic lymphatic filariasis and occult filariasis (tropical pulmonary eosinophilia). It is also used to treat loiasis. It has been replaced by ivermectin in the treatment of onchocerciasis (Rosenthal 2012), as it may accelerate blindness and cause severe Mazzotti reaction.

Diethylcarbamazine may also be used for chemoprophylaxis – 300 mg weekly or 300 mg on 3 successive days each month for loiasis, and 50 mg monthly for lymphatic filariasis (Rosenthal 2012). It is usually given with albendazole 400 mg for prevention of lymphatic filariasis (Martin 2015).

10.1.4 Dosage and Administration

The standard dose of diethylcarbamazine is 6 mg/kg/per day for 12 days for *W. bancrofti* infection, and for 6 days for *B. malayi* infection. The children under 10 years of age should receive half of the adult dose. If given early in the course of disease, the lymphatic damage may be prevented, but it does not reverse the damage already occurred.

DEC is the drug of choice for the treatment of tropical pulmonary eosinophilia where it is given for a longer period of 3–4 weeks.

In all cases, the treatment is best initiated with a smaller dose for initial 2–3 days in order to avoid the danger of immunological reactions, i.e., 50 mg on day 1 (1 mg/kg in children), three 50 mg doses on day 2, and three 100 mg doses on day 3 (2 mg/kg in children) which is continued to complete a 2- to 3-week course. It should not be given on empty stomach.

It is the best available drug for the therapy of loiasis. It is no longer recommended for initial treatment of onchocherciasis because of severe reactions (Mazzotti reaction) related to microfilarial destruction.

In loiasis, the treatment is initiated with test doses of 1 mg/kg daily for 2–3 days, escalating to maximally tolerated daily dose 8–10 mg/kg for a total of 2–3 weeks.

Must Remember: Diethylcarbamazine

- DEC is most effective, safest, and most commonly used antifilarial drug.
- It is a good microfilaricidal also a partial macrofilaricidal.
- It must not be used in areas where onchocerciasis occurs with lymphatic filariasis.

10.1.5 Toxicity and Side Effects

If a daily dose of 8–10 mg/kg is exceeded, the direct toxic reaction to this drug is rarely severe and usually disappears spontaneously within a few days despite continuation of treatment. These reactions are fever, anorexia, nausea, headache, vomiting, arthralgia, and dizziness.

Immunological reaction similar to Mazzotti reaction in onchocerciasis may be induced by disintegrating microfilariae and dead adult worms. The incidence and severity of these reactions are correlated both with the degree of microfilaremia and dose of diethylcarbamazine. The reactions to dying microfilariae are usually mild in *W. bancrofti*, more intense in *B. malayi*, and occasionally severe in *Loa loa* infection (Rosenthal 2012). Fever, headache, dizziness, anorexia, malaise, urticaria, vomiting, and asthmatic attacks may occur within a few hours of the first dose and usually subside by the fifth day of treatment. Reversible proteinuria may occur.

In bancroftian and brugian filariasis, nodular swellings may occur along the course of lymphatics and often accompanying lymphadenitis. This reaction usually subsides within a few days. It is due to killed adult worms in the lymphatics, and lymph nodes.

This drug is safe during pregnancy. It does not have any specific contraindication except when the patient cannot tolerate it. In order to prevent reactions, antihistaminics may be given with each dose. For this reason, some preparations are available with a combination of antihistaminics with this drug. Caution is exercised when using this drug in patients with hypertension or renal disease.

10.1.6 Preparations and Availability

Diethylcarbamazine is usually marketed as Banocide, Hetrazan, or Unicarbazan in Indian market. It is available in the form of tablets (50 or 100 mg), liquid, and injections. It is stable even under conditions of high temperature and humidity.

Combination preparations are available along with antihistaminics and steroids.

10.2 Ivermectin

Isolation of the anthelmintic components from cultures of soil actinomycete, *Streptomyces avermitilis* led to the discovery of avermectins, a novel class of 16-membered macrocylic lactones (Campbell 1989).

Ivermectin (mectizan), a semisynthetic macrocyclic lactone, is a mixture of avermectin B_{1a}, and avermectin$_{1b}$. It is derived from soil actinomycete *Streptomyces avermitilis*. It is an insecticide that was developed for crop management.

10.2.1 Pharmacologic Action

Ivermectin acts on parasite-specific inhibitory glutamate-gated chloride channel receptors. It causes hyperpolarization of the parasite cell membrane with muscle paralysis and death of worms. At higher doses, it can potentiate GABA-gated chloride channels. It does not cross blood–brain barrier and therefore has no paralytic action on mammals (Pong et al. 1980; Wang and Pong 1982).

Infections caused by gastrointestinal nematodes, e.g., strongyloidiasis, ascariasis, trichuriasis, and enterobiasis show good response to ivermectin but the hookworms (ankylostomiasis) are affected to a lesser extent (Naquira et al. 1989). The cestodes and trematodes are not sensitive to ivermectin as they do not have high affinity to avermectin receptors.

Ivermectin is a safe and highly effective broad-spectrum antiparasite in humans and is the drug of first choice in the treatment of filarial infections (Rang et al. 2007a). It is more effective than diethylcarbamazine in bancroftian filariasis where it reduces the microfilaremia to near zero levels. In brugian filariasis, diethylcarbamazine-induced clearance may be superior.

A single dose kills the immature microfilariae of *Onchocerca volvulus* but not the adult worms. The microfilarial counts are reduced to low levels over a few weeks and remain severely depressed for up to 12 months.

10.2.2 Absorption, Fate, and Excretion

Ivermectin is administered by oral and subcutaneous routes. After oral administration, it is rapidly absorbed from the bowel and the peak plasma levels are achieved within 4–5 h of oral administration. It is about 93 % bound to plasma proteins (Klotz et al. 1990) and virtually none appears in urine (Krishna and Klotz 1993). The highest concentrations are seen in liver and fat, and extremely low levels in brain. The half-life is approximately 16 h. The drug and its metabolites are excreted in feces (Rosenthal 2012).

Must Remember: Ivermectin

- Safe and highly effective microfilaricidal drug, especially bancroftian filariasis
- Ideal for use in areas where onchocerciasis coexists with filariasis
- Commonly used in filarial elimination program
- Diethylcarbamazine and ivermectin are first choice drugs

10.2.3 Therapeutic Uses

- *Onchocerciasis* – A single oral dose of 150 μg/kg given every 6–12 months is considered effective and safe in adults and children 5 years or older (Goa et al. 1991). No food or alcohol should be taken for at least 2 h before or after its administration. It results in reversal of lymphadenopathy and acute inflammatory changes in ocular tissues, and marked reduction of microfilariae in the skin and ocular tissues, but cure is not obtained as the ivermectin has little effect on adult worms.
- *Lymphatic filariasis* – Ivermectin is as effective as diethylcarbamazine for controlling lymphatic filariasis and can be used in the regions where onchocerciasis, loiasis, or both infections are endemic with lymphatic filariasis. Single annual dose (400 μg/kg) is both effective and safe in lymphatic filariasis (Ottsen and Ramchandran 1995).
- *Intestinal nematode infection* – A single dose of 150–200 μg/kg of ivermectin can cure strongyloidiasis which is also effective against co-existing ascariasis, trichuriasis, and enterobiasis (Naquira et al. 1989).
- It is also the drug of choice in cutaneous larva migrans, and also useful in the treatment of pediculosis (lice) and scabies (Martin 2015).

10.2.4 Side Effects and Toxicity

Ivermectin should not be given to children less than 5 years of age and during pregnancy, and also in conditions associated with an impaired blood–brain barrier, e.g., meningitis.

Ivermectin is generally well tolerated, but its toxicity occurs nearly always from Mazzotti-like reactions to dying microfilariae, the symptoms of which are usually mild and include mild itching and swollen tender lymph nodes. They last for a few days and are relieved by aspirin and antihistaminics.

Rarely more severe reactions occur which include high fever, tachycardia, hypotension, prostration, dizziness, headache, myalgia, arthralgia, diarrhea, and facial and peripheral edema. They respond to corticosteroids (Martin 2015).

Rarely postural hypotension occurs within 12–24 h of drug administration. It responds to rest and oral fluids.

10.3 Benzimidazole Derivatives

The benzimidazoles consisting of mebendazole and albendazole are broad-spectrum anthelmintic agents that are highly effective in ascariasis, intestinal capillariasisis, enterobiasis, trichuriasis, and hookworm infection. These agents are active against both larval and adult stages of nematodes. They are ovicidal for Ascaris and Trichuris.

Albendazole is better than mebendazole in curing hookworm infection in children, strongyloidiasis, cystic hydatid disease and neurocysticercosis, and larval forms of *Taenia solium* (Liu and Weller 1993; Horton 1989).

The primary action of these drugs is inhibition of microtubule polymerization by binding to helminth β-tubulin (Lacey 1990), thus interfering with microtubule-dependent functions such as glucose uptake (Rang et al. 2007a).

10.3.1 Absorption, Fate, and Excretion

Both these drugs are poorly and erratically absorbed after oral administration. The absorption of albendazole is increased when given with a fatty meal (Rosenthal 2012). Their metabolic products appear in urine. Both these drugs have an excellent safety profile. Overall, the incidence of side effects, primarily mild gastrointestinal symptoms occur only in 1 % of patients (Urbani and Albonico 2003).

10.3.2 Therapeutic Uses

- *Albendazole* – It is safe and very effective in the control of gastrointestinal nematode infections which include mixed infections of Ascaris, Trichuria, and Ankylostoma with cure rates of about 97 %. It is administered 400 mg as a single dose. In heavy infection, it may have to be given for 3 days, i.e., three doses. It is the drug of choice to treat inoperable patients of hydatid cyst, and also for prevention of spread of infection during surgical excision of cyst. It is also the drug of choice to treat cysticercosis.

Lymphatic Filariasis Albendazole kills adult filarial worms when administered 400 mg twice daily for 14 days. The dead adult worms produce several local reactions at the sites where they are lodged, e.g., in the scrotum is bancroftian filariasis. It does not kill microfilariae, hence the microfilarial count is not reduced immediately. But if a single dose of albendazole 400 mg is administered with diethylcarbamazine (DEC) or ivermectin, the killing of microfilariae by these agents is markedly enhanced. Therefore, albendazole combined with diethylcarbamazine or ivermectin is recommended in global program of elimination of lymphatic filariasis (Molyneux and Zagaria 2002). The most suitable dosage schedule recommended for elimination of lymphatic filariasis in India is the administration of a single annual dose of albendazole 400 mg combined with diethylcarbamazine 6 mg/kg body weight for 4–6 years. It will prevent the transmission of filariasis in a community by lowering the microfilarial count. Also, it has the additional benefit of clearing a variety of intestinal worms. The benefits of adding albendazole to DEC or ivermectin for elimination of lymphatic filariasis are now doubted (Addiss et al. 2004).

Albendazole has excellent tolerability than mebendazole and has the advantage of single-dose administration in many intestinal infections (Tripathi 2013a).

Mechanism of Action Albendazole inhibits the polymerization of parasitic β-tubulin into microtubules (Prichard 1994). It results in impaired uptake of glucose by the larval and adult forms of the parasite which causes their immobilization and death. A secondary effect of albendazole may be inhibition of enzyme fumarate reductase that is helminth specific.

Adverse Effects It has few side effects when used for a short period and they include nausea, vomiting, headache, and abdominal pain. Rare toxicity includes pyrexia, skin rash, itching, sore throat, thinning or loss of hair, and unusual weakness. The serious toxicity includes acute kidney failure, pancytopenia, agranulocytosis, thrombocytopenia (rare), and hepatotoxicity with elevated liver enzymes. Therefore, blood counts and liver function tests should be done repeatedly during prolonged albendazole treatment (Rosenthal 2012).

Must Remember: Albendazole

- Broad-spectrum anthelmintic
- Macrofilaricidal
- Used in filarial eradication programme with DEC or ivermectin

- *Mebendazole* – Mebendazole is a potent anthelmintic-like albendazole with a wide range of activity against both nematodes and cestodes, and against both tissue stages of the parasite as well as in the lumen of the gut. It acts by inhibiting the assembly of the microtubules in the parasite and also by irreversibly blocking glucose uptake (Martin 2015). It is poorly absorbed from the gastrointestinal tract; hence, high doses must be used when treating tissue infections like filarial infection.

It stops the development of the embryos of onchocerciasis, and when given with levamisole, it has both microfilaricidal and embryostatic effects. The microfilarial counts in the blood fall slowly and the effects may last for up to 6 months.

Dose – 100 mg twice daily orally for 3 days or 500 mg as a single dose.

Adverse Effects The side effects are unusual at lower doses but common when high doses are given and even death can occur with very high doses. It should not be given during pregnancy.

10.4 Doxycycline

Like minocycline, doxycycline is a semisynthetic broad-spectrum antibiotic (a tetracycline) which possesses a wide range of antimicrobial activity against aerobic and anaerobic gram-positive and gram-negative bacteria.

It is the antibiotic of first choice to treat *Brucella*, *Vibrio cholerae*, *Ureaplasma urealyticum*, *Rickettsiae*, *Calymmatobacterium granulomatis*, *Borrelia*, *Mycoplasma pneumoniae*, and *Chlamydia* spp. infections.

It has a longer half-life and does not have any nephrotoxic activity because of biliary excretion. It is the drug of choice for early stage lime disease and in the prophylaxis of anthrax (Sharma and Sharma 2011).

Doxycycline has recently been shown to have significant macrofilaricidal activity against *W. bancrofti* which seems to be better than any other drug available against adult worms (Rang et al. 2007b; Rosenthal 2012). It acts indirectly by killing *Wolbachia*, an intracellular bacterial symbiont of the filarial worms. This bacterium is essential for worm fertility and survival. It is given 100–200 mg daily orally for 4–6 weeks to kill *Wolbachia* thereby controlling acute filariasis. By killing *Wolbachia* it makes the adult female *W. bancrofti* and *Onchocerca* worms sterile (Taylor and Hoerauf 2001). Hence, it may be an important drug for filariasis, both for treatment of active disease and mass chemoprophylaxis compaigns. One study has shown that the *Wolbachia* depletion is associated with the reduction of levels of vascular endothelial growth factors (VEGFs) essential for lymphangiogenesis.

Doxycycline treatment results in 78 % reduction of macrofilarial activity. It does not happen early (within days) as seen with diethylcarbamazine. Hence, its use does not result in adverse reactions related to the death of worms, e.g., scrotal pain, abscesses, etc. It may be associated with antibiotic-related diarrhea.

Recently, doxycycline has been shown to be effective in *B. malayi* infection.

Another unique feature of doxycycline is reduction of diameter of scrotal lymphatics which is increased due to toxins produced by filarial worms (a marker of lymphangiogenesis induced by filarial worms). This effect is absent in diethylcarbamazine. This effect of doxycycline may be responsible for reduction of size of small to medium hydroceles after doxycycline therapy. It may be used in mass chemotherapy campaigns (Rosenthal 2012).

Must Remember: Doxycycline

- Broad-spectrum antibiotic
- Kills adult worms by killing intracellular endosymbiont *Wolbachia* bacteria
- Strong macrofilaricidal effect without microfilarial death-induced adverse reactions

Doxycyline has a strong microfilaricidal effect without mircofilarial death-related toxic reactions with reversal of pathological changes seen in this disease.

Hence, doxycycline treatment is ideal for paticnts who seek treatment that targets the disease-producing adult worms as well as the disease, e.g., scrotal hydrocele.

Side Effects Similar to other tetracyclines the side effects include gastrointestinal irritation, hepatic toxicity, brown discoloration of teeth in children, and hypersensitivity reaction. These reactions are uncommon. It should not be given during pregnancy (Tripathi, 2013b).

10.5 Metrifonate (Trichlorfon)

It is an organophosphate which is a strong inhibitor of cholinesterases that was first used as an insecticide. It has a high anthelmentic activity which was proved in 1960s.

It is commonly used as an alternative to praziquantel to treat *Schistosoma haematobium* infection. It is effective, cheap, and well tolerated in urinary schistosomiasis.

It is also used in bancroftian filariasis as it is an effective microfilaricide. Its dose is 10 mg/kg body weight for 3 consecutive days. It also kills the microfilariae of *Onchocerca volvulus* partially.

Side Effects Although plasma cholinesterase levels fall and remain low for several weeks after treatment, the side effects are not severe. If the dose is increased above 10 mg/kg nausea, vomiting and abdominal pain are frequent.

Must Remember
- Two microfilaricides – Diethylcarbamazine and ivermectin
- Two macrofilaricides – Albendazole and Doxycycline

10.6 Levamisole (Ergamisol)

It acts by interfering with the carbohydrate metabolism and inhibiting the production of succinate dehydrogenase resulting in muscular paralysis of worms. It is most commonly used in the treatment of round worm (*Ascaris lumbricoides*) infection (Rang et al. 2007a).

Levamisole is also a non-humoral immunostimulant in immunosuppressed patients. It increases delayed hypersensitivity and/or T-cell-mediated immunity. Hence it has been used in Hodgkin's lymphoma, rheumatoid arthritis, and more recently in adjuvant chemotherapy of colorectal carcinoma (Chirigos 1992). The mechanism of immune stimulation is not known.

Antifilarial Activity In a study, a single dose of levamisole, 3 mg/kg body weight, had significant microfilaricidal effect in some patients of bancroftian filariasis though there was a significant variation in the response. In some patients, the blood remained negative or at a low level for microfilariae for several months. The patients with high pretreatment microfilaremia responded less to this treatment than those with low counts. Diethylcarbamazine–levamisole combined treatment appears to have no benefit over the use of diethylcarbamazine alone. Levamisole has significant activity against microfilariae of *W. bancrofti* and *B. malayi*, but it is not as effective as diethylcarbamazine, and the side effects are more.

Levamisole does not have significant action on adult worms and microfilariae of *Onchocerca volvulus*, but its local application may find a place in the treatment of ocular onchocerciasis.

Side Effects The side effects of this drug are uncommon and include fever, nausea, emesis, abdominal pain, dizziness, diarrhea, cutaneous rash, and transient neutropenia.

10.7 Suramin

Suramin is also known as Antrypol. It kills adult *W. bancrofti* and other filarial parasites. It has some effect on microfilariae also. It was introduced to treat African trypanosomiasis in the 1920s, and it is its drug of choice. It was subsequently found to be effective in filarial infection also. However, because of its high toxicity and availability of better filaricides, it is not usually used to treat filariasis. Further, it has to be administered by a slow intravenous injection as it is not absorbed from gastrointestinal tract. It is excreted slowly in urine and is detectable in urine up to 3 months after the last dose.

Side Effects The side effects occur due to innate toxicity of the drug or from its filaricidal action. The toxic side effects include fatal collapse during injection, significant albuminuria, oral ulceration, exfoliative dermatitis, severe diarrhea, prolonged high fever, and prostration. The less severe toxicity include tiredness, anorexia, malaise, polyuria, and increased thirst and tenderness in palms and soles.

The side effects from its filaricidal action include urticaria, swelling, tenderness and abscess formation around dead adult worms, painful immobilization of hip joint due to inflammatory reaction to worm bundles adjacent to joint capsule; intensely itchy urtico-papular rash associated with death of microfilariae; inflammatory and subsequent degenerative changes in the optic nerve and retina due to death of intraocular microfilariae; and swollen painful joints, particularly of hands and feet, possibly due to formation of immune complexes.

Contraindications Suramin is a very toxic drug, hence it must always be given under medical supervision in a hospital. It should not be given to old and infirm and patients with severe liver disease, children below 10 years of age, totally blind patients asking for relief from intensely itchy lesions; mild or moderate asymptomatic onchocerciasis when eyes are not at risk, and pregnant women.

10.8 Amodiaquine

It is a congener of chloroquine that is no longer recommended for the chemoprophylaxis of falciparum malaria due to its toxicity, like hepatotoxicity and agranulocytosis. In a total dose of 40 mg/kg, it appears to be macrofilaricidal but is not used for this purpose because of its toxicity. Some amodiaquine congeners may have a higher chemotherapeutic index and may be used in chemoprophylaxis against *W. bancrofti* infection in man (McMahon 1979).

The summary of commonly used antifilarial drugs are given in the following table (Table 10.1 and 10.2):

10.9 Herbal Remedies

There are several herbs which have been used traditionally by local practitioners to treat lymphatic filariasis for centuries. Following are some of the herbs having antifilarial activity (Chandy et al. 2011):

1. *Vitex negundo* L (roots) (Sahare et al. 2008)
2. *Butea monosperma* L (roots and leaves) (Sahare et al. 2008)
3. *Ricinus communis* L (leaves) (Sahare et al. 2008)
4. *Aegle marmelos* Corr (leaves) (Sahare et al. 2008)
5. *Canthium mannii* (Rubiaceae) (Wabo Pone et al. 2010)
6. *Boerhaavia diffusa* L (whole plant) (Jain and Singh 2010)
7. Asperzine B (Pani 2013) – It is an herbal product manufactured by Phyto Pharma of Odisha (India) which is used by tribal population of Koraput and Sambalpur. It is a mixture of *Streblus asper*, *Argyreia speciosa*, *Symplocos*, and liquorice. It is available in capsule and syrup form.

It results in disappearance of microfilariae and macrofilariae from the body within 6 weeks of treatment. It irritates the stomach hence should be used with precaution in peptic ulcer patients. Sometimes Jarisch–Herxheimer type of reaction consisting of increase in edema, itching, fever, and sweating from limbs occur. It is transient and disappears after the use of antihistaminics.

The common side effects of this product include anorexia, epigastric pain, hyperacidity, nausea, vomiting, and constipation. Less common side effects are diarrhea, reeling headache, insomnia, and heaviness in chest.

Dose–10 ml of syrup or 1 capsule is given three times daily after meals for 6 weeks. Another course can be given after 15 days interval.

Table 10.1 Most commonly used antifilarial drugs

Drug	Antifilarial action	Clinical uses	Dose and administration	Side effects
Diethylcarbamazine	Antimicrofilarial – Quick and complete Adult worms – Killed slowly and incompletely	Treatment of lymphatic filariasis	6 mg/kg body weight orally after meals in 3 divided doses for 10–14 days	Usually well tolerated Immunological reaction similar to Mazzotti reaction in onchocerciasis may occur in the beginning of treatment
		Treatment of tropical pulmonary eosinophilia	4–6 mg/kg body weight orally for 3–4 weeks	
		Prevention of lymphatic filariasis	A single dose of 6–mg/kg body weight with albendazole 400 mg annually for 4–6 years	
Ivermectin	Microfilariae – Most are eliminated Adult worms – No effect	Onchocerciasis	A single oral dose of 150 μg/kg every 6–12 months in adults and children 5 years of older	Mild ocular irritation and somnolence Mazzotti reaction may occur due to death of microfilariae consisting of headache, rash, pruritus, arthralgia, myalgia, and lymphadenopathy
		Lymphatic filariasis	A single oral dose of 400 μg/kg annually	
		Intestinal nematode infection	A single oral dose of 150–200 μg/kg	
		Prevention of lymphatic filariasis	A single annual oral dose of 400 μg/kg of body weight with 400 mg of albendazole for 4–6 years	

(continued)

Table 10.1 (continued)

Drug	Antifilarial action	Clinical uses	Dose and administration	Side effects
Albendazole	Microfilariae – No direct effect Adult worms – Most are eliminated	As a broad-spectrum anthelmintic	400 mg orally as a single dose	Usually well tolerated Usually mild side effects Headache, nausea, vomiting, and abdominal pain Rarely fever, skin rash or itching Not given during pregnancy
		Echinococcosis	400 mg twice daily orally for 4 weeks	
		Prevention of lymphatic filariasis	A single dose of albendazole 400 mg with 6 mg/kg body weight of diethylcarbamazine or 400 μg/kg of ivermectin is once a year for 4–6 years	

Table 10.2 Effective antifilarial drug but not yet commonly used

Drug	Pharmacological action	Clinical uses	Dose	Side effects
Doxycycline	Antibiotic action	As a broad-spectrum antibiotic in a variety of infections	100 mg twice daily orally for 10–14 days	Usually well tolerated Adverse reactions include gastrointestinal irritation, hepatic and renal toxicity and pigmentation of teeth
	Antifilarial action Mircofilariae – No direct action Adult worms – Killed due to killing of Wolbachia	Lymphatic filariasis	100–200 mg daily orally for 4–6 weeks	

(This chapter is based on an article, "Antifilarial drugs," sent by Dr IP Jain, Former Professor and Head of Department of Pharmacology, GSVM Medical College, Kanpur).

References

Addiss DG, Critchley J, Ejere H, et al. International Filariasis Review Group. Cochrane Database Syst Rev. 2004;CD0037553.

Awadzi K, Adjapon-Yomoah KK, Edwards G, et al. The effect of moderate urine alkalinization on diethylcarbamazine therapy in patients with onchocerciasis. Br J Clin Pharmacol. 1986;27:669–76.

Campbell WC. Ivermectin and abamectin. New York: Springer; 1989. http://www.springer.com/in/book/9781461281849.

Chandy A, Thakur AS, Singh MP, Manigauha A. A review of neglected tropical disease: filariasis. Asian Pac J Trop Med. 2011;4:581–6.

Chirigos MA. Immunomodulator: current and future development and application. Thymus. 1992;19:S7–20.

Edwards G, Breckenridge AM, et al. The effect of variations in urinary pH on the pharmacokinetics of diethylcarbamazine. Br J Clin Pharmacol. 1981;12:807–12.

Faulkner JK, Smith KJ. Dealkylation and N-oxidation in the metabolism of 1-diethyl-carbamyl-4-methyl piperazine in the rat. Xenobiotica. 1972;2:59–68.

Goa KL, McTavish D, Clissold SP. Ivermectin: a review of its antifilarial activity, pharmacokinetic properties and clinical efficacy in Onchocerciasis. Drugs. 1991;42:640–58.

Hawking F. Diethylcarbamazine and new compounds for the treatment of filariasis. Adv Pharmacol Chemother. 1979;16:129–94.

Horton RS. Chemotherapy of Echinococcus infection in man with albendazole. Trans R Soc Trop Med Hyg. 1989;83:97–102.

Jain SP, Singh J. Traditional medicinal practice among the tribal people of Raigarh (Chhattisgarh, India). Indian J Nat Product Resour. 2010;1:109–15.

Klotz U, Qgbuokiri JE, Okonkwo PO. Ivermectin binds avidly to plasma proteins. Eur J Clin Pharmacol. 1990;39:607–8.

Krishna DR, Klotz U. Determination of Ivermectin in human plasma by high performance liquid chromatography. Arznei Mittelforshung. 1993;43:609–11.

Lacey E. The mode of action of benzimidazoles. Parasitol Today. 1990;6:112–5.

Liu LX, Weller PF. Strogyloidiasis and other intestinal nematode infections. Infect Dis Clin North Am. 1993;7:655–82.

Mackenzie CD, Kron MA. Diethylcarbamazine: a review of its action in onchocerciasis, lymphatic filariasis and inflammation. Trop Dis Bull. 1985;82:R1–37.

McMahon JE. Preliminary screening of antifilarial activity of levamisole and amodiaquine on Wuchereria bancrofti. Ann Trop Med Parasitol. 1979;73(5):465–72.

Martin LC. Anthelmintic drugs. In: Whalen K, editor. Illustrated reviews: pharmacology. 6th ed. New Delhi: Wolters Kluwer; 2015. p. 561–2.

Molyneux DH, Zagaria N. Lymphatic filariasis elimination, progress in global programme development. Ann Trop Med Parasitol. 2002;98:515–40.

Naquira C, Jimenez G, Guerra JG, et al. Ivermectin for human strongyloidiasis and other intestinal helminths. Am J Trop Med Hyg. 1989;40:304–9.

Ottsen EA, Ramchandran CP. Lymphatic filariasis infection and disease. Control strategies. Parasitol Today. 1995;11:129–31.

Pani S. Pani's filariasis. 3rd ed. New Delhi: Jaypee Brothers; 2013.

Pong SS, Wang CD, Fritz LC. Studies on the mechanism of action of avermectin B1a: stimulation of release of gamma-aminobutyric acid from brain synaptosomes. J Neurochem. 1980;34:351–8.

Prichard R. Anthelmintic resistance. Vet Parasitol. 1994;54:259–68.

Rang HP, Dale MM, Ritter JM, Flower RJ, Henderson G. Anthelminthic drugs. In: Pharmacology. 7th ed. Edinburgh: Elsevier Churchill Livingstone; 2007a. p. 668–72.

Rang HP, Dale MM, Ritter JM, Flower RJ, Henderson G. Antibacterial drugs. In: Pharmacology. 7th ed. Edinburgh: Elsevier Churchill Livingstone; 2007b. p. 629.

Rosenthal PJ. Clinical pharmacology of the antihelminthic drugs. In: Katzung BG, Masters SB, Trevor AJ, editors. Basic & clinical pharmacology. 12th ed. New Delhi: Tata McGraw Hill; 2012. p. 937–42.

Sahare KN, Anandharaman V, Meshram VG, Meshram SU, Gajlakshmi D, Goswami K, et al. In vitro effect of four herbal plants of the motility of Brugia malayi microfilariae. Indian J Med Res. 2008;127:467–71.

Sharma HL, Sharma KK. Broad-spectrum antibiotics: tetracyclines and chloramphenicol. In: Principles of pharmacology. 2nd ed. Hyderabad: Paras Medical Publisher; 2011. p. 749.

Spiro R, Parsons WG. Inhibition of post-translational modification and surface expression of a melanoma-associated chondroitin sulfate proteoglycan by diethylcarbamazine or aminonium chloride. J Biol Chem. 1986;216:5121–9.

Taylor MJ, Hoerauf A. A new approach to the treatment of filariasis. Curr Opin Infect Dis. 2001;14:727–31.

Tripathi KD. Anthelmintic drugs. In: Essentials of medical pharmacology. 7th ed. New Delhi: Jaypee; 2013a. p. 849–56.

Tripathi KD. Tetracyclines and chloramphenicol. In: Essentials of medical pharmacology. 7th ed. New Delhi: Jaypee; 2013b. p. 732–9.

Urbani C, Albonico M. Anthelminthic drug safety and drug administration in the control of soil-transmitted helminthiasis in community compaigns. Acta Trop. 2003;86:215–23.

Wabo Pone J, Bilong Bilong CF, Mpoame M. In vitro nematicidal activity of extracts of Canthium mannii (Rubiaceae) on different life cycle stages of Heligmosomomoides polygyrus (Nematoda, Heligomosomatidae). J Helminthol. 2010;84:156–65.

Wang CC, Pong SS. Actions of avermectin B1a on GABA nerves. Prog Clin Biol Res. 1982;97:373–95.

Wartman WB. Filariasis in American armed forces in World War II. Medicine. 1947;26:334–94.

Clinical Manifestations of Filariasis 11

The lymphatic filariasis manifests itself in a variety of subclinical and clinical manners.

11.1 Subclinical or Asymptomatic Microfilaremia

In filarial endemic areas, many people do not have any symptoms or signs of filariasis, yet the examination of blood shows a large number of microfilariae. These people are carriers of infection and reservoirs of ongoing transmission. The microfilarial burden may exceed 10,000 microfilariae in 1 mL of blood. These patients were further studied, and the following are the findings:

- *Lymphoscintigraphy* – The lymphatics of these individuals have profound changes, including marked dilatation and tortuosity with collateral channeling, increased flow, and abnormal patterns of lymph flow (Friedman et al. 1994; Freedman et al. 1995).
- *Ultrasonography* – Ultrasonography of scrotal lymphatics showed motile adult worms in dilated lymphatics in 50 % of these men having bancroftian infection. It is known as "filarial dance sign" (Noroes et al. 1996).
- *Superficial skin punch biopsy* of limbs shows abnormally dilated lymphatic vessels.

In addition to above, 40 % of asymptomatic microfilaremic individuals reveal microscopic hematuria and/or proteinuria indicative of renal damage (Dreyer et al. 1992).

11.2 Acute Clinical Disease

Acute clinical filariasis is characterized by recurrent attacks of fever with or without rigors associated with inflammation of lymph nodes (lymphadenitis) and lymphatics (lymphangitis) and related structures. In brugian infection, attacks of fever,

T.C. Goel, A. Goel, *Lymphatic Filariasis*, DOI 10.1007/978-981-10-2257-9_11

lymphadenitis, and lymphangitis are common, while in bancroftian filariasis, the attacks are few and occur insidiously (Pani et al. 1990). The inguinal, axillary, and epitrochlear lymph nodes are commonly involved. In bancroftian filariasis, the lymphatics of male genitals are commonly involved, leading to funiculitis, epididymitis, and/or orchitis (Pani and Srividya 1992).

Acute filarial attacks are known to occur in infants as young as 3 months of age but are usually more common in older children and continue throughout life (Dasgupta 1984; Nanduri and Kazura 1989). Acute filariasis occurs in people living in endemic areas but it can also occur in filaria-infected expatriates (Melrose et al. 2000).

11.3 Chronic Filarial Disease

The chronic manifestations of lymphatic filariasis are postulated to develop nearly 10–15 years after initial infection (Partono 1987).

In bancroftian filariasis, the main clinical manifestations include scrotal hydrocele, lymphedema, elephantiasis, and chyluria. The chronic lymphedema, elephantiasis, involves entire lower extremity, scrotum, penis, entire upper extremity, vulva, and breast.

In brugian filariasis, the lower extremity below the knee and the upper extremity below the elbow are commonly involved and the genitals are rarely involved (Pani et al. 1990).

Tropical pulmonary eosinophilia (TPE) occurs in some persons infected with *Wuchereria bancrofti* and *Brugia malayi*. It is characterized by paroxysmal cough and wheezing that are usually nocturnal (and probably related to nocturnal periodicity of microfilariae) and pronounced blood eosinophilia, i.e., more than 300 eosinophils/mL. The sitewise clinical manifestations are given in Table 11.1 (Shenoy and Shenoy 2010).

The acute filarial fever is the commonest acute clinical manifestation. It is caused by microfilaremia. The scrotal hydrocele is the commonest chronic manifestation (Chandy et al. 2011).

11.4 Classification of Clinical Manifestations

- *Common manifestations*
  (a) Inflammatory manifestations
    1. Filarial fever
    2. Acute lymphangitis (AFL)
    3. Acute lymphadenitis
    4. Acute dermatolymphangioadenitis (ADLA)
    5. Funiculitis
    6. Epididymo-orchitis
    7. Cellulitis

8. Abscess
(b) Obstructive manifestations
1. Scrotal hydrocele
2. Chronic lymphedema–elephantiasis
3. Chyluria
(c) Tropical pulmonary eosinophilia
- *Less common manifestations*
(a) Inflammatory manifestations
1. Ulceration
2. Gangrene
3. Salpingo-oophoritis
(b) Obstructive manifestations
1. Lymphangiovarix
2. Lymphadenovarix
3. Chylocele
4. Lymph scrotum
5. Chylous ascites
- *Rare manifestations*
(a) Inflammatory manifestations – cystitis, peritonitis, thrombophlebitis, synovitis, arthritis, myositis
(b) Obstructive manifestations – chylous diarrhea, chylothorax, lymphuria, hematuria, pericardial effusion, constrictive pericarditis, chylous arthritis
- *Very rare manifestations* – eosinophilic lymphadenopathy, solitary coin lesions of the lung, subcutaneous nodules – most of these manifestations are isolated case reports.

11.5 Anatomical Classification of Clinical Manifestations

- *Lymphatic system*
1. Acute lymphangitis (AFL)
2. Acute lymphadenitis
3. Acute dermatolymphangioadenitis (ADLA)
4. Lymphangiovarix
5. Lymphadenovarix
6. Chronic lymphadenitis, lymphadenopathy
- *Lower extremity*
1. Acute lymphangitis (AFL)
2. Acute lymphadenitis
3. Acute dermatolymphangioadenitis
4. Chronic lymphedema–elephantiasis
5. Cellulitis, abscess
6. Lymphorrhea, chylorrhea
7. Ulceration

8. Gangrene
9. Synovitis, arthritis of knee joint

- *Male external genitalia*
  1. Funiculitis
  2. Epididymo-orchitis
  3. Hydrocele
  4. Lymphangiovarix
  5. Chronic lymphedema–elephantiasis, of scrotum and/or penis
  6. Chylocele
  7. Lymph scrotum
  8. Chylorrhea, lymphorrhea
  9. Pyocele
  10. Gangrene of scrotum
- *Female genital tract*
  1. Cellulitis, abscess
  2. Chronic lymphedema–elephantiasis
  3. Chylorrhea-lymphorrhea
  4. Salpingo-oophoritis
- *Female breast*
  1. Cellulitis, abscess
  2. Chronic lymphedema–elephantiasis
  3. Subcutaneous nodules, lump
  4. Lymph varix
- *Thorax*
  1. Chylothorax
  2. Chylopericardium, chronic pericarditis
- *Abdomen, including kidneys*
  1. Retroperitoneal lymphangitis
  2. Chyluria
  3. Hematuria
  4. Lymphuria, proteinuria
  5. Chylous ascites
  6. Chylous diarrhea
  7. Nephrotic syndrome
  8. Glomerulonephritis
- *Neurological manifestations* – there are no neurological manifestations as this parasite does not cross blood–brain barrier (Pani 2013). Further, there are no lymphatics in the central nervous system – it may be another cause.

Table 11.1 Sitewise clinical manifestations

Site – structure/part affected	Acute manifestations	Chronic manifestations
Extremities, mostly the lower	Lymphangitis (AFL) Lymphadenitis Acute dermatolymphangioadenitis (ADLA) Abscess	Chronic lymphadenitis – lymphadenopathy Lymphedema Elephantiasis Lymphadenovarix
Scrotum	Lymphangitis Abscess	Hydrocele Chylocele Lymphedema Elephantiasis Lymph scrotum Lymphorrhea, chylorrhea
Spermatic cord	Acute funiculitis Abscess	Chronic funiculitis Lymphangiovarix/cyst
Epididymis and testis	Acute epididymo-orchitis	Chronic/recurrent epididymo-orchitis
Abdomen	Acute retroperitoneal lymphangitis	Chyluria Chylous ascites Chylous diarrhea Chylous cyst
Breast	Lymphangitis Abscess	Lymphedema Varicose lymphatics Elephantiasis Nodule/mass
Vulva	Acute lymphangitis Abscess	Lymphedema Elephantiasis
Lungs	–	Tropical pulmonary eosinophilia

11.6 Manifestations of Lymphatic Filariasis in Children

In endemic areas, filariasis is first acquired during childhood and manifests as acute dermatolymphangioadenitis attacks, scrotal hydrocele, and lymphedema of extremities.

11.7 Geographic Variation in Clinical Manifestations

Clinical manifestations of filariasis differ significantly between different geographic areas, e.g., tropical pulmonary eosinophilia (TPE) and chyluria commonly occur in South and Southeast Asian countries while they occur less commonly in Africa. In Tanzania, which is a highly endemic lymphatic filariasis area, TPE is rare (Magnussen et al. 1995).

Table 11.2 Clinical manifestations of filariasis (Ghooi and Khanna 1976)

Manifestation	Number of cases
Eosinophilia	30
Filarial fever	55
Elephantiasis	45
Scrotal hydrocele	40
Lymphadenopathy	40
Abscess	25
Epididymo-orchitis	16
Lymph varix	4
Hematuria	3
Varicose groin glands (lymphadenovarix)	2
Chyluria	0

In Papua New Guinea, the bancroftian microfilarial prevalence can be very high reaching up to 60–80 % in the population while the clinical prevalence rates of hydrocele and elephantiasis tend to be similar or lower than those noted in highly endemic areas, i.e., 15–30 % of microfilarial prevalence elsewhere in the world (Kazura et al. 1997).

11.8 Relative Frequency of Clinical Manifestations

Many workers have described the clinical manifestations of lymphatic filariasis (Chatterjee 1959; Beaver et al. 1971; Chatterjee 1971; Madhavan et al. 1972; Babu et al. 2001). The relative incidence of clinical manifestations among 90 cases of lymphatic filariasis as reported by Ghooi and Khanna (1976) is shown in Table 11.2.

Babu et al. (2001) reported the occurrence of filariasis from Khurda district of Odisha among 5357 patients, including 2806 males and 2551 females. The following were the findings:

Manifestation	Male	Female	Total
ADL	175	119	294
Scrotal hydrocele	115	–	115
Elephantiasis	69	115	184
ADL + elephantiasis	16	14	30
ADL + hydrocele	32	–	32
Elephantiasis + hydrocele	5	–	5
ADL + elephantiasis + hydrocele	1	–	1
Arm elephantiasis	2	5	7
Breast swelling	-	5	5
Total manifestations	415	256	671

11.9 Our Experience

Out of a total of 50,224 patients admitted in the Surgical Indoors of King George's Medical College, Lucknow, during 1979–1984, 1539 patients had lymphatic filariasis (more than 3 % of all admissions). Approximately 35,000 patients attend surgical outdoor every year; 2–3 % of these patients come with some filarial manifestation.

The relative frequency of clinical manifestations of admitted patients is given in the following table (Goel 1986):

Manifestation	1979	1980	1981	1982	1983	1984
Filarial hydrocele	185	178	180	184	182	208
All hydroceles	209	190	197	206	204	215
Chronic lymphedema–elephantiasis						
Lower extremity	19	11	9	18	15	19
Scrotum/penis	6	5	4	7	4	6
Upper extremity	0	1	0	0	0	0
Breast	1	0	1	0	0	1
Vulva	1	0	0	0	0	0
Funiculitis	14	9	9	9	11	14
Epididymo-orchitis	18	19	9	4	9	13
Chyluria	2	9	6	14	8	10
Filarial abscess	2	4	6	5	2	15
Lymph varix	2	0	0	0	1	2
Hematuria	4	8	7	3	2	4
Lymph scrotum	2	0	0	1	1	2
Scrotal gangrene	5	4	3	2	2	2
Lymphadenopathy	5	4	3	3	2	7
Hematochezia	0	0	0	0	2	0
Total	266	252	237	250	241	303
Total indoor admissions	7783	8347	8358	8344	8447	8945
Total outdoor attendance	33,932	24,178	36,074	37,097	39,326	40,103

References

Babu BV, Acharya AS, Mallick G, et al. Lymphatic filariasis in Khurda district of Orrisa, India: an epidemiological study. Southeast Asian J Trop Med Public Health. 2001;32(2):240–3.

Beaver PC, Fallon M, Smith GH. Pulmonary nodule caused by a living B malayi-like filaria in an artery. Am J Trop Med Hyg. 1971;20:661–6.

Chandy A, Thakur AS, Singh MP, Manigauha A. A review of neglected tropical diseases: filariasis. Asian Pac J Trop Med. 2011;4:581–6.

Chatterjee KD. Parasitology. 2nd ed. Calcutta: Published by Author; 1959. p. 162.

Chatterjee BP. A short textbook of surgery, vol. 1. 1st ed. Calcutta: New Central Book Agency; 1971. p. 40–1.

Dasgupta A. Cursory survey of lymphatic filariasis. An overview. Indian J Pathol Microbiol. 1984;27:273–80.

Dreyer G, Ottesen EA, et al. Renal abnormalities in microfilaremic patients with bancroftian filariasis. Am J Trop Med Hyg. 1992;46:745–51.

Freedman DO, de Almeido Filho PJ, Besh S, Silva MC M e, Braga C, Maciel A, Furtado AF. Abnormal lymphatic function in presymptomatic bancroftian lymphatic filariasis. J Infect Dis. 1995;171:997–1001.

Friedman DO, Filho PJA, Besh S, et al. Lymphoscintigraphic analysis of lymphatic abnormalities in symptomatic and asymptomatic human filariasis. J Infect Dis. 1994;70:927–33.

Ghooi AM, Khanna T. Surgical manifestations of filariasis. Indian J Surg. 1976;38:150.

Goel TC. Clinical manifestations of lymphatic filariasis. In: Sen AB, Katiyar JC, editors. Perspectives of parasitology, vol. 1. Lucknow: Print House; 1986. p. 89–123.

Kazura JW, Bockarie M, Alexander N, et al. Transmission intensity and its relationship to infection and disease due to Wuchereria bancrofti in Papua New Guinea. J Infect Dis. 1997;176:242–6.

Madhavan M, Sankaran V, Chandra K, Reddy DJ. Atypical manifestations of filariasis in Pondicherry. Indian J Surg. 1972;34:362.

Magnussen P, Makunde W, Simonsen PE, et al. Chronic pulmonary disorders including tropical pulmonary eosinophilia, in villages with endemic lymphatic filariasis in Tanga region and in Tanga town, Tanzania. Trans R Soc Trop Med Hyg. 1995;89:406–9.

Melrose WD, Usurup J, et al. Development of antifilarial antibodies in a group of expatriate mine-site workers with varying exposure to the disease. Trans R Soc Trop Med Hyg. 2000;94: 706–7.

Nanduri J, Kazura JW. Clinical and laboratory aspects of filariasis. Clin Microbiol Rev. 1989;2:39–50.

Noroes J, Addiss D, Amaral F, Coutinho A, Medeiros Z, Dreyer D. Occurrence of adult Wuchereria bancrofti in the scrotal area of men with microfilaremia. Trans R Soc Trop Med Hyg. 1996;90:55–6.

Pani S. Pani's filariasis. 3rd ed. New Delhi: Jaypee Brothers; 2013.

Pani SP, Srividya A. Clinical manifestations of bancroftian filariasis with special reference to lymphedema grading. Indian J Med Res. 1992;102:114–8.

Pani SP, Krishnamoorty K, et al. Clinical manifestations in Malayan filariasis infection with special reference to lymphedema grading. Indian J Med Res. 1990;91:200–7.

Partono F. The spectrum of disease in lymphatic filariasis. Ciba Found Symp. 1987;127:15–31.

Shenoy KR, Shenoy A. Manipal manual of surgery. 4th ed. New Delhi: CBS; 2010. p. 110–8.

Part II

Acute Clinical Manifestations

12 Filarial Fever

It is the most common symptom of clinical lymphatic filariasis and may occur alone or may be associated with some other clinical manifestation of filariasis. Fever associated with elephantiasis is called as "elephantoid fever."

12.1 Etiology

It is certain that adult filarial worms are responsible for nearly all the clinical manifestations of filariasis. The fever is usually due to subclinical sterile lymphangitis and lymphadenitis caused by toxins and allergens produced by this parasite. Secondary streptococcal infection of affected lymphatics may contribute in the etiology of fever.

Pani (2013) has described filarial fever in great detail in his monograph on filariasis.

12.2 Clinical Features

The attack begins with rigor and tremor. It starts suddenly and persists for about 1–3 h. The patient feels shivery throughout the whole body but more marked in the extremities and back. It may be associated with flushing of the face and conjunctival congestion with lacrimation and nasal discharge. The mucosa of pharynx, larynx, and nose is congested.

The temperature is subnormal during the rigor, i.e., 96 °F or 97 °F. Hence, the patient asks for heavy cover by thick blankets and feels better if pressure is put over the back (Pani 2013).

Etiologically, the rigor is related to the excessive production of histamine and H-like substances in response to liberation of toxins and allergens from dead adult worms.

T.C. Goel, A. Goel, *Lymphatic Filariasis*, DOI 10.1007/978-981-10-2257-9_12

The patient may vomit, especially if the attack comes after a heavy meal. It is a specific symptom of retroperitoneal lymphatic involvement.

As soon as the rigor subsides the fever supervenes. It starts with headache and body ache. The fever remains high (101–104 °F) for 2–3 days. It is continuous and may be lowered in the morning and may even become normal in a few patients. It may be associated with coated tongue and halitosis. There may be cough with or without expectoration. The pulse and respiration rate may increase during the attack of fever.

When the fever subsides, the local signs of filariasis may become obvious, and the related lymph nodes may become painful and tender.

The fever tends to recur and the recurrences may go on for years. It may come sometimes as late as 20 years after leaving the endemic area.

12.3 Differential Diagnosis

The filarial fever must be differentiated from other such types of fevers seen in clinical practice.

1. *Malaria* – It is another important cause of fever with rigor seen in endemic areas. The differential diagnosis of filarial fever from malarial fever is given in the following table:

Features	Filariasis	Malaria
Fever	Rigor followed by fever not followed by sweating Temperature remains elevated for 2–3 days	Rigor followed by fever followed by sweating with relief of fever Temperature is normal between the attacks of malaria
Liver and spleen	Not palpable	Likely to be palpable
Blood	Shows eosinophilia, may be microfilariae found in night blood smear	Malarial parasite (BT and MT rings) may be seen in red blood cells during an attack

2. *Subphrenic abscess* – It may present with fever with rigor and sweating without any other obvious symptoms and signs; hence, it is said about subphrenic abscess – signs of "pus somewhere, pus nowhere else, and pus under diaphragm" (Barnard aphorism). Hence, the patient should be examined and investigated accordingly. The displaced liver may be palpable in right upper abdomen, and four zones of altered resonance on percussion may be present on the back of right lower chest Radiography shows elevated right diaphragm with gas and fluid level under the right diaphragm (Bhat 2013).
3. *Enteric fever* – It is also a common cause of fever in filarial infested regions. Hence, the filarial fever has to be differentiated from enteric fever, which is characterized by continuous fever, discomfort or pain in abdomen, enlarged spleen (may be liver also), relative bradycardia, rose spots on the skin, and leukopenia

with relative lymphocytosis (Schwartz 2015) – leukopenia, bradycardia, and splenomegaly are not found in filariasis. The diagnosis of enteric fever is excluded by negative blood culture or immunological tests for enteric fever.

12.4 Investigations

- The blood shows leukocytosis, especially eosinophilia. The night blood smear is likely to be positive for microfilariae.
- Further investigations are done to rule out other possible causes of fever, for example, blood smear for malarial parasite, and blood culture for enteric fever.

12.5 Treatment

The patient is given bed rest and symptomatic and supportive treatment. Antifilarial drugs are not given in the beginning of treatment as they may aggravate the symptoms. Antibiotics are usually given, e.g., penicillin, amoxicillin, amoxiclav, or tetracycline. Many experts do not like to give streptomycin as it produces perilymphatic fibrosis, which may aggravate lymphedema in future.

References

Bhat Sriram M. Subphrenic abscess. In: SRB's manual of surgery. 4th ed. New Delhi: Jaypee Brothers; 2013. p. 810.

Pani S. Pani's filariasis. 3rd ed. New Delhi: Jaypee Brothers; 2013.

Schwartz BS. Enteric fever (typhoid fever). In: Papadakis MA, McPhee SJ, editors. Current medical diagnosis & treatment. 54th ed. New York: McGraw Hill; 2015. p. 1437–8.

Acute Filarial Lymphangitis (AFL) 13

Recently, two syndromes of acute filarial attacks in the extremities are described, and they include acute filarial lymphangitis (AFL) and acute dermatolymphangioadenitis (ADLA) (Dreyer et al. 1999). The details of these two syndromes are given in this chapter.

Acute filarial lymphangitis (AFL) is acute inflammation of lymphatics that occurs in lymphatic filariasis due to death of adult filarial worms in the lymphatics spontaneously or following administration of diethylcarbamazine. It is one of the early manifestation of this disease and rare as compared to acute dermatolymphangioadenitis (ADLA).

13.1 Clinical Features

It is characterized by a circumscribed inflammatory nodule or a cord centered on degenerating adult worms with red streaks of lymphangitis spreading in a descending fashion (centrifugal fashion) from the nodule or cord. There is no fever. The affected lymphatic may be tender and enlarged and feel like a cord. It usually has a mild clinical course without any secondary infection and rarely causes lymphedema. The pathogenesis and clinical consequences of AFL are given in the following Flow Chart 13.1:

The lymphatics of lower extremity, external genitalia, and retroperitoneum are commonly involved. Rarely, the lymphatics of breast and upper extremity are affected.

Lower Extremity It starts as a "focal spot" of sharp circumscribed pain and tenderness below one of the malleolus followed by ascending lymphangitis originating in this area. It may start higher up in the thigh with descending lymphangitis. In fair skinned people, the inflamed lymphatics may be visible as red streaks.

Scrotum The scrotal lymphatics is a preferred site of localization of adult filarial worms as confirmed by "filarial dance sign" (FDS) detected during Doppler

T.C. Goel, A. Goel, *Lymphatic Filariasis*, DOI 10.1007/978-981-10-2257-9_13

Dead adult worm in a lymphatic vessel
Usually of the lower extremity, may be inguino-scrotal region or breast
(Died spontaneously or following drug treatment of filariasis)

↓

Acute inflammation

↓

Acute filarial lymphangitis (AFL)

↓

- Malaise and chills
- Painful enlarged local lymph nodes
- Circumscribed inflammatory nodule or cord around degenerating worm with streaks of acute inflammation (lymphangitis) spreading in a descending fashion (opposite to bacterial lymphangitis)

↓

May cause lymphatic obstruction when inflammation heals but it is a localized obstruction

↓ ↓

Lymphedema (Rare sequel of AFL) | Scrotal hydrocele (Common cause of hydrocele)

Flow Chart 13.1 Pathogenesis and result of acute filarial lymphangitis (AFL)

ultrasonography in many asymptomatic microfilaremic males (Amaral et al. 1994). Their presence is correlated with higher microfilarial blood levels, but they have been detected even in amicrofilaremic males (Amaral et al. 1994). Scrotal lymphangitis is characterized by scroto-inguinal pain, redness, heat, and tenderness.

Inguinal lymph nodes are usually enlarged and tender in acute filarial lymphangitis of lower extremity and scrotum. The disease subsides spontaneously in most of the patients, but the recovery is incomplete with some thickening of the lymphatics and related skin.

Complications of above two anatomical types of acute filarial lymphangitis include cellulitis, abscess formation, and ulceration. The lymphangitis of inguino-scrotal lymphatics may be followed by scrotal hydrocele, but that of lower extremity may rarely cause lymphedema.

Retroperitoneal Lymphangitis Sometimes lymphatics of retroperitoneum are involved, which results in "acute abdomen-like" clinical picture. It is characterized by acute abdominal pain, fever with rigor, vomiting, and abdominal distension. It is a quite serious condition as the patient may rapidly develop peritonitis with fatal consequences. Other manifestations of filariasis may be present. The blood may show eosinophilia and microfilaremia.

Ultrasonography and other investigations may be required to rule out other important causes of acute abdomen. The treatment includes nothing orally, intravenous fluids and parenteral diethylcarbamazine.

Lymphadenitis and lymphangitis can involve both upper and lower extremities in both bancroftian and brugian lymphatic filariasis, but involvement of the genital and mammary lymphatics occurs almost exclusively in Wuchereria bancrofti infection. The genital involvement may manifest as funiculitis and epididymo-orchitis, which presents as scrotal pain and tenderness (Nutman and Weller 2012).

References

Amaral F, Dreyer G, Figueredo-Silva J, et al. Live adult worms detected by ultrasonography in human bancroftian filariasis. Am J Trop Med Hyg. 1994;50(6):753.

Dreyer G, Dreyer P, Piessens WF. Extralymphatic disease due to bancroftian filariasis. Braz J Med Biol Res. 1999;32:1467–72.

Nutman TB, Weller PF. Filarial and related infections. In: Longo DL, Fauci AS, Kasper DL, Hauser SL, Jameson JL, Loscalzo J, editors. Harrison's internal medicine. 18th ed. New York: McGraw Hill; 2012. p. 1745–8.

Acute Lymphadenitis (ADL) 14

Lymphadenitis and lymphangitis are common inflammatory manifestations of filariasis and are complimentary to each other (Pani 2013), as lymphadenitis always has some element of lymphangitis, which may not be clinically detected. Similarly, lymphangitis is always associated with involvement of draining lymph nodes.

It is one of the most common clinical presentations of filariasis as the adult filarial worms reside in the lymph sinuses of the lymph nodes. It is a reactive inflammatory reaction to dead adult worms.

The inguinal and iliac group of lymph nodes is commonly affected as the lower extremity is the most common site of mosquito bite. The axillary, epitrochlear, popliteal, and abdominal lymph nodes may also be involved. It occurs both in bancroftian and brugian type of filarial infection Fig. 14.1.

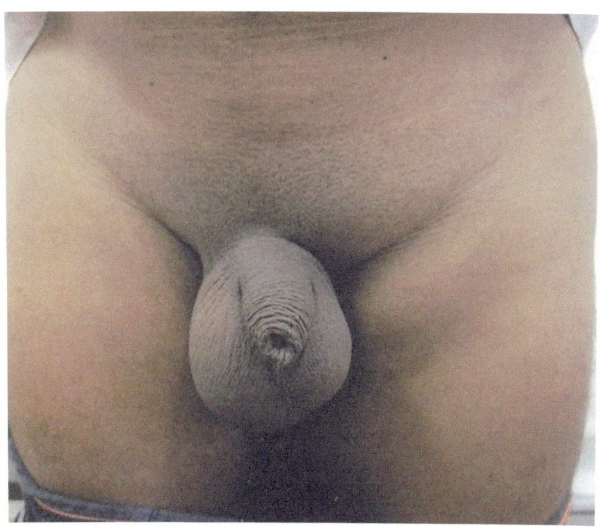

Fig. 14.1 Filarial left ilioinguinal lymphadenopathy with groove sign separating the enlarged external iliac lymph nodes from enlarged inguinal lymph nodes with right-sided hydrocele

T.C. Goel, A. Goel, *Lymphatic Filariasis*, DOI 10.1007/978-981-10-2257-9_14

14.1 Clinical Features

The patient presents with local pain, fever with rigors, and enlarged tender lymph nodes in this sequence. As the local signs develop, the fever subsides gradually due to the localization of disease. The lymphadenopathy is associated with retrograde lymphangitis extending peripherally from the involved lymph node. The lymph nodes are grossly enlarged, hot, tender, discrete, and firm or soft (boggy) in consistency. The epitrochlear lymph nodes are enlarged early in subperiodic form of filariasis while it is relatively less common in the periodic form. A single abscess may develop along the involved lymph node or vessel. Concomitant local thrombophlebitis can occur.

It usually runs a mild clinical course and rarely causes residual lymphedema. Some lymphedema may be present during the acute phase of this disease.

Iliac Lymphadenitis Sometimes, patient presents with iliac lymphadenitis with local pain and fever. On the right side, it may be confused with acute appendicitis. The inflamed lymph nodes may cause spasm of iliopsoas muscle leading to fixed flexion deformity of hip joint. The enlarged lymph nodes may be palpable as a fixed mass to the pelvic wall. Untreated patient may present with an iliac abscess.

14.2 Pathology

The lymph nodes are enlarged and reveal granulomatous inflammation, proliferation of reticuloendothelial cells, and eosinophilic infiltration. The sinuses are dilated with a wide zone of macrophages with a variable number of eosinophils, lymphocytes, and foreign body giant cells at the periphery. In serial sections, segments of adult filarial worms may be seen in some cases.

In acute disease, small necrotic areas may be seen with acute inflammatory cells in the surrounding tissues. In chronic disease, fibrous scarring is noted.

14.3 Chronic Filarial Lymphadenitis

Recurrent attacks of filariasis may turn this disease into chronic one. It commonly affects the inguinal lymph nodes when the patient presents with inguinal lymphadenopathy, may be with some inguinal pain. The lymph nodes remain chronically enlarged, often significantly, i.e., 5–7.5 cm in size without much tenderness.

As time passes, the chronic lymphadenitic lymph nodes may undergo calcification, which gives irregular mottled appearance on radiography with calcification more at the periphery than at the center. It is a healed lesion and is unlikely to have reinfection.

14.4 Differential Diagnosis

1. *Tuberculous lymphadenitis* – The differences between tuberculous and filarial lymphadenitis are given in the following Table 14.1:
2. *Syphilitic lymphadenitis* – In syphilis, the lymph nodes are involved in primary (usually inguinal) and secondary stage of syphilis (generalized lymphadenopathy especially epitrochlear and suboccipital). The lymph nodes are mildly enlarged, discrete, hard, nontender, and mobile (shotty). A history of extramarital sexual exposure is available. In primary syphilis, the discharge of the primary sore may be examined for spirochaetes. The serologic tests for syphilis are usually positive 10 days after exposure.
3. *Lymphogranuloma venereum* – It is an acute and chronic sexually transmitted disease caused by *Chlamydia trachomatis* types L1–L3 (Schwartz 2015). It is characterized by an evanescent genital lesion followed by inguinal lymph node enlargement (usually bilateral) 1–4 weeks after exposure. The enlarged lymph nodes have a tendency to fuse, soften (bubo), and rupture to form multiple draining sinuses with marked scarring. Anorectal manifestations may be present in women. The diagnosis is confirmed by a positive compliment fixation test.
4. *Nonspecific lymphadenitis or reactive lymph nodes* – This type of inguinal lymphadenopathy is usually seen in barefoot walkers or persons with chronic foot or perianal infection. The lymph nodes are enlarged, mild to moderate in size, firm, nontender, and mobile. Biopsy shows chronic inflammation without segments of adult filarial worm.

14.5 Treatment

The acute disease is treated with antibiotics with relief of pain and fever and other symptoms. Antihistaminics may be of help. As soon as the acuteness comes under control antifilarial drugs, e.g., diethylcarbamazine may be given.

Table 14.1 Differences between Tuberculous lymphadenitis and Filarial lymphadenitis

Features	Tuberculous lymphadenitis	Filarial lymphadenitis
Age	Commonly young people	More common in middle aged people
Site	Can affect any group of lymph nodes but the cervical lymph nodes are commonly involved	Inguinal lymph nodes are most commonly involved
Signs	Matting of lymph node is an early and specific sign	Matting of enlarged nodes may be seen in late stage of disease
Fever	Low-grade fever in the evening is a common symptom	Recurrent attacks of fever with rigor is a specific symptom
Biopsy	Shows tubercles having central caseous necrosis	Shows chronic inflammation may be with eosinophilic infiltration and segments of dead adult filarial worms

In chronic disease, residual symptomatic lymph nodes may be excised if they do not respond to antifilarial treatment continuously given for 3 months (Pani 2013).

The flexion deformity following iliac lymphadenitis is corrected by traction to lower extremity for 3 weeks or more as required.

References

Pani S. Pani's filariasis. 3rd ed. New Delhi: Jaypee Brothers; 2013.

Schwartz BS. Enteric fever (typhoid fever). In: Papadakis MA, McPhee SJ, editors. Current medical diagnosis & treatment. 54th ed. New York: McGraw Hil; 2015. p. 1437–8.

Acute Dermatolymphangioadenitis (ADLA)

15

It is acute inflammation of skin, subcutaneous tissue, lymphatics, and lymph nodes of the affected part seen in lymphatic filariasis. It is the most common acute clinical manifestation of lymphatic filariasis (Shenoy 2008).

15.1 Etiology

It is not caused by filarial infection per se but caused by secondary bacterial infection in the leg and foot predisposed by the presence of live adult worm in a lymphatic vessel dilated by "toxins" secreted by the worm or exposure to fresh infection with entry of stage 3 larvae in the lymphatics (Ottesen 1980; Partono 1987). It is now accepted without doubt that these acute episodes are caused by bacterial infection (Shenoy et al. 1999). The entry of infection, i.e., streptococci, most commonly occurs through fungal lesions in the interdigital spaces, injuries, other infective lesions (e.g., paronychia), and eczema or fissures in the feet. The fungal infection of web spaces of toes gets aggravated during rainy season or due to household work when the feet are soaked in water. The fungal infections of foot act only as entry points for the bacteria, and the fungi themselves do not invade and cause ADLA.

15.2 Clinical Features

It is usually characterized by severe pain, fever, chills, headache, vomiting, and pain in the affected part, usually lower extremity, less commonly scrotum, or upper extremity. In severe cases, there may be toxemia, altered sensorium, and urinary incontinence. These episodes are more frequent as the lymphedema progresses. The affected part (extremity) is diffusely swollen, red, tense, warm, and very tender. Red streaks may be visible along the inflamed lymphatics. Edematous inflammatory plaques, clearly demarcated from normal skin, are seen (Nutman and Weller 2012). The local lymph nodes of the groin or axilla may be enlarged and tender. It may result in abscess formation or ulceration.

T.C. Goel, A. Goel, *Lymphatic Filariasis*, DOI 10.1007/978-981-10-2257-9_15

15.3 Course and Sequelae

It occurs several times in a year more so in rainy season. It is considered as an important cause of chronic lymphedema–elephantiasis. About 4 such attacks per year occur in bancroftian filariasis and 2 in brugian filariasis (Panicker and Sebasan 1990).

The lymphatic obstruction following attacks of ADLA is marked, diffuse, and multiple, hence commonly resulting in chronic lymphedema–elephantiasis. See the flow chart given below Flow Chart 15.1.

15.4 Investigations

The blood shows polymorphonuclear leukocytosis and may be microfilariae in the night smear. It may be sent for culture. Specimens for culture may be taken from the infective lesions of the toes or web spaces. The dilated lymphatics with live adult worms may be seen by Doppler ultrasonography in earlier attacks ("filarial dance sign") (Amaral et al. 1994), but this sign is absent when the secondary bacterial infection or lymphedema is established.

Live adult worm in a lymphatic vessels most commonly of lower extremity

↓

Secretion of 'toxins'

↓

Lymphangiectasia (dilated local lymphatics)

↓

Entry of microbes through the web space or digital lesions
(secondary bacterial invasion)

↓

Acute diffuse inflammation of skin, subcutaneous tissue,
lymphatics and lymph nodes of the extremity
(acute dermatolymphangioadenitis, ADLA)

↓

Diffuse acute inflammation with redness, tenderness and
diffuse swelling with enlarged tender local lymph nodes

↓

Subsidence of acute inflammation following treatment or
spontaneously with time

↓

Adenolymphatic obstruction (marked, diffuse or multiple)

↓

Chronic lymphedema-elephantiasis
(common consequence)

Flow Chart 15.1 Pathogenesis and result of acute dermatolymphangioadenitis (ADLA) due to lymphatic filariasis

15.5 Treatment

Bed rest, elevation of affected extremity, pain relief, and treatment with local antibiotic or antifungal ointment of entry lesions of foot, toes, or web spaces may be enough in mild disease.

Moderate or severe attacks require oral or parenteral administration of antibiotics. The commonly used antibiotics like penicillin, doxycycline, ampicillin, amoxicillin, or cotrimoxazole may be given till the infection is controlled (Shenoy 2008). On receipt of culture and sensitivity report, suitable changes are made in the antibiotic therapy.

15.6 Prevention

The most distressing aspect of attacks of ADLA is that they prevent the victim from attending his daily activities for several days during each episode leading to financial loss. These attacks are preventable and hence must be prevented. They are prevented by a simple, effective, and cheap method of looking after the local hygiene of the affected limb (Dreyer et al. 1999), i.e., the foot. The foot care program to prevent ADLA attacks consists of the following (Shenoy et al. 1999):

1. The extremity, especially the interdigital clefts and deep skin folds, should be washed with soap and water twice a day or at least once before going to bed and wiping dry with a clean cloth or drying it with a hair dryer.
2. The nails should be kept clean and clipped at intervals as required.
3. Injuries to the foot are prevented and treated promptly if they occur.
4. Infections are controlled by local use of antibiotic or antifungal ointments as indicated in the webs of toes, skin folds, and sides of the feet.
5. The patient should use a comfortable foot wear, neither tight nor loose.

In endemic areas, the regular foot care should be taught and encouraged from early age as the filarial infection is frequently acquired during childhood.

The differences between acute filarial lymphangitis (AFL) and acute dermatolymphangioadenitis (ADLA) are given in the following table:

Features	Acute filarial lymphangitis (AFL)	Acute dermatolymphangioadenitis (ADLA)
Definition	Acute inflammation of a lymphatic around a dead filarial worm with death occurring spontaneously or after antifilarial treatment	Considered to occur due to secondary bacterial infection of compromised lymphatics (lymphangiectasis) due to the presence of a live adult worm in lymphatic vessels and secreting "toxins"
Etiology	Probably an immunological phenomenon	Secondary infection of lymphangiectatic vessels

Features	Acute filarial lymphangitis (AFL)	Acute dermatolymphangioadenitis (ADLA)
Clinical features	Episodic attacks of malaise, fever and chills, and painful enlarged lymph nodes draining the affected part usually the lower extremity Presents as circumscribed inflammatory nodule or a cord centered around a degenerating adult worm with streaks of inflamed lymphatics spreading in a descending fashion (centrifugal)	Diffuse spreading cutaneous inflammation with or without ascending lymphangitis usually of the lower extremity Limb is swollen, red, hot, and tender Pitting edema present Inflammation is usually due to secondary bacterial infection entering from web spaces of toes or nails
Course	The attack usually resolves spontaneously after about a week followed by excessive exfoliation of skin	The attack may resolve spontaneously or following antibiotic therapy but with difficulty and takes more time May result in an abscess formation or ulceration
Lymphatic damage	Minimal and localized	Significant and diffuse or multiple
Lymphedema	Mild and transient	Severe, persistent, or recurrent and may be progressive
In males	External genitalia is commonly affected and may present as acute funiculitis or epididymo-orchitis or scrotal hydrocele	External genitalia is less commonly affected

References

Amaral F, Dreyer G, Figueredo-Silva J, et al. Live adult worms detected by ultrasonography in human bancroftian filariasis. Am J Trop Med Hyg. 1994;50(6):753.

Dreyer G, Figueredo-Silva J, Neafie RC, Addiss DG. Lymphatic filariasis. In: Nelson AH, Horsburg RC, editors. Pathology of emerging infections 2. Washington: American Society of Microbiology; 1999. p. 317–42.

Nutman TB, Weller PF. Filarial and related infections. In: Longo DL, Fauci AS, Kasper DL, Hauser SL, Jameson JL, Loscalzo J, editors. Harrison's internal medicine. 18th ed. New York: McGraw Hill; 2012. p. 1745–8.

Ottesen EA. Immunopathology of lymphatic filariasis in man. Springer Semin Immunopathol. 1980;2:373–85. http://link.springer.com/article/10.1007%2FBF01857174#page-1.

Panicker KN, Sebasan S. Socioeconomic properties – miscellaneous publications of VCRC. Miscellaneous publications of Vector Control Research Center. 1990;16:42–7.

Partono F. The spectrum of disease in lymphatic filariasis. Ciba Found Symp. 1987;127:15–31.

Shenoy RK. Clinical and pathological aspects of filarial lymphedema and its management. Korean J Parasitol. 2008;46(3):119–25.

Shenoy RK, Kumaraswami V, Suma TK, et al. A double-blind placebo controlled study of the efficacy of oral penicillin, diethylcarbamazine or local treatment of the affected limb in preventing acute adenolymphangitis in lymphedema caused by brugian filariasis. Ann Trop Med Parasitol. 1999;93(4):367–77.

Filarial Funiculitis 16

Inflammation of spermatic cord, epididymis, and testis is known as funiculitis, epididymitis, and orchitis, respectively. Usually, the involvement of one structure invites the involvement of other as these three structures are anatomically continuous and are provided with common lymphatics and lymph nodes (Pani 2013). These manifestations are seen in bancroftian filariasis and not in brugian filariasis.

Filarial funiculitis is the inflammation of spermatic cord, which is one of the most frequent (second) clinical presentations of lymphatic filariasis.

16.1 Pathology

The spermatic cord is swollen and acutely inflamed. It contains inflamed "wiry" lymphatics. The veins of the cord are also inflamed (thrombophlebitis) with involvement of other structures of cord to produce one mass. One or more nodules may be present.

Although the lower or intrascrotal portion of the cord is the preferred site of involvement, the inguinal or even the abdominal part may be involved. Adult filarial worms may be present in the lesion. Small (micro) abscesses may form in the cord around degenerating worms or segments of worms. Such changes may be present in the spermatic cord without any clinical symptom (silent funiculitis).

16.2 Clinical Features

Most of the patients are 20–40 years of age. The onset of the disease is usually sudden with inguinoscrotal pain and fever with rigors and may be vomiting. Hence, it may mimic an attack of ureteral colic or torsion of testis.

On examination, the spermatic cord is swollen, firm ("rope-like"), and tender. The epididymis and testis are commonly involved with inflammation of cord (funiculitis with epididymo-orchitis).

T.C. Goel, A. Goel, *Lymphatic Filariasis*, DOI 10.1007/978-981-10-2257-9_16

16.3 Differential Diagnosis

1. *Ureteral colic*—Usually, the pain starts suddenly after midnight in the loin and radiates to the groin. It is gripping in nature, and the patient tosses over the bed in agony often associated with profuse sweating and nausea. It may be referred to the testis, which may be retracted up due to reflex spasm of cremaster. There may be tenderness and rigidity along the course of ureter (Das 2013). Radiography usually shows a vertically oval radio-opaque shadow along the line of ureter. The diagnosis can be confirmed by intravenous or CT urography.
2. *Torsion of testis*—The patient is usually an adolescent male 12–18 years of age who presents with agonizing pain of sudden onset in the groin and lower abdomen with vomiting without fever. It may follow straining at stool, lifting heavy weight, coitus, or jumping off a bicycle (Das 2013). The testis is pulled up and very tender. Hence, it is difficult to palpate. Elevation of scrotum increases the pain (Prehn's sign). The loss of testicular arterial pulsation can be seen by color Doppler study.
3. *Strangulated inguinal hernia*—The patient presents with an inguinal or inguino-scrotal swelling of acute onset with pain and signs of acute intestinal obstruction. The swelling is irreducible, tense, and tender and does not have cough impulse (Das 2013).

16.4 Investigations

The blood shows leukocytosis and may have increased eosinophil count. Microfilaremia is usually present.

The motile adult worms may be visible in dilated inguinal lymphatics ("filarial dance sign," Amaral et al. 1994) during Doppler ultrasonography.

16.5 Treatment

The patient is given symptomatic treatment including analgesics and antibiotics. Use of a suspensory bandage helps in relief of pain. After 2–3 days a full course of diethylcarbamazine may be given.

References

Amaral F, Dreyer G, Figueredo-Silva J, et al. Live adult worms detected by ultrasonography in human bancroftian filariasis. Am J Trop Med Hyg. 1994;50(6):753.

Das S. A manual on clinical surgery. 10th ed. Kolkata: Published by the Author; 2013. p. 582, 605, 629.

Pani S. Pani's filariasis. 3rd ed. New Delhi: Jaypee Brothers; 2013.

Filarial Epididymo-Orchitis

17

It is inflammation of epididymis and testis due to the death of filarial worms, which may be precipitated by secondary bacterial infection. It is one of the common manifestation of filariasis (Das 2013; Pani 2013).

17.1 Pathology

Epididymis and testis are enlarged and inflamed. The sinus of the epididymis is obliterated. Microscopic examination shows acute inflammation with portions of dead adult filarial worms in various sections. The scrotal sac has a small amount of inflammatory exudate (secondary hydrocele).

17.2 Clinical Features

The patient presents with severe pain in the scrotum, fever with rigors and swelling of acute onset. The scrotum is swollen, red, hot, and tender and has a smooth surface. The globus major is affected first. The testis enlarges very rapidly. It is smooth and very tender. The epididymis is affected more than the testis. A small secondary hydrocele is a frequent accompaniment.

17.3 Investigations

The blood may reveal leukocytosis, eosinophilia, and microfilaremia. The worms in the epididymis can be visualized by ultrasonography (Amaral et al. 1994).

T.C. Goel, A. Goel, *Lymphatic Filariasis*, DOI 10.1007/978-981-10-2257-9_17

17.4 Termination

The first attack may disappear spontaneously or following treatment in which the epididymis and testis return to normal or near normal, or the lesion may progress to pyocele formation. Recurrent attacks are very common and may be followed by subacute inflammation.

17.5 Subacute Epididymo-Orchitis

It is characterized by mild enlargement of epididymis and testis. The epididymis is tender and may have one or more nodules.

Microscopic examination shows evidence of chronic inflammation with extensive fibrosis, which blocks vasa efferentia leading to sterility. Parts of dead and calcified filarial worms are frequently seen.

17.6 Treatment

Patient is given bed rest, plenty of fluids, pain relief, elevation of scrotum, and antibiotics. As soon as the acute symptoms are relieved, diethylcarbamazine is added to the treatment.

If there is doubt regarding the diagnosis or the patient is not relieved within 24–48 h, exploration is indicated for careful examination of testis, epididymis, and lower end of the spermatic cord. The scrotal wound is closed around a drain.

References

Amaral F, Dreyer G, Figueredo-Silva J, et al. Live adult worms detected by ultrasonography in human bancroftian filariasis. Am J Trop Med Hyg. 1994;50(6):753.

Das S. A manual on clinical surgery. 10th ed. Kolkata: Dr S Das; 2013. p. 582, 605, 629.

Pani S. Pani's filariasis. 3rd ed. New Delhi: Jaypee Brothers; 2013.

Filarial Cellulitis–Abscess

18

18.1 Cellulitis

Cellulitis is an acute diffuse inflammation of subcutaneous cellular tissue usually caused by streptococci or staphylococci. In filariasis, acute inflammation of lymphatics and adjacent tissue is caused by dying adult worms. It is aggravated by the secondary bacterial invasion – in the lower extremity from the lesions of web spaces of toes or nails and in the scrotum and breast by scratching trauma.

The patient presents with local pain, redness, and diffuse swelling without a definitive edge. Fever with rigors is usually present.

The patient is given symptomatic treatment with analgesics and antibiotics. Diethylcarbamazine is given after the subsidence of acute symptoms. Local application of magnesium sulfate cream may give relief in symptoms.

18.2 Filarial Abscess

It is a common manifestation of lymphatic filariasis. Of the 90 patients of filariasis reported by Ghooi and Khanna (1976), the filarial abscess was present in 25 patients – 20 in lower extremity, 4 in the scrotum, and 1 in the upper extremity. Abscess may occur in any type of filarial infection, but the infection with *Brugia timori* appears to result in more abscesses than infection with *Brugia malayi* (Edesen 1962) or *Wuchereria bancrofti* (Okon et al. 2010).

Pathology A filarial abscess usually occurs around a dead adult worm or its degenerating segments. Hence, the abscess cavity contains a dead or fragmented worm and a small amount of sterile pus. It may have intercommunicating pockets. Secondary invading bacteria may be present in the pus.

T.C. Goel, A. Goel, *Lymphatic Filariasis*, DOI 10.1007/978-981-10-2257-9_18

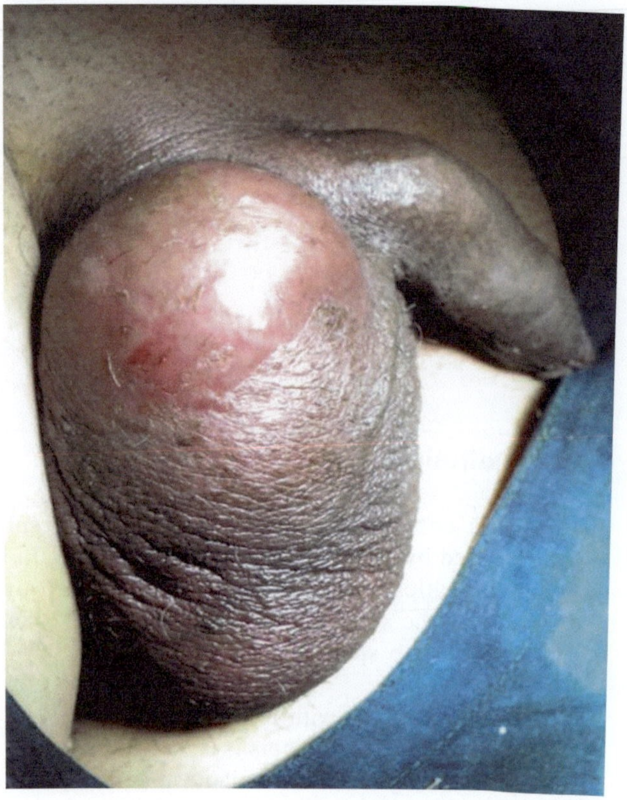

Fig. 18.1 Scrotal abscess having a localized superficial swelling of right side of scrotum. Left-sided filarial hydrocele is also present (Photo courtesy of Professor D. Dalela)

Clinical Features It usually starts suddenly with extreme local pain with prolonged rigor followed by high fever and toxemia. It may be associated with or preceded by an attack of lymphangitis or cellulitis. It has all the signs of an abscess, i.e., swelling, redness, heat, tenderness, and bogginess Fig. 18.1.

It usually occurs in the subcutaneous tissue planes of lower extremity, scrotum, inguinal region, breast, upper extremity, and at the sites of lymph nodes of the inguinal, axillary, epitrochlear, and propliteal regions.

Filarial abscess may occur deep to deep fascia in the intermuscular fascial planes of thigh, popliteal fossa, or leg. Rarely, it may occur in the thorax or abdomen – these two are dangerous sites as it may rupture into pleural or peritoneal cavity.

Pyocele It is an accumulation of pus in tunica vaginalis of scrotum, which may follow acute filarial epididymo-orchitis or may occur due to secondary infection in a filarial hydrocele. It rarely occurs in a previously normal testis and epididymis.

The patient presents with severe scrotal pain and swelling associated with fever with rigors and toxemia of acute onset. The hemiscrotum of one side is swollen, red, hot, and tender. The spermatic cord is also swollen and tender (Fig. 18.2).

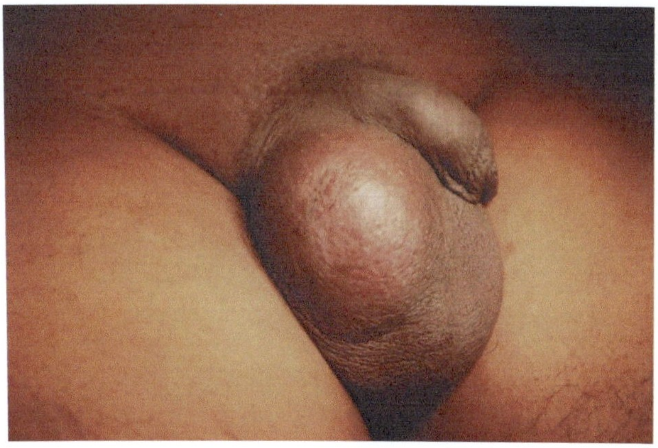

Fig. 18.2 Right-sided pyocele with left-sided filarial hydrocele

The blood will show leukocytosis, may be eosinophilia and microfilaremia. It must be sent for culture and sensitivity. The local lesion can be imaged by ultrasonography, CT scan, or MRI.

It is treated with analgesics, antibiotics and drainage of pus (Pani 2013). Diethylcarbamazine is started after subsidence of acute symptoms.

References

Edesen JF. The epidemiology and treatment of infection due to Brugia malayi. Bull WHO. 1962;27(4–5):529–41.

Ghooi AM, Khanna T. Surgical manifestations of filariasis. Indian J Surg. 1976;38:150.

Okon OE, Iboh CI, Opara KN. Bancroftian filariasis among the Mbembe people in Cross River State, Nigeria. J Vector Borne Dis. 2010;47(2):91–6.

Pani S. Pani's filariasis. 3rd ed. New Delhi: Jaypee Brothers; 2013.

Part III

Chronic Clinical Manifestations

Hydrocele of Tunica Vaginalis Testis 19

The word hydrocele is made of two Greek words: "hydro," which means water, and "kele," which means tumor (swelling). It is an accumulation of excessive amounts of transudate or watery (serous) fluid in the sac of tunica vaginalis. It is the most commonly observed chronic clinical manifestation of lymphatic filariasis caused by *Wuchereria bancrofti* (Figs. 19.1 and 19.2) (Ahorlu et al. 2001), and more than 80 % hydroceles in tropical countries are due to filarial infection. It is not usually seen in brugian filariasis (both *Brugia malayi* and *Brugia timori*).

It is an important public health problem in many developing countries (Michael and Bundy 1997). There are 26.79 million cases of hydrocele worldwide, and 48 % of these cases are in India (Michael et al. 1996). In Africa, 20–30 % or more of adult males have hydrocele (Gyapong et al. 1994; Dunyo et al. 1996).

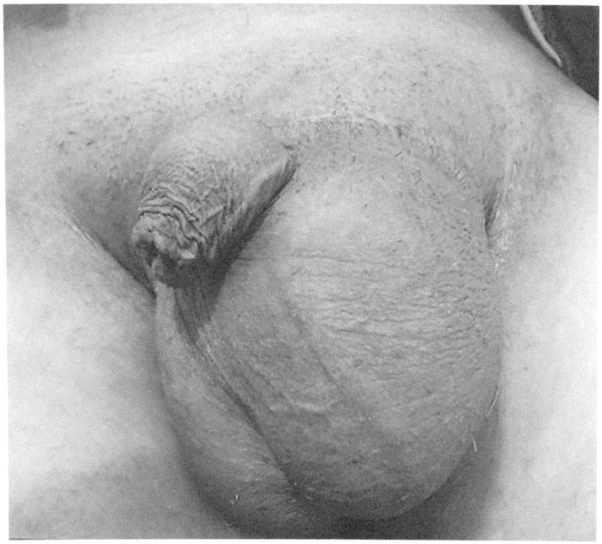

Fig. 19.1 Left-sided scrotal hydrocele (Courtesy – Professor D. Dalela)

T.C. Goel, A. Goel, *Lymphatic Filariasis*, DOI 10.1007/978-981-10-2257-9_19

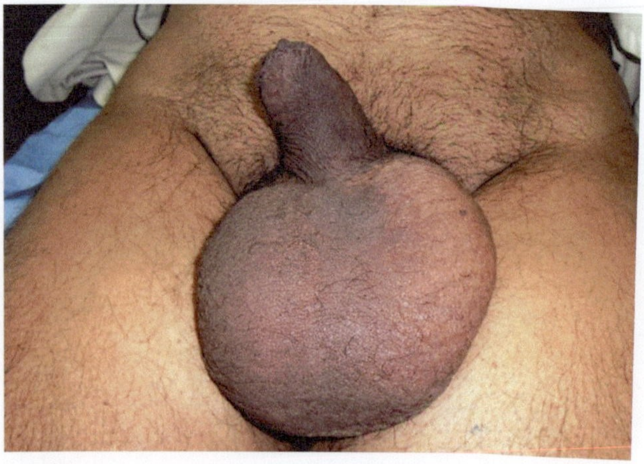

Fig. 19.2 Bilateral scrotal hydrocele. The skin of the scrotum has mild elephantiatic changes (Courtesy – Professor D. Dalela)

19.1 Etiopathogenesis

Normally, a thin film of serous fluid (capillary fluid) is present in the tunica vaginalis. It is generated by serous surfaces of tunica and reabsorbed through the venous and lymphatic system of the spermatic cord. Thus, there is a dynamic equilibrium between the production and the reabsorption of tunica vaginalis fluid (Kinmonth 1982).

The filarial worms commonly inhabit the inguinal lymphatics and in the epididymis producing inflammation and adenolymphatic obstruction. Thus, the fluid accumulation is due to the following:

1. Excessive production of fluid due to repeated attacks of filarial epididymitis and/or funiculitis producing inflammatory exudation and subsequent adenolymphatic obstruction which results in transudation of fluid in the tunica.
2. Interference in the reabsorption and drainage of fluid due to damage to endothelium of tunica and obstruction of lymphatics of spermatic cord and inguinal region. The lymphatic obstruction seems to be the main factor.
3. Rarely, a lymph varix of spermatic cord may rupture into scrotal sac leading to a lymphocele, which is one type of hydrocele.
4. Persistent processus vaginalis may have a role in the pathogenesis of hydrocele as hydroceles are still found in Leogane, Haiti, despite successful eradication of filariasis with mass drug administration program (McAlister and Trottier 2013).

Apart from lymphatic filariasis, other causes of hydrocele are as follows:

1. Congenital
2. Primary or idiopathic
3. Secondary hydrocele due to epididymo-orchitis, tuberculous epididymitis, and malignancy

19.2 Pathology

Fluid Its volume is increased, but the increase is variable. In early hydrocele, the fluid resembles that of idiopathic hydrocele. It is clear, amber-colored (like urine) with a specific gravity of 1022–1024. It contains inorganic salts, albumin 6 %, and fibrinogen and no leukocytes. The fluid as such does not clot, but if mixed even with a trace of blood, it clots to form a gel due to conversion of fibrinogen into fibrin.

The fluid in a late hydrocele is rich in cholesterol and contains a variable amount of protein with an average of 5.7 g percent.

Microfilariae may be present and Demarquay (1863) recognized them for the first time in the hydrocele fluid. However, most hydroceles do not have microfilariae unless contaminated by blood during aspiration (Dreyer et al. 1996).

Tunica Vaginalis It shows signs of chronic inflammation and may have yellowish cholesterol plaques. In a long-standing case, it may be thickened markedly. It may be calcified at places and may have calcified remnants of adult filarial worms. Calcification of tunica is very rare in idiopathic hydrocele.

Microscopically, it shows chronic inflammatory changes, interstitial edema, lymphatic dilatation, and follicular and perivascular lymphoid cell aggregation.

Epididymis It may be normal or may be enlarged due to chronic inflammation, interstitial fibrosis, and lymphatic dilatation. Remnants of dead filarial worms may be present.

Testis Testis may be normal or may show changes similar to those of epididymis. The seminiferous tubules may show some changes. Tunica albuginea is thickened and may show chronic inflammatory cell infiltration and multiple adhesions. In long-standing cases, there may be some evidence of testicular atrophy due to persistently increased intrascrotal pressure.

Other Changes Compensatory hypertrophy of cremaster muscle may be seen due to increased weight of scrotum. Skin of the scrotum loses its elasticity and there is hypertrophy of dartos muscle though it becomes functionally weak (Pani 2013).

19.3 Anatomical Types of Hydrocele

1. *Vaginal hydrocele* – The collection of fluid in the tunica is confined to scrotum only. This type of hydrocele is most common.
2. *Infantile hydrocele* – It is an inguinoscrotal hydrocele where the hydrocele extends up to the internal ring but does not communicate with peritoneal cavity.

3. *Congenital hydrocele* – It is just like infantile hydrocele that is communicating with the peritoneal cavity at internal ring with a narrow hole, which does not permit herniation of bowel. Hydrocele is of minimum size in the morning and maximum in the evening. It may have a cough impulse.
4. *Encysted hydrocele* – It is localized collection of fluid in the processus vaginalis usually in the lower part of cord above the testis. If the testis is pulled down, the swelling moves down correspondingly and on leaving it returns to its original position (traction test).
5. *Abdominoscrotal hydrocele or hydrocele-en-bisac* – It is a biloculated hydrocele having a scrotal hydrocele and an extraperitoneal inguinal hydrocele sac both communicating with each other by a narrow isthmus at the neck of scrotum (Fig. 19.3).

19.4 Clinical Features

In tropical countries where the lymphatic filariasis is rife, more than 80 % of hydroceles are due to filarial infection. If a hydrocele is associated with scrotal lymphangiectasis or nodules in the cord in a patient in an endemic area, it is highly suggestive of filarial etiology (DeVries 2002). It has been observed that the incidence of hydrocele in a population increases with microfilaremia and the filarial density in that area. It commonly follows one or repeated attacks of epididymo-orchitis. In early acute hydrocele following first attack of filariasis the swelling may disappear completely following treatment or spontaneously. However, a past history of filariasis is not present in a large number of patients.

It can occur at any age from birth to old age but commonly seen in adult age group (Pani 2013). The patient usually presents with a unilateral often, painless scrotal swelling of insidious onset. It may enlarge gradually and may attain a big size with burial of penis in the anterior wall of scrotum. Bilateral hydrocele often with different sizes on two sides is not uncommon (Simonsen 2009).

Sometimes, the patient complains of heaviness or dragging discomfort in the scrotum.

The upper limit of the swelling is reachable (Fig. 19.4) except in abdominoscrotal and congenital hydrocele. It is smooth, nontender, fluctuant, and translucent (Fig. 19.5). In a long-standing hydrocele, the translucency may be lost due to increased thickening or calcification of tunica and may be increased turbidity of hydrocele fluid due to it being a chylocele, hematocele, or pyocele.

In a small hydrocele, the testis is palpable even if the fluid surrounds it from all rounds, but in a large hydrocele, it is not palpable.

The penis is central in bilateral hydrocele but may be deviated to opposite and in unilateral hydrocele. In a large hydrocele, it may be buried in the anterior wall of scrotum.

A small hydrocele does not have any bad social or economic impact, but a large hydrocele may have significant socioeconomic implications. Studies in some villages

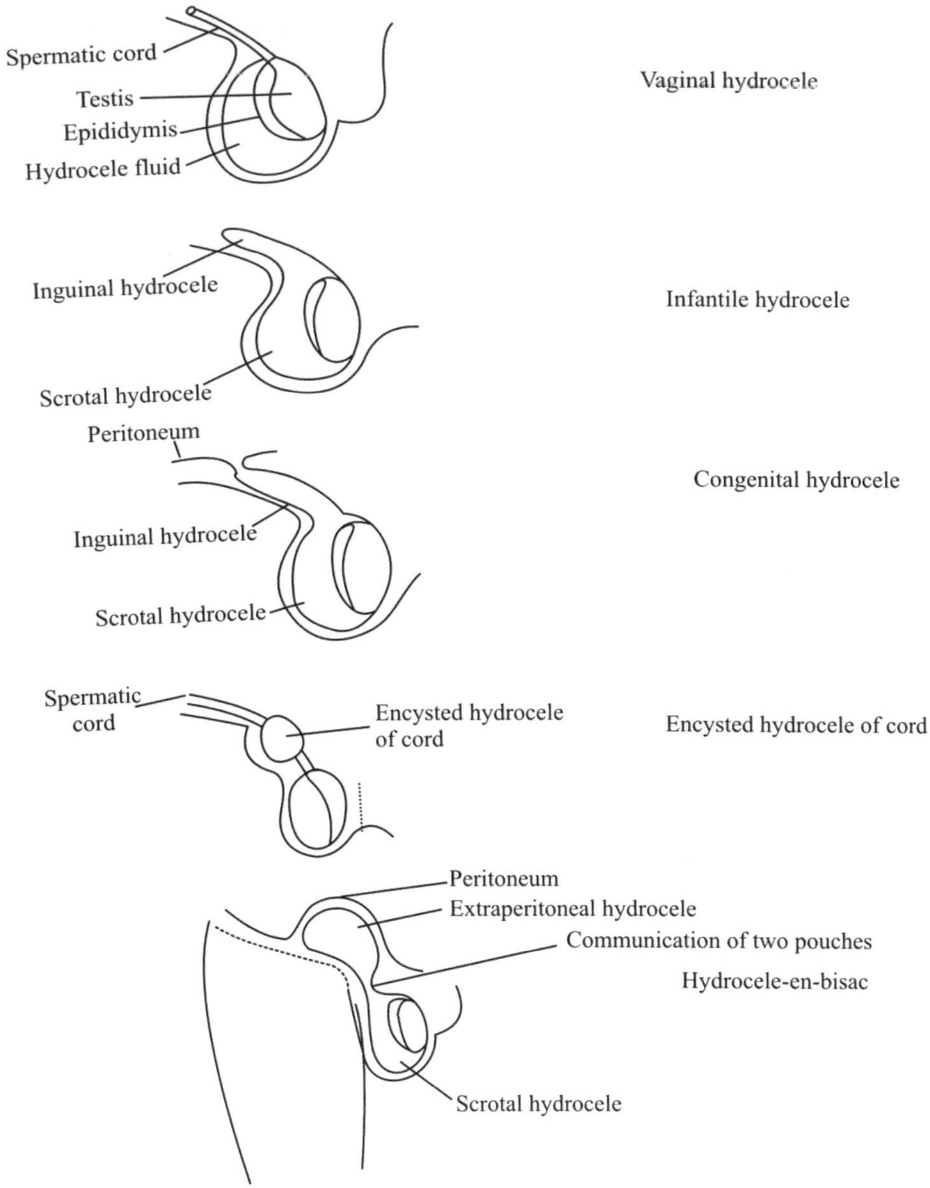

Fig. 19.3 Anatomical types of hydrocele

in Ghana revealed a negative impact of hydrocele in terms of work performance and sexual activity and fear of public ridicule (Ahorlu et al. 2001; Babu et al. 2009).

A filarial hydrocele (secondary hydrocele) should be differentiated from primary hydrocele as given in the following table:

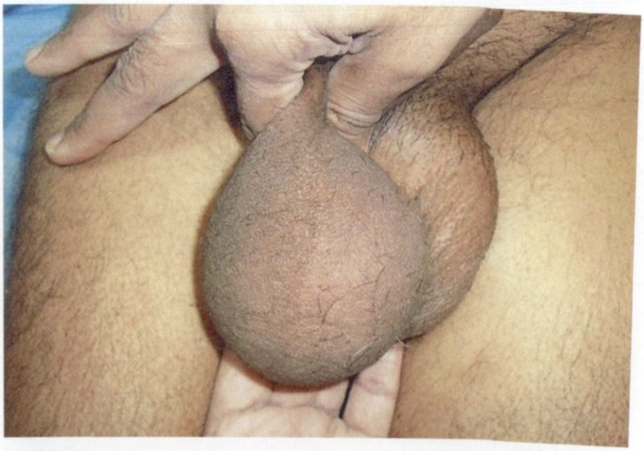

Fig. 19.4 Reaching the upper limit of a scrotal swelling. It is right-sided scrotal hydrocele (Courtesy – Professor D. Dalela)

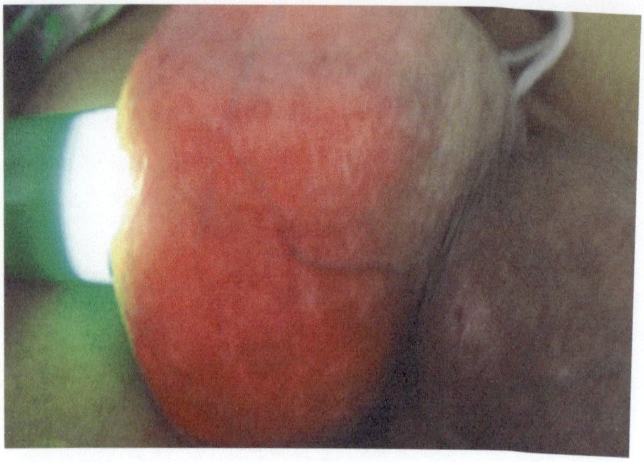

Fig. 19.5 Eliciting transillumination in a scrotal hydrocele (Courtesy – Professor D. Dalela)

Table 19.1 Differences between filarial hydrocele and Primary hydrocele

Features	Filarial hydrocele	Primary hydrocele
Etiology	Inguinal adenolymphatic obstruction or epididymo-orchitis due to bancroftian filariasis	Cause not known exactly, may be due to defective absorption of normal fluid of tunica vaginalis
Size	Moderate to big or very big	Small to big
Palpability of testis	Chances of impalpability are more	Chances of impalpability are less
Skin and subcutaneous tissue	May be normal or may be lymphedematous or elephantoid	Normal
Translucency	Early and small – may be positive Late and big – lost	Usually positive
Past history	Recurrent attacks of fever with rigors usually present	Nothing significant
Treatment	Antifilarial drugs and excision of sac	Partial excision and eversion, or Lord's plication

Rarely, a hydrocele can occur in a female in the inguinal canal. It is known as hydrocele of canal of Nuck.

19.5 Clinical Classification of Hydroceles

Capuano and Capuano (2012) have described a clinical classification of hydrocele, which is based on four clinical criteria:

1. Type of hydrocele – unilateral or bilateral
2. Side of hydrocele – right or left side of scrotum
3. Size of hydrocele
   - Stage I – size of hydrocele less than that of tennis ball
   - Stage II – size of hydrocele more than that of a tennis ball and the lower pole of scrotum does not reach halfway down the thigh (between the lower border of greater trochanter and mid thigh)
   - Stage III – the lower pole of scrotum goes below the mid thigh between the mid thigh and upper edge of patella
   - Stage IV – the lower pole of scrotum reaches between the upper border of patella and tibial tuberosity
   - Stage V – the lower limit of scrotum reaches between tibial tuberosity and mid leg
   - Stage VI – the lower limit of scrotum reaches between mid leg and ankle
4. Burial of penis
   - Grade 0 – no apparent burial with normal length of penis
   - Grade 1 – partial burial with length of visible part of penis more than 2 cm
   - Grade 2 – partial burial of penis in anterior wall of scrotum with visible part less than 2 cm
   - Grade 3 – total burial of penis with prepuce or glans penis (in circumcised patients) visible
   - Grade 4 – total burial of penis with stretched and lengthened prepuce causing micturition problems

The higher-grade filarial hydroceles are usually associated with some element of filarial lymphedema of scrotum, which contributes to the size of hydrocele and burial of penis in the anterior wall of scrotum.

Stage I and stage II hydrocele associated with grade 0 or 1 penis burial could be labeled "simple hydrocele" and can be managed at WHO level II health care center as the surgical treatment is simple with no anticipated complication. Stage III and stage IV hydrocele associated with grade 2, 3, or 4 penis burial could be labeled complicated hydrocele and should be treated at level III health care facility as the operation requires more facilities and skill and may be followed by some complications.

As there is a strong feeling of shame and embarrassment among hydrocele patients, the problem of sexual disability is usually not acknowledged unless the patients are specifically probed by health care team.

Further, it is difficult for a filarial hydrocele patient to get a girl of choice for marriage. Hence, he marries a girl of lower socioeconomic status. The parents offer their daughters to such a man under compulsive situations (with little or no dowry) (Babu et al. 2009).

19.6 Complications

1. *Rupture* – a hydrocele may rupture following minor injury, or at times spontaneously. It requires immediate intervention. It may sometimes result in cure of hydrocele due to absorption of fluid via dartos.
2. *Hematocele* – it may be traumatic or spontaneous. The traumatic hematocele results in pain of sudden onset and increase of the swelling of hydrocele, which loses its translucency. Spontaneous hemorrhage into the hydrocele sac occurs gradually. The blood clots and the hydrocele becomes old clotted hematocele (Pani 2013), which may be difficult to differentiate from malignancy of testis. Acute hematocele requires urgent intervention. Old clotted hematocele usually ends up in orchiectomy.
3. *Pyocele* – It is the result of secondary infection of hydrocele and characterized by pain; fever may be with rigor, redness, and sudden increase in size of the scrotal swelling (Fig. 19.6). The treatment includes antibiotics and drainage
4. *Calcification* – Repeated attacks of filariasis cause fibrosis and thickening of tunica which may undergo calcification with time. In an old-standing filarial

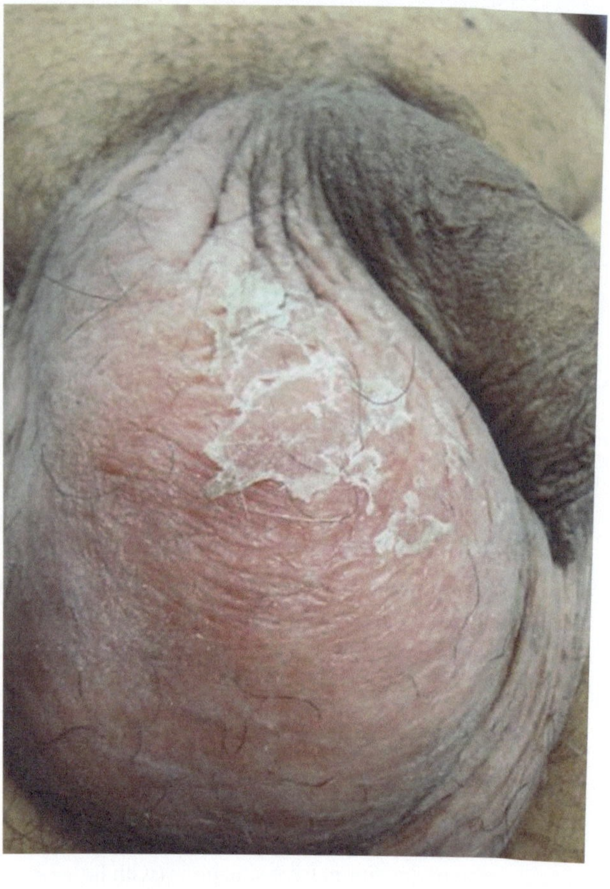

Fig. 19.6 Right-sided pyocele with red desquamating overlying skin (Courtesy – Professor D. Dalela)

hydrocele, the testis, epididymis, and vas may undergo calcification, which may result in obstructive azoospermia and sterility (Pani 2013).

19.7 Investigations

- Blood may show eosinophilia. Microfilaremia is usually absent but the microfilariae may be present in the hydrocele fluid. However, the scrotal puncture should be avoided for fear of secondary infection. The immunological tests for filariasis are usually positive.
- Ultrasonography confirms the presence of fluid and gives information about the condition of testis (Fig. 19.7), e.g., a testicular tumor with secondary hydrocele (Fig. 19.8). CT scan can also be done (Fig. 19.9).
- Immunologic examination of hydrocele fluid – The filaria-related antigens (Og4C3 assay) and antibodies found in serum (ELISA) can be detected with equal sensitivity in hydrocele fluid. Hence, this test can be used as an alternative in the immunodiagnosis of filarial etiology of hydrocele (Mishra et al. 2014), and also to monitor filaria elimination program.

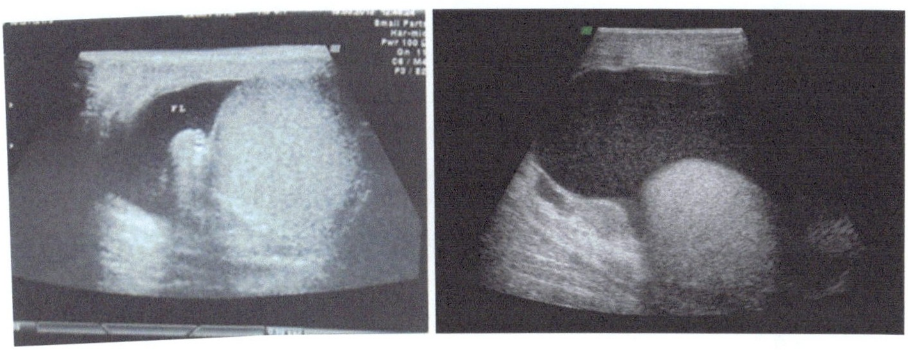

Fig. 19.7 Ultrasonography of scrotum showing normal testis, epididymis, and fluid accumulation due to hydrocele

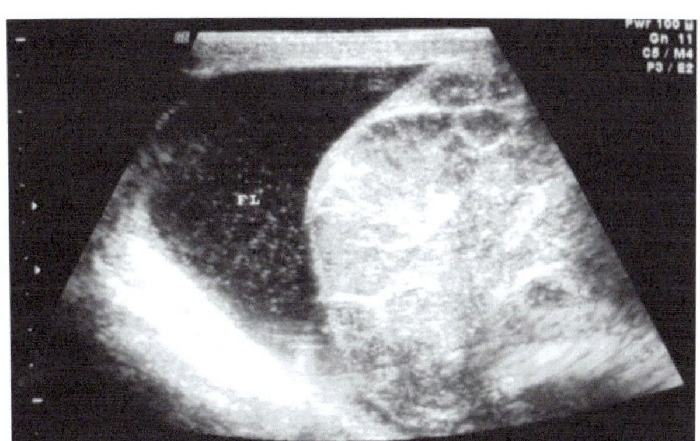

Fig. 19.8 Ultrasound examination of scrotum shows hydrocele with a septated testicular mass which turned out to be a spermatocytic seminoma

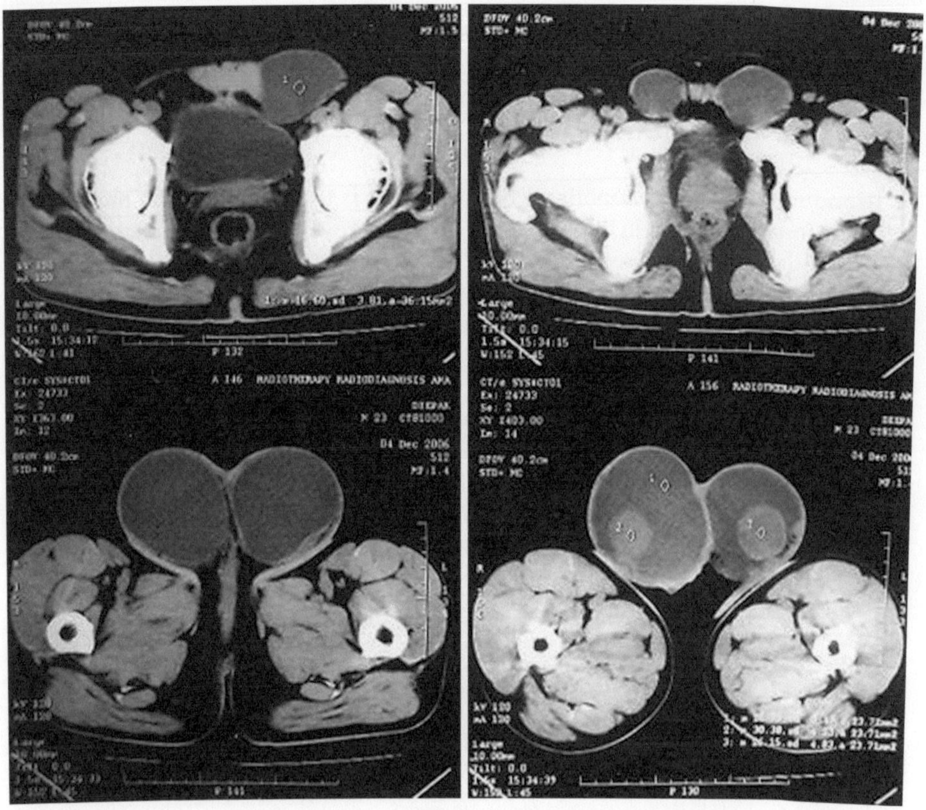

Fig. 19.9 Axial CT scan at the scrotal level showing bilateral hydrocele. Both the testes are normal (Courtesy – Professor D. Dalela)

19.8 Treatment

Although this disease is not painful and not a threat to life, it should be treated because of its bad social and economic consequences in those afflicted (Dreyer et al. 1997; Coreil et al. 1998; Ahorlu et al. 2001; Gyapong et al. 2000).

- A small hydrocele of short duration (acute hydrocele) may disappear spontaneously or following diethylcarbamazine and/or doxycycline therapy (Addiss and Dreyer 2000).
- A large hydrocele usually requires an operation, the indications for operation are as follows:
  1. Interference in work, sexual function, and/or micturition as the penis may be buried in the scrotum of a large hydrocele
  2. Symptomatic hydrocele with dragging pain and heaviness
  3. Medically disqualified people who want to join public services

Anesthesia The operation is usually done under local anesthesia with injection of lignocaine (1 %) into the spermatic cord and then into the line of incision.

Further, a hydrocele can be operated under spinal, epidural, or general anesthesia. The choice of the anesthesia depends upon surgeon and patient's preference and the facilities available.

The operative procedures include Lord's operation (Lord 1964), **eversion of sac** (Jaboulay 1902), and excision of sac. Before the surgery, it is necessary to ensure that all superficial skin inflammation, bacterial infections, and fungal infections are fully controlled (DeVries 2002). The scrotal hygiene is ensured by whole body bath and scrotal washing with soap and water twice daily for 3 days. It is very important to reduce the operative wound infection rate (Ananthakrishnan and Pani 2005). Diabetes mellitus must be excluded by proper investigations. If it is present, it must be fully controlled before operation.

Lord's Operation This operation is indicated in early thin-walled hydroceles. The aim of operation is to reduce the area of secretion without leaving any space in the scrotum for collection of blood.

A small scrotal incision is given just large enough to deliver the testis out. The parietal layer of tunica, which is recognized by its bluish hue, is exposed without much dissection of dartos layer and opened. The cut edges of tunica are held in Allis forceps, and the testis is brought out. The everted tunica is plicated circumferentially with interrupted 2/0 or 3/0 absorbable sutures placing them 1 cm apart with a 1-cm distance between two passes. As the sutures are tied, the sac gathers (like an accordion) around the circumference of testis and epididymis like the rim of a bicycle wheel (Fig. 19.10). It reduces the secreting area of tunica.

This operation is not possible to do in a large thick-walled hydrocele.

EVERSION OF SAC (Jaboulay 1902) After delivering the testis, the redundant tunica is excised leaving a small cuff along the posterior border of testis. The cut edges of tunica are everted and stitched together behind the epididymis by a running absorbable suture to control bleeding and avoiding strangulation of cord (Fig. 19.11). After the eversion is completed, the junctional region of testis with lower end of the cord looks like the neck of a bottle. Hence, it is called "bottle operation." Now some workers recommend use of one or two interrupted sutures instead of a continuous suture as it will prevent accumulation of blood between the epididymis and everted tunica. A great effort should be made to prevent postoperative hematoma, which is a dangerous complication.

The aim of this procedure is to expose the secreting surface of tunica to the outer layers of scrotal wall including dartos which absorb all the secretion of exposed tunica.

This operation is best avoided in a filarial hydrocele because of the following reasons (Ananthakrishnan and Pani 2005):

1. In hydrocele larger than tennis ball, the everted tunica makes a significant swelling behind the testis.

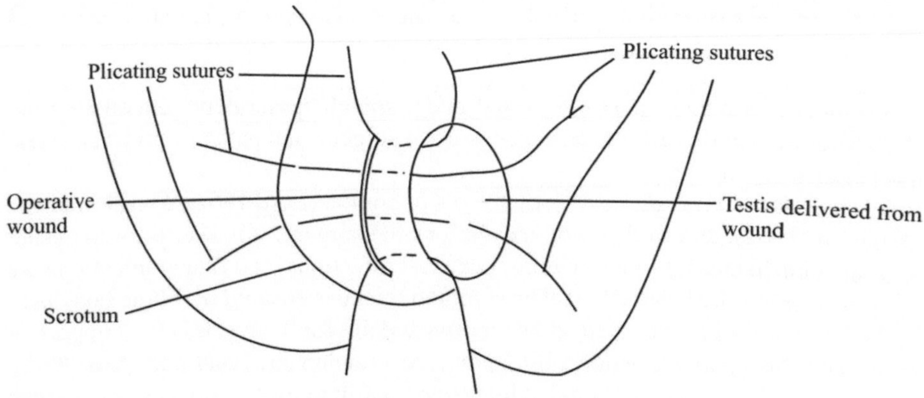

Fig. 19.10 Lord's operation for an early hydrocele with thin-walled sac

Fig. 19.11 Eversion of sac (Jaboulay)

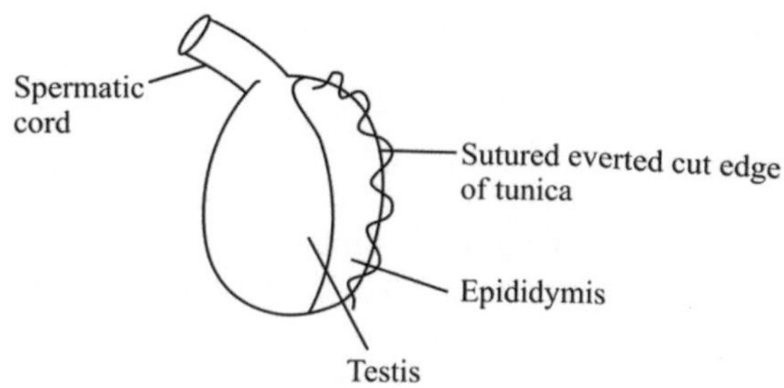

2. The tunica in filarial hydrocele in abnormal. Hence, it is better to excise it. Leaving it may result in elephantiasis of scrotum or lymph scrotum, the latter being a troublesome complication. However, the reports of occurrence of these complications are insufficient to avoid **eversion of sac**.
3. If the eversion is not done properly, it may result in recurrence of hydrocele, as the tunica of upper pole may escape eversion if a large hydrocele is operated with a relatively small incision placed lower down (Goel et al. 1987).

Excision of Sac A large hydrocele with a thick tunica is treated by complete excision of tunica with the help of a cutting diathermy. It removes or reduces the secretory surface of the tunica. The cut edge of tunica around the testis is underrun with a continuous interlocking hemostatic suture for meticulous hemostasis (Fig. 19.12). As there is significant risk of scrotal hematoma, suction drainage is required at least for 48 h.

Following operation, there occur significant improvements in the patient's ability to walk and work (and sexual performance if obstructed by a large hydrocele). However, the surgical services need to scale up and expand to reach the patients where they are and have poor access to currently available treatment facility (Santon et al. 2015).

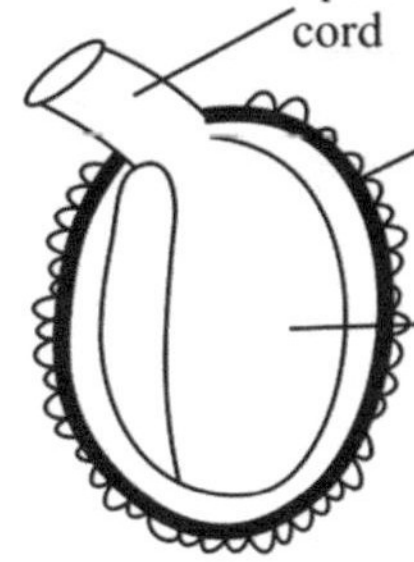

Fig. 19.12 Excision of sac

The operation is preferably done with a vertical incision to preserve the already damaged superficial lymphatics of skin and subcutaneous tissue to prevent secondary obstruction from scarring and subsequent lymph scrotum (DeVries 2002).

Excision of Skin Pani (2013) has recommended excision of redundant skin of scrotum at the time of hydrocele operation. It has the following advantages:

1. The postoperative pain is less as the testis does not hang much downward.
2. The patient is less prone to develop elephantiasis of scrotum.

No other author has described excision of skin with hydrocele operation, and we also do not do it as we do not find any extra advantage with this extra work.

For all the three operations synthetic absorbable suture, e.g., vicryl is ideal but chromic catgut may be used to minimize the cost (Ananthakrishnan and Pani 2005).

- *Aspiration and sclerotherapy* – It may be done in symptomatic patients who are poor surgical risks. The hydrocele is aspirated dry by needle puncture and a sclerosant, e.g., tetracycline, is injected in the hydrocele sac to prevent fluid from reaccumulating. The results of this treatment are variable, but it is very painful. Usually, three treatment sessions are required. It has a high recurrence and complication rate, and the complications include infection and testicular loss (Thompson and Odell 1979). Other sclerosants that can be used include polidocanol, sodium tetradecyl sulfate, and phenol.

Due to so many problems, sclerotherapy is not an appropriate treatment for young otherwise healthy males.

19.9 Problems Encountered During Operation

1. Injury to testis – The testis may be injured when the sac is being opened. It must be prevented by confirming the "feel" of testis, which is firm and solid. The tunica looks bluish and glistening and feels soft and cystic. Even then if the testis is injured, it must be repaired before doing anything else.

2. Hemorrhage – There is a real risk of scrotal hematoma in the postoperative phase, which is a bad complication. It must be avoided by ligation and electrocoagulation of the bleeders. Both these methods leave areas of devitalized tissue in the scrotum, increasing the risk of wound infection. It can be reduced by ligating or coagulating the bleeding points only and no extra tissue.
3. Sometimes, a part of tunica near the upper pole escapes eversion. It is more likely to happen if the tunica is high type and going up to the lower part of spermatic cord. It must be avoided as it will lead to recurrence of hydrocele.
4. Injury to cord structures and epididymis
5. Sometimes, the hydrocele is multiloculated when it should be excised carefully to prevent injury to testis, epididymis, and lower spermatic cord. If a loculus escapes excision, it may enlarge and behave later on like a hydrocele.
6. Pus may be encountered instead of serous fluid. If it is found it is drained. If the testis is found diseased, it should be excised.
7. Chyle may be found (chylocele). It is treated just like a hydrocele by excision of sac.
8. Hematocele – If an old clotted hematocele is found, it is completely evacuated and the testis is examined, which is usually atrophic when it may be excised.

19.10 Postoperative Complications of Hydrocele Surgery

1. *Hemorrhage* – It is the most common complication that has some serious implications. It is of three types – primary, reactionary, and secondary.

   Primary hemorrhage occurs immediately after operation and may be due to slipping of ligature from a ligated vessel or dislodgement of clot. The wound is explored, hematoma is evacuated, and the bleeding points are ligated or electrocoagulated as required.

   Reactionary bleeding occurs within 48 h after operation on recovery of intraoperative hypotension (rare). It is treated like primary hemorrhage.

   Secondary hemorrhage occurs a few days after operation and is due to wound infection. There is local pain and the penis swells up. It is treated with antibiotics, evacuation of exudate, and hemostasis.
2. *Retention of urine* – It occurs in 2–3 % of patients. The etiological factors include fluid overload, use of morphine for pain relief, trying to pass urine while in bed with inadequate privacy, and extrinsic pressure on urethra due to tight bandage. The cause is removed and the patient is given psychic support, pain relief, suprapubic hot and cold compresses early ambulation, and help to go to urinal to pass urine in private. If still the urine is not passed, catheterization is done.
3. *Wound infection* – The scrotum is heavily contaminated by fecal and other bacteria due to proximity with anus. Hence, in spite of proper aseptic precautions, infection of wound may occur, especially if there is hematoma formation in the wound. Diabetic patients are more prone to wound infection. The patient is given broad spectrum antibiotics, and the pain and fever are relieved. The wound may drain pus or exudate if one or two stitches are removed, which is

sent for culture and sensitivity. On receipt of report the antibiotics are changed accordingly.

4. *Hypospermia or azoospermia* – It may rarely follow hydrocele operation due to accidental ligation or division of vas during operation or its involvement in post-operative fibrosis. It might have been there before operation but detected after operation and marriage when the wife of the patient does not conceive. Hence, its legal aspects must be kept in the mind. It is treated with recanalization.
5. *Lymph scrotum* – This crippling complication may follow after the operation of a hydrocele in filarial endemic areas, especially if operation is done with a cosmetic transverse incision and **eversion of sac** (Aguiar-Santos et al. 2009). To prevent this complication, the operation should be done with a longitudinal incision with complete excision of tunica vaginalis and meticulous hemostasis by electrocauterization of cut edge and a running suture.
6. *Recurrence* – Recurrence after operation is very rare but can occur. The causes of recurrence include failure to do complete eversion or excision of sac and regeneration of tunica from the cut edge after excision of sac. The possibility of incomplete eversion is strong when eversion is done with a low small incision in a relatively large scrotal hydrocele (Goel et al. 1987) Flow chart 19.1.

19.11 Prevention

The annual mass drug administration (MDA) of WHO (1997) consisting of a single dose of albendazole-diethylcarbamazine or albendazole-ivermectin may reduce the incidence of hydrocele as reported from Papua New Guinea (Bockarie et al. 2002)

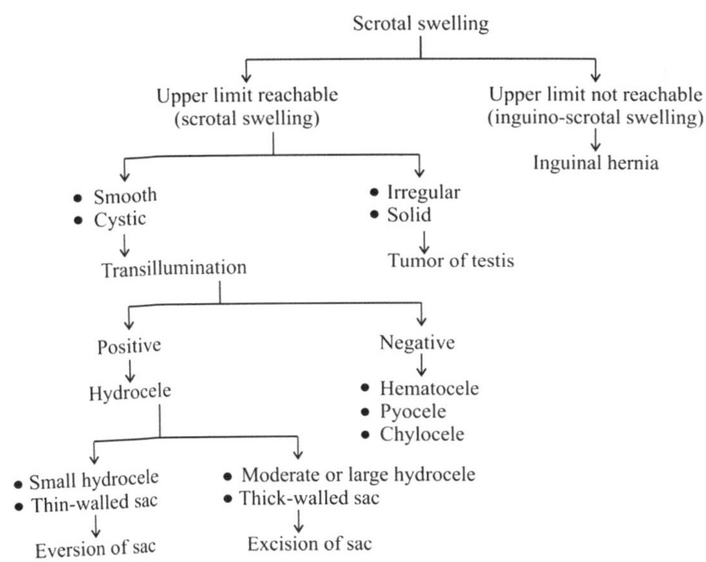

Flow Chart 19.1 Management of a scrotal hydrocele

and India (Yuvaraj et al. 2008). However, even then, it is seen to occur in these areas, of course less frequently. Hence, the program's second arm, i.e., disability management, must go hand in hand.

References

Addiss DG, Dreyer G. Treatment of lymphatic filariasis. In: Nutman TB, editor. Lymphatic filariasis: tropical medicine: science and practice. London: Imperial College Press; 2000. p. 151–99.

Ahorlu C, Dunyo SK, Asamoah G, Simonsen PE. Consequences of hydrocele and benefits of hydrocelectomy: a qualitative study in lymphatic filariasis in endemic communities on the coast of Ghana. Acta Trop. 2001;80:215–21.

Aguiar-Santos AM, Leal-Cruz M, Netto MJ, Carrera A, Lima G, Rocha A. Lymph scrotum: an unusual urological presentation of lymphatic filariasis, a case series study. Rev Int Med Trop Sao Paulo. 2009;51(4):179–83.

Ananthakrishnan N, Pani SP. Surgery for vaginal hydrocele: an update. Indian J Urol. 2005;21: 35–8.

Babu BV, Mishra S, Nayak AN. Marriage, sex and hydrocele: an ethnographic study on the effect of filarial hydrocele on conjugal life and marriageability from Orissa, India. PLoS Negl Trop Dis. 2009;3(4):e414. doi:10.1371/journal.pntd.0000414.

Bockarie MJ, Tisch DJ, Kastens W, et al. Mass treatment to eliminate filariasis in Papua New Guinea. N Engl J Med. 2002;347:1841–8.

Capuano GP, Capuano C. Surgical management of morbidity due to lymphatic filariasis. The usefulness of a standardized international clinical classification of hydroceles. Trop Biomed. 2012;29(1):24–38.

Coreil J, Mayard G, Louis-Charles J, Addiss D. Filarial elephantiasis among Haitian women: social context and behavioural factors in treatment. Trop Med Int Health. 1998;3(6):467–73.

Demarquay JN. Note sur une tumeur des bourses contenant un liquide laiteux (galactocèle de Vidal) et referment des petits etres verrneformes que l'on peut considerer comme des helminthes hematordes a l'état d'embryon. Gaz Med Paris 1863;18:665–67.

DeVries CR. The role of the urologist in the treatment and elimination of lymphatic filariasis worldwide. BJU Int. 2002;89 Suppl 1:37–43.

Dreyer G, et al. Studies on the periodicity and intravascular distribution of Wuchereria bancrofti microfilariae in paired samples of capillary and venous blood from Recife, Brazil. Trop Med Int Health. 1996;1:264–72.

Dreyer G, Noroes J, Addiss D. The silent burden of sexual disability associated with lymphatic filariasis. Acta Trop. 1997;63:57–60.

Dunyo SK, Appawu M, Nkrumah FK, Baffoe-Wilmot A, Pedersen EM, Simonsen PE. Lymphatic filariasis on the coast of Ghana. Trans R Soc Trop Med Hyg. 1996;90:634–8.

Goel TC, Chandra H, Dalela D. Recurrent scrotal hydroele. Surgery. 1987;1:28–9.

Gyapong JO, Magnussen P, Binka FN. Parasitological and clinical aspects of bancroftian filariasis in Kassena Nankana District, Upper East Region, Ghana. Trans R Soc Trop Med Hyg. 1994;88:555–7.

Gyapong M, Gyapong JO, Weiss M, Tanner M. The burden of hydrocele in North Ghana. Acta Trop. 2000;77:287–94.

Jaboulay: Lyon Strock. 1902;2:192.

Kinmonth JB. The lymphatics. 2nd ed. London: Edward Arnold; 1982. p. 211.

Lord PH. Bloodless operation for the radical cure of idiopathic hydrocele. Br J Surg. 1964;51:914.

McAlister VC, Trottier V. Role of persistent processus vaginalis in hydroceles found in tropical population. Can J Surg. 2013;56:e29–31.

Michael E, Bundy DAP, Grenfell BT. Reassessing the global prevalence and distribution of lymphatic filariasis. Parasitology. 1996;112:409–28.

Michael E, Bundy DAP. Global mapping of lymphatic filariasis. Parasitol Today. 1997;13:472–6.

Mishra S, Achary KG, Mandal NN, Tripathy A, Kar SK, Bal MS. Hydrocele fluid: can it be used for immuno-diagnosis of lymphatic filariasis. J Vector Borne Dis. 2014;51:188–93.

Pani S. Pani's filariasis. 3rd ed. Jaypee Brothers: New Delhi; 2013.

Santon MC, Smith EL, Martindale S, Mkwanda SZ, Kelly Hope LA. Exploring hydrocele surgery accessibility and impact in a lymphatic filariasis endemic area of Southern Malawi. Trans R Soc Trop Med Hyg. 2015;109(4):252–61.

Simonsen PE. Filariases. In: Cook GC, Zumla AI, editors. Manson's tropical diseases. 22nd ed. Philadelphia: Saunders Elsevier; 2009. p. 1–15.

Thompson H, Odell M. Sclerosant treatment for hydroceles and epididymal cysts. Br Med J. 1979;2:704.

Yuvaraj J, Pani SP, Vanamail P, Ramaiah KD, Das PK. Impact of seven rounds of mass administration of diethylcarbamazine and ivermectin on prevalence of chronic lymphatic filariasis in South India. Trop Med Int Health. 2008;13:737–42.

World Health Organization. Elimination of lymphatic filariasis as a Public health Problem. Resolution no. 50.29 of World Health Assembly, May 1997.

Chronic Lymphedema–Elephantiasis 20

The term lymphedema, which is synonymous with lymphatic edema, means a swelling of some part of the body due to a fault in the local lymphatic system (Kinmonth 1982).

Chronic lymphedema–elephantiasis is one of the most common chronic manifestation of lymphatic filariasis. It is the most troublesome manifestation that represents the end stage of disease. It is especially prevalent in India, Africa, and South America where 5–10 % of population may be affected with this problem. It is the result of an inability of the existing lymphatics to accommodate the protein and fluid entering the interstitial space at the tissue level (Browse and Steward 1985).

The first recorded case of elephantiasis dates back to prebiblical times. Sushruta in sixth century BC described it as "Shleepada" (श्लीपद), where "Shlee" (श्ली) means elephant and "Pada"(पद)means leg (Bhishagratna 1963). Celsus (30 BC–AD 50) is credited with the first use of the term elephantiasis in modern medicine, which was also known as satyriasis, leontiasis, and sarcocele. This term was accepted by many workers of that time, including Ben Abbas (930–994) and Avicenna (980–1037), and it is being used even today (Hadju 2002).

20.1 Etiology

The causes of chronic lymphedema–elephantiasis are as follows:

- The most important cause of secondary lymphedema all over the world (90 %) especially tropical and subtropical countries is bancroftian filariasis. Brugian filariasis (*Brugia malayi* and *Brugia timori*) is responsible for about 10 % of patients that too confined below the knee and elbow in lower and upper extremities, respectively.
- Primary lymphedema is due to congenital abnormalities of the lymphatics.

T.C. Goel, A. Goel, *Lymphatic Filariasis*, DOI 10.1007/978-981-10-2257-9_20

- Destruction of regional lymph nodes by malignant invasion, radical node dissection, and/or radiotherapy is the most common cause of secondary lymphedema in developed countries.
- Infectious processes such as tuberculosis and lymphogranuloma venereum (Pipinos and Baxter 2012) are less common causes and are usually seen in developing countries.
- Podoconiosis – In some parts of Africa, e.g., Ethiopia, the lymphatics may be damaged by bare foot walking in fields having soil with volcanic ash. It results in elephantiasis of lower extremity (Yimer et al. 2015).

20.2 Pathogenesis

In filarial disease, the third stage larvae enter the superficial lymphatics most commonly of the lower extremity following an infected mosquito bite. The larvae become adult worms and procreate to produce microfilariae. There is no reaction till the worms are alive, but when the worms die spontaneously or due to drugs, there is severe inflammatory reaction in the containing lymphatics and lymph nodes (adenolymphangitis).

It is followed by fibrous scarring and fibrous adenolymphatic obstruction. As a result of this, the patient gradually develops distal swelling due to accumulation of lymph (lymphedema). The immune response to dead filarial worms may play some role in adenolymphangitis and subsequent lymphatic obstruction.

The recurrent attacks of filarial inflammation increase severity and extent of obstruction, leading to increase in edema and making the edema fluid progressively protein-rich, which causes fibrosis in the lymphedematous tissue.

The recurrent attacks of inflammation (acute dermatolymphangioadenitis, ADLA) cause thickening, black discoloration, and drying of the overlying skin. Thus, the affected part of limb looks like the limb of an elephant. Hence, this filarial manifestation is called elephantiasis. The following flow chart shows the pathogenesis of filarial elephantiasis Flow Chart 20.1.

20.3 Sites of Chronic Lymphedema Elephantiasis (Khanna 1970)

- Commonly involved sites
  1. Lower extremity
  2. Scrotum
  3. Penis
- Less commonly involved sites
  1. Breast
  2. Vulva
  3. Upper extremity
- Very rare sites – Localized and pedunculated form of elephantiasis (Manson-Bahr 1960)
  1. Scalp

Mosquito (having third stage filarial larvae) bite, most commonly in the lower extremity

↓

Entry into local lymphatics and lymph nodes

↓

Death of worms spontaneously or due to drugs

↓

Filarial adenolymphangitis

↓

Adenolymphatic obstruction

↓

Accumulation of interstitial fluid or lymph in the tissues

↓

Lymphedema

↓

Recurrent attacks of acute dermatolymphangioadenitis (ADLA)

↓ (branches into two)

- Further progression of obstruction (multiple levels or sites)
- Addition of inflammatory exudate to edema fluid → Activation of keratinocytes to produce collagen

↓ (both converge)

Fibrous proliferation including subdermal fibrosis

↓

Lymphedema and fibredema

↓

Elephantiasis

Flow Chart 20.1 The etiopathogenesis of chronic lymphedema–elephantiasis

2. Face
3. Buttocks
4. Lower limb

20.4 Pathology

All the elephantoid process is outside the deep fascial envelope of the extremity, the deep fascia, and the deeper tissues being normal. It is due to the entry and activity of the infective larvae in the subcutaneous plane following mosquito bite.

The skin is markedly thickened (looks like rind of an orange) and firm and cuts like an unripe pear. There is excessive deposition of fibrous tissue, which is maximum in the dermis and becomes less and less as one goes towards the deep fascia.

The subcutaneous fatty tissue is replaced by fibrous tissue superficially and blubbery tissue toward the deep fascia with a lot of watery fluid exuding out from the dilated spaces and dilated lymphatics.

It must be stressed that elephantiasis is by no means the inevitable consequence of lymphatic filarial infection. Even in endemic areas where most of the people are exposed to infection during their entire life do not acquire it. Even all the people who develop microfilaremia, lymphadenopathy, and recurrent attacks of fever and lymphangitis do not develop elephantiasis.

References

Bhishagratna KKL. An English translation of Shusruta Samhita based on the original Sanskrit text, vol. 2. Varanasi: Chowkamba Sanskrit Series Office; 1963. p. 439–49.

Browse NL, Steward G. Lymphoedema: pathophysiology and classification. J Cardiovasc Surg (Torino). 1985;26:91–106.

Hadju SI. A note from history: elephantiasis. Ann Clin Lab Sci. 2002;32(2):207–9.

Khanna NN. Surgical treatment of elephantiasis of male genitalia. Plast Reconstr Surg. 1970; 46(5):481.

Kinmonth JB. The lymphatics. 2nd ed. London: Edward Arnold; 1982. p. 83–104.

Manson-Bahr P. Tropical diseases. 15th ed. London: Cassell; 1960.

Pipinos II, Baxter BT. The lymphatics. In: Townsend Jr CM, Beauchamp RD, Evers BM, Mattox KL, editors. Sabiston textbook of surgery, vol. 2. 19th ed. Philadelphia: Elsevier Saunders; 2012. p. 1819.

Yimer M, Hailu T, Mulu W, Abera B. Epidemiology of elephantiasis with special emphasis on podoconiosis in Ethiopia: a literature review. J Vector Borne Dis. 2015;52:111–5.

Chronic Lymphedema-Elephantiasis of Lower Extremity

21

Chronic lymphedema–elephantiasis of lower extremity is one of the most common chronic obstructive manifestations of filariasis (Fig. 21.1). It is a very old problem as Manu in Manusmriti says that a priest having this problem should not be invited to perform the religious rites in annual remembrance festivities (श्राद्धकर्म). Sushruta (सुश्रुत), father of Indian Surgery (fourth century BC), described it as "Shleepada" (श्लीपद) (Bhishagratna 1963).

21.1 Etiology

It is postulated that the elephantiasis is the end stage of filariasis and results from cell-mediated immune reaction to dead adult worms leading to recurrent adenolymphangitis, which causes adenolymphatic obstruction.

A patient will not develop clinical lymphedema after the first attack, as there is enough lymphatic reserve for drainage, and because of lymphatic regeneration. However, the repeated attacks of inflammation lead to more and more adenolymphatic damage and laying down of more and more scar tissue where the lymphatic regeneration is no more possible.

Recent histological and lymphoscintigraphic studies have shown dilatation and proliferation of lymphatic endothelium associated with abnormal lymphatic function leading to lymphedema (and hydrocele) in the absence of overt inflammatory response. The immunity system during the development of this noninflammatory pathology is downregulated through the production of contra-inflammatory immune molecules.

21.2 Pathogenesis

- *Lymphedema* – Following adenolymphatic obstruction, the lymph accumulates in the lymphatics distal to the obstruction leading to closure of the valves due to back pressure or fluid recoil starting at the segment of lymphatic vessel nearest

T.C. Goel, A. Goel, *Lymphatic Filariasis*, DOI 10.1007/978-981-10-2257-9_21

the obstruction and going to the most distal segment. The extracellular fluid around the end of the vessel would now have to accumulate sufficiently to open the valves at the proximal end of each segment against the pressure closing the valve from the lymph already held back in each segment. The lymphatics holding more than normal amount of fluid dilate resulting in valvular failure and regurgitation. Thus, the extracellular fluid fails to be reabsorbed and accumulates around the distal end of lymphatics heralding the onset of lymphedema.

The accumulation of lymph (extracellular fluid) gradually spreads to the adjacent sites. Thus, the lymphedema marches on and on.

- *Fibredema* – As the extracellular fluid starts to accumulate, there is no fibrous proliferation as the fluid is low in protein content. As the time passes, the protein content of edema fluid increases. The main contributor to increase in the protein content is recurrent attacks of acute inflammation resulting in exudation of proteins of high molecular weight which cannot be drained out because of adenolymphatic obstruction.

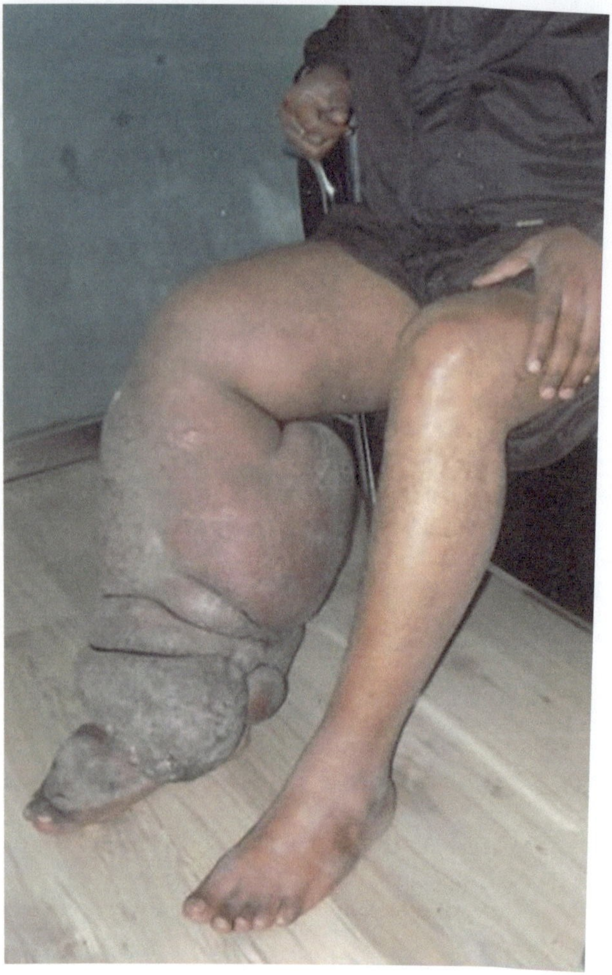

Fig. 21.1 Massive filarial chronic lymphedema–elephantiasis of right lower extremity involving the thigh also. The skin of lower part is pigmented, rough, and dry and has multiple deep skin folds (Courtesy of Dr. RK Mishra of SIPS)

The protein in the tissue fluid is an ideal medium for the proliferation of fibroblasts which gradually replace the adipose tissue.
The change from edema to fibredema occurs first at the site of onset of edema (usually below the medial malleolus), and the elephantiasis spreads directly into the adjacent areas after they have become edematous.

- *Elephantiasis* – The secondary and recurrent bacterial or fungal infections act to give the black pigmented, rough, and dry appearance to the skin of the affected part like that of an elephant.

21.3 Pathology

The filarial lymphedema–elephantiasis involves mostly the foot and leg. Mild lymphedema may extend into the thigh, but there is no distinct line of demarcation between the normal and lymphedematous skin.

The sole of foot escapes because of firm attachment of the skin with the plantar fascia; it may partly be due to weight bearing.

The total disease process occurs outside the deep fascial envelope, the deeper tissues being normal (Fig. 21.2). It may be because of the entry of infective larvae and development into the adult worms in the superficial lymphatic system of the extremity especially lower extremity as it is the most common site of the mosquito bite.

In early disease (lymphedema), the limb is swollen to a varying degree with nearly normal skin. As the elephantoid changes occur, the skin becomes thick, rough, and dry. Near the ankle joint, many grooves may develop in the swelling probably due to movements of the joint which become deeper and deeper as the swelling increases. Later on, the skin may develop many nodular excrescences on the toes and foot.

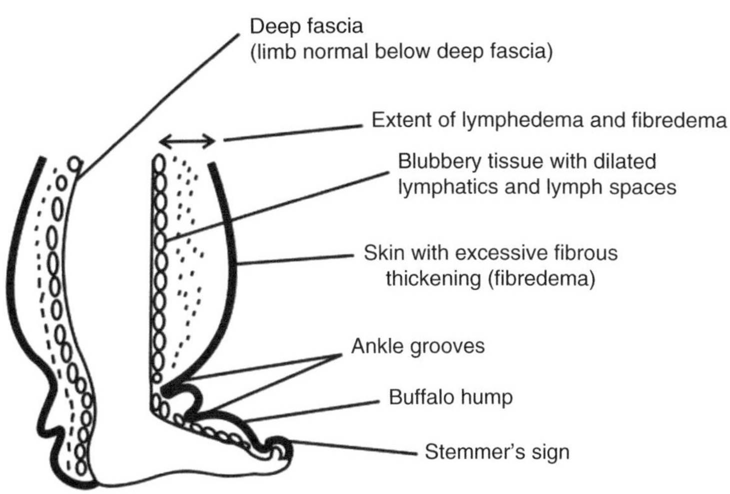

Fig. 21.2 Pathology of elephantiasis of leg

Gross Pathology The skin cuts like an unripe pear, and the subcutaneous tissue shows a blubbery appearance with a lot of watery fluid exuding out from divided dilated lymphatics and tissue spaces. The subcutaneous fat is replaced by connective tissue. The vascularity of the tissues has increased, especially the venous component. Peripheral lymphovenous shunts have been observed by some workers.

Micropathology There is excessive deposition of fibrous tissue, which is maximum in the dermis and becoming less and less towards the deep fascia. Matas (1913) described it as "chronic inflammatory fibromatosis or hypertrophy of the hypodermal and dermal connective tissue." The elephantoid tissue is infiltrated by eosinophils, plasma cells, and mononuclear cells around the segments of dead or calcified worms. The lymphatics show obliterative endolymphangitis with scarring.

The extent and the degree of lymphedema–elephantiasis depend upon two factors – the level of lymphatic obstruction and the stretchability of skin:

1. If the obstruction is inguinal and the skin of the limb is relatively normal, the subcutaneous type of lymphedema of any degree can occur (Fig. 21.6).
2. If the lymphatic obstruction is peripheral and at multiple levels with secondary infection (repeated attacks of ADLA), the swelling is not marked and the skin is blackish, thick, rough, and dry (Fig. 21.8).

21.4 Clinical Features

Chronic lymphedema–elephantiasis commonly manifests between 30 and 45 years of age and a little more common in males than in females. It is usually unilateral. The disease develops through a series of events:

- Recurrent attacks of fever with rigor with adenolymphangitis with mild pitting edema of extremity – the swelling reduces on keeping the limb elevated for some time.
- With subsidence of attack, the swelling reduces but the "status quo ante" is seldom attained.

With subsequent attacks, there is further increase in the lymphedema with every attack adding to the swelling. Chronic lymphedema may develop in the absence of overt inflammatory reaction. In bancroftian filariasis, the edema may extend above the knee or elbow to involve the thigh or upper arm respectively. In brugian disease, the swelling is limited below the knee or elbow.

- Gradually, the skin becomes black, thick, rough, and dry with loss of elasticity. It cannot be pinched or moved on deeper tissue. The hairs become sparse.
- The lymphedema starts around the ankle filling the perimalleolar depressions (tree trunk pattern) and then making the dorsum of the foot swell up giving a

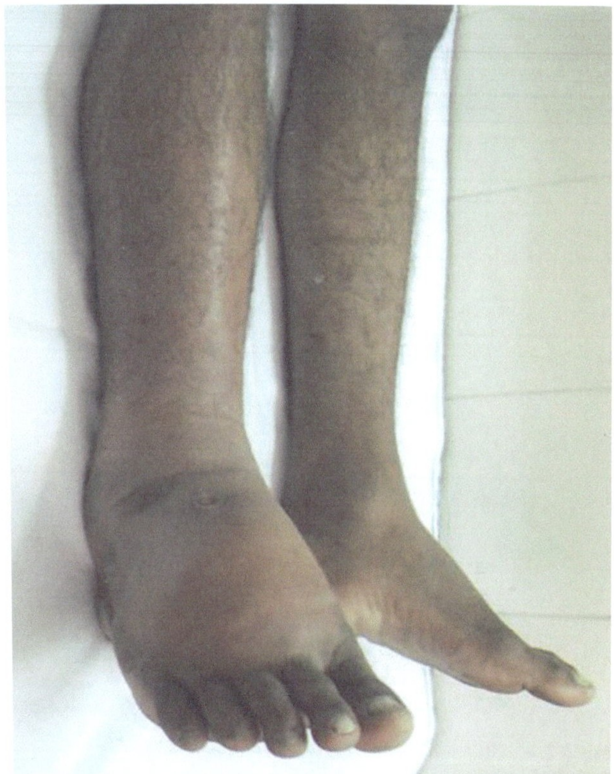

Fig. 21.3 Filarial elephantiasis of right lower limb with buffalo hump on dorsum of foot (Courtesy of Dr. MK Srivastava)

buffalo hump appearance. The skin of the dorsum of foot cannot be pinched because of subcutaneous fibrosis (Stemmer's sign). The dorsum of the toes is also swollen (Figs. 21.3, 21.4, 21.5, 21.6, 21.7, and 21.8), and the swollen toes assume a square shape because of pressure of adjacent toes in the shoe (squaring of the toes).

- The edema pits on pressure, and gradually as it changes into fibredema, it pits less and less till it stops pitting. The skin is lichenified and looks like peau d'orange (Pipinos and Baxter 2012).
- There is usually no pain, but heaviness is a common symptom. Severe pain is indicative of acute attack of filariasis or secondary infection, which is usually associated with fever with rigor.
- In the advanced stage of disease, the skin is thickened and thrown into folds often with depigmentation, nodules, warty growths, intertrigo of webs of toes, or chronic nonhealing ulcers (Burri et al. 1996). The swelling may be huge and grotesque, incapacitating the patient requiring help even for personal needs. Fungal infection in interdigital region and deep folds is common, from where bacteria can enter and cause lymphangitis. The fungi do not invade the tissues. The patients with large ugly limbs are often ostracized from their communities, unable to socialize and to attend school or find work (Venkata Phani Deepathi et al. 2011).

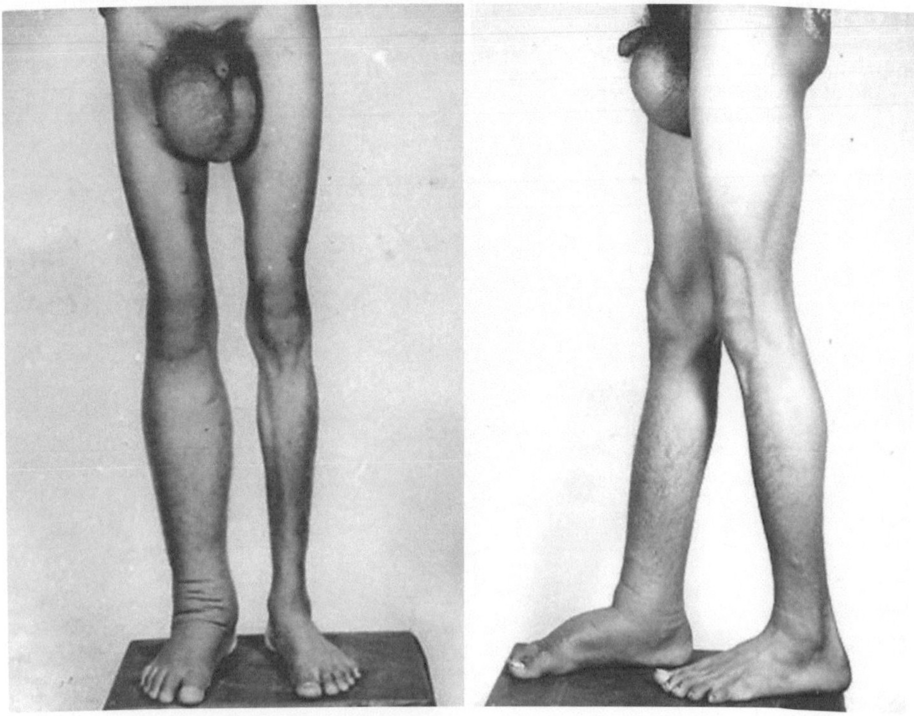

Fig. 21.4 Mild chronic filarial lymphedema of right lower extremity extending up above the knee. This patient has bilateral filarial hydrocele also

21.5 Brunner's Grading of Lymphedema

Table 21.1 presents Brunner's grading of lymphedema.

21.6 Assessment of Lymphedema: Fibredema (Lymphedema/Fibrous Proliferation Indices)

For assessment of relative proportion of lymphedema and fibredema, the following measurements are taken (Goel 1985):

1. Depth of a pit left after 2 min of sustained digital pressure (or by the rounded end of a pen) at midpoint of swollen leg and foot
2. Circumference of both diseased and normal limbs at the midpoints of feet and legs
3. Volume of both the limbs up to the tibial tuberosity by water displacement method

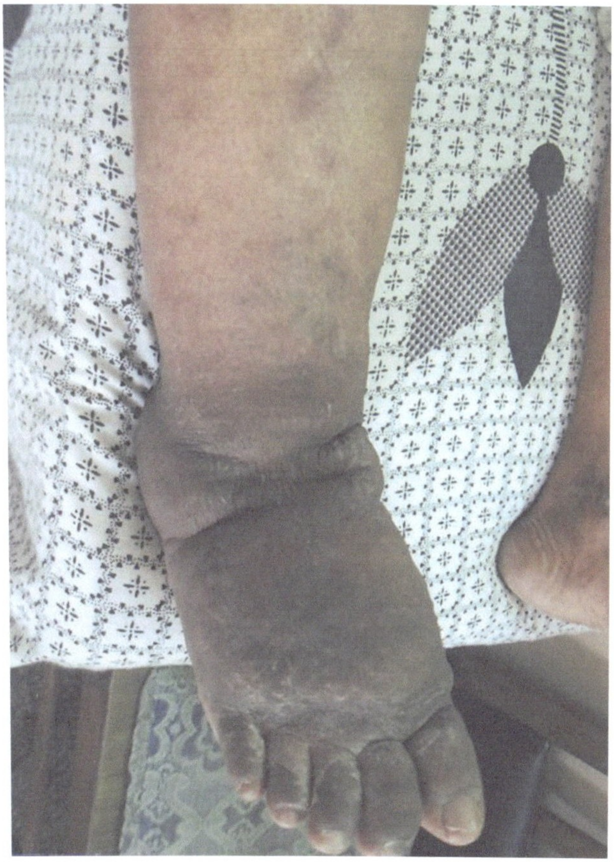

Fig. 21.5 Filarial elephantiasis of right leg and foot. The skin is rough, dry and pigmented

Now the diseased limb is given a pressure bandage and put on full-time elevation of 6 in. or above the level of heart for 24 h for reducing the edema, and the above measurements are taken again.

From these measurements, the extent of lymphedema and fibredema are assessed fairly accurately.

21.7 Differential Diagnosis

(a) *From primary lymphedema* – The differences between the primary and secondary lymphedema are given in Table 21.2.

(b) *From other causes of secondary lymphedema*

1. Infections other than filariasis causing cellulitis, lymphangitis, and lymphadenitis, especially when there are recurrent attacks that destroy lymphatics and lymph nodes followed by fibrosis. They also result in lymphedema.

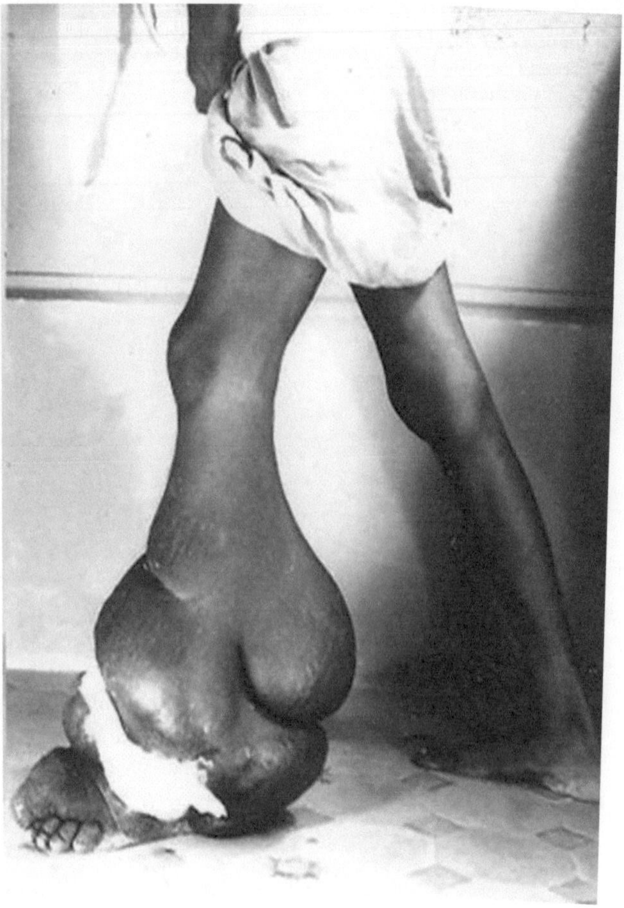

Fig. 21.6 Massive filarial lymphedema of left lower extremity with grooves and hanging lymphedematous skin around the ankle

2. Malignancy – Advanced or extensive lymph node metastases and primary lymphatic malignancy of inguinal lymph nodes may cause lymphedema by invasion of lymphatics and lymph nodes.

   Extrinsic pressure of large tumors may cause lymphedema. For example, large tumors of pelvis can cause lymphedema of both lower limbs by pressure on pelvic veins and lymphatics. Hence, if a middle-aged person presents with lymphedema of recent onset of lower limbs, he/she must be investigated for large pelvic masses. Such lymphedema often commences proximally in the thigh rather than distally in the foot and leg.

   The block dissection of inguinal lymph nodes for carcinoma of penis, scrotum, or vulva may be followed by lymphedema of lower limb. It is more likely if it is combined with postoperative radiotherapy.
3. Trauma may be followed by lymphedema, e.g., degloving injuries, circumferential wounds, and full thickness burns may produce distal lymphedema due to loss of lymphatics. The etiology of traumatic lymphedema is

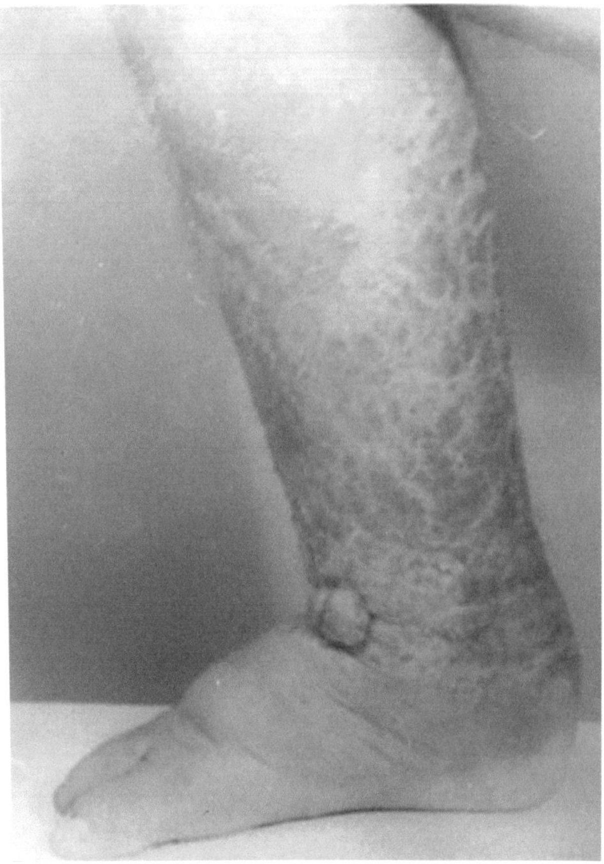

Fig. 21.7 Chronic filarial lymphedema of right lower extremity with vesicles, fistulae lymphorrhea, and a verrucous nodule on the front of ankle

multifactorial, including lymphatic injury or destruction and local venous thrombosis.

4. Exposure to foreign material, e.g., silica particles (endemic elephantiasis, podoconiosis) – It is a common problem of tropical countries which affects more than 5,00,000 people in Africa, especially in Ethiopia where 192 million people are at risk. It occurs due to barefoot cultivation in the soil composed of particles of silica from alkaline volcanic rocks (red volcanic soil) and absorption of ultrafine particles through the skin of feet. They destroy the peripheral lymphatics and can be seen in the macrophages in the local lymph nodes. The edema starts in the sole and spreads rapidly upwards (Yimer et al. 2015) and may extend up to the knee.
5. Factitious lymphedema is due to tying a tourniquet or belt. The mark or cutoff can be seen just above the swelling, which pits on pressure. The patient may be a psychopath.
6. Phlebedema – It is diffuse swelling of lower limb due to accumulation of transudate caused by congestive heart failure or renal failure (Cho and

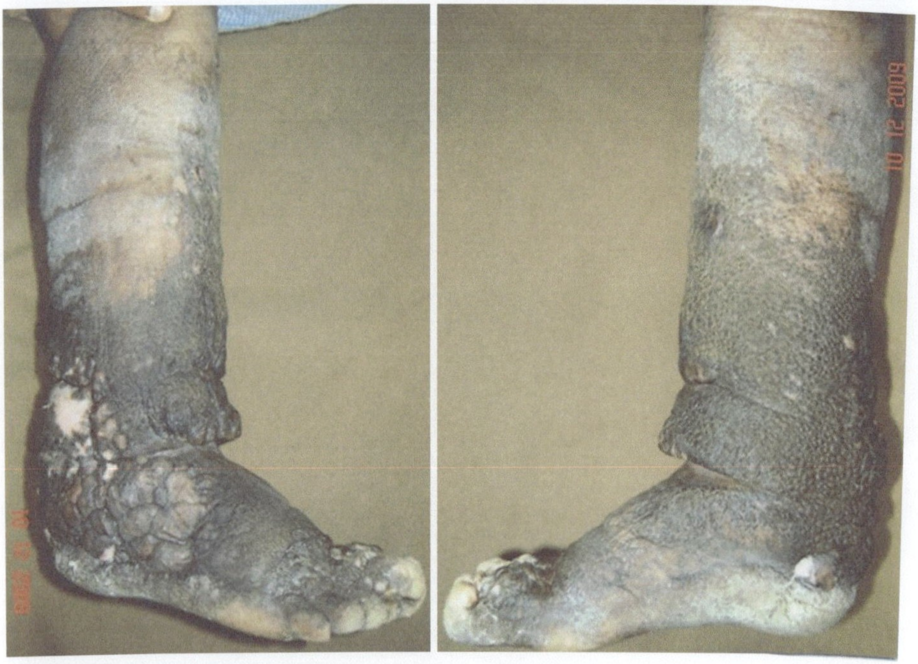

Fig. 21.8 Filarial elephantiasis of right lower limb with not much swelling of lymphedema but marked skin changes, i.e., pigmentation, depigmentation, nodularity, thickening, and grooves (Courtesy of Dr. Surajit Bhattacharya)

Table 21.1 Brunner's grades of chronic lymphedema

Grade	Pitting on pressure	Effect of elevation over night	Skin changes
Grade I	Present Complete pitting	Disappears more or less completely	No skin changes
Grade II	Present Not full pitting	Disappears partially on elevation	No skin changes
Grade III	Nonpitting edema	Not relieved on elevation	Early changes present
Grade IV	Nonpitting edema	Not relieved on elevation	Late changes present including papillae, fissuring and other irreversible changes

Atwood 2002) (bilateral), or venous obstruction or chronic venous insufficiency of lower limb (unilateral). The differences between phlebedema and lymphedema are given in Table 21.3.

(c) *From solid swelling of lower extremity*

1. Lipedema (lipodystrophy) – This problem begins at puberty in females and is characterized by bilateral, usually symmetrical swelling of lower limbs

Table 21.2 Differences between primary and secondary lymphedema

Features	Primary lymphedema	Secondary lymphedema
Etiology	Congenital aplasia and hypoplasia of lymphatics	Filarial adenolymphatic obstruction is the most common cause
Occurrence	Less common	More common
Age	At birth, during adolescence, and during 35–50 years of age	Middle ages
Sex	Females are more often affected	Males are more often affected
Onset and progress	Gradual and slowly progressive	Starts acutely and then progresses with repeated attacks of acute filariasis
Family history	Likely to be positive	Negative
Precipitating factor	Absent	Acute infection or reinfection
Regional lymph nodes	Absent	Often enlarged
Capillary hemangioma	May be present	Absent
Drainage operations (lymphangioplasty)	May be of help	Usually do not help

due to excessive deposition of subcutaneous fat. The buttocks, thighs, and legs are affected, and the feet are not affected. The trunk may be involved. It gives an inverse shouldering effect at the malleoli (Fig. 21.9). The swelling is soft, does not pit on pressure, and does not reduce on elevation of limb. The overlying skin is normal. The diagnosis can be confirmed by MRI, which shows excessive fat in the subcutaneous plane and no fluid accumulation

2. Congenital arteriovenous fistula – It causes diffuse enlargement of the limb (local gigantism) in which all the component tissues of the limb are enlarged (hypertrophied). It is characterized by dilated tortuous pulsating veins, non-pitting swelling, and continuous murmur.
3. Elephantiasis neuromatosa – It is diffuse enlargement of the limb due to excessive thickening of sheaths of subcutaneous nerves. The skin is markedly thickened, tender, and soft or firm and may be edematous.

21.8 Complications

Common complications include recurrent cellulitis, abscess, chronic eczema, fungal infections of skin (dermatophytosis) and nail (onychomycosis), fissuring and verrucae, and papillae (warts). Cellulitis is potentially a life-threatening complication (Schook et al. 2014).

- Ulceration may occur due to repeated trauma caused by scratching to satisfy itching of eczema. It is unusual unless associated with damage to the blood circulation of skin of leg due to attacks of infection, inflammation, or trauma (Kinmonth

Table 21.3 Differences between phlebedema and lymphedema

Features	Phlebedema	Lymphedema
Definition	Accumulation of transudate in the lower limb due to venous obstruction and stasis	Accumulation of lymph in the tissues of lower limb due to adenolymphatic obstruction
Etiology	Congestive cardiac failure Chronic venous insufficiency	Filarial adenolymphatic obstruction
Onset	Rapid	Slow
Duration	Short	Long
Progress	Fluctuating	Steady with recurrent attacks
Side	Bilateral in CHF, unilateral in chronic venous disease	Usually unilateral
Severity	Moderate	Moderate to severe
Toes	Unaffected or slightly swollen	Affected, squared off in late disease May have papillomatosis
Overlying skin	Normal in congestive cardiac failure May be lipodermatosclerotic in chronic venous insufficiency	Coarse, thickened, and hyperkeratotic
Subcutaneous veins	May be prominent	Not prominent
Pitting on pressure	Present	Early disease present, late disease absent
Lymphorrhea	Not present	May be present
Consistency of swelling	Soft pitting edema	Firm rubbery and may pit with difficulty
Elevation of limb	Rapid and complete or near complete reduction of swelling	Slow and incomplete reduction or no reduction of swelling
Signs of deep vein thrombosis	May be present	Absent
Ulceration	Common manifestation of chronic venous insufficiency	Rare occurrence
	Bluish red ulcer with pigmentation around	Pale ulcer with lymphorrhea
Lymphoscintigraphy	Decreased lymph nodes	Increased or enlarged lymph nodes

1982). The lymphatic obstruction does not disturb the supply of oxygen and nutrients to the tissues; hence, ulceration in lymphatic obstruction is very rare.

- Lymphangioma – It consists of dilated dermal lymphatics that "blister" on the skin surface containing clear or blood-stained fluid. With passage of time, it thromboses and fibroses resulting in the formation of hard nodules. If it is less than 5 cm across, it is termed lymphangioma circumscriptum. If it is more widespread, it is called lymphangioma diffusum. If it forms a reticulate pattern of ridges, it is termed lymphedema ab igne. It may weep on skin surface causing lymphorrhea and open portals for infection to enter (cellulitis).

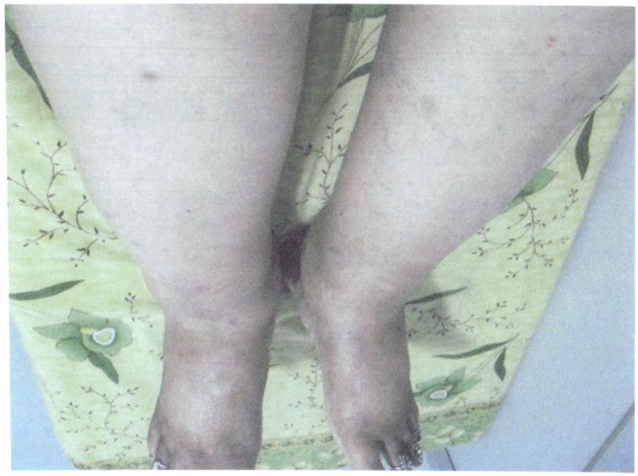

Fig. 21.9 Bilateral lipedema of both lower extremities in a woman of 47 years of age with proximal swelling more than the distal

- Lymphangiosarcoma – It is a malignant tumor that occurs in long-standing lymphedema. It was originally described to occur in postmastectomy lymphedema (Stewart–Treves syndrome) and affects about 0.5 % of patients at a mean duration of onset of 10 years. In other lymphedemas, it usually takes about 20 years to manifest. The patient presents with single or multiple bluish-red cutaneous and subcutaneous nodules, which spread to form satellite lesions that may become confluent. The diagnosis can be confirmed by biopsy. It usually requires amputation and has a poor prognosis.

Muller et al. (1987) has described a case of 19-year-old inhabitant of South India with chronic filarial lymphedema of 15-year duration who developed lymphangiosarcoma. They reviewed two further cases of lymphangiosarcoma occurring on filarial lymphedema and reported in the literature (Devi and Bahuleyan 1977; Sordillo et al. 1981).

Other malignancies, which may be associated with chronic lymphedema, are Kaposi's sarcoma (HIV), squamous cell carcinoma, liposarcoma, malignant melanoma, malignant fibrous histiocytoma, basal cell carcinoma, and lymphoma. This association may be due to impairment of surveillance.

21.9 Investigations

Blood The blood is sent for counts, urea, creatinine, electrolytes, total protein, sugar, and liver function tests if indicated.

In filarial lymphedema, the blood may show eosinophilia and microfilariae in the night blood smear. The serologic tests for filariasis, including bentonite flocculation, indirect hemagglutination, ELISA, and indirect fluorescent antibody tests, may be helpful, but they cannot differentiate between past and active infection.

Urine The urine is sent for routine examination, especially for chyle. Rarely, it may reveal microfilariae.

Lymphangiography It is the radiographic visualization of regional lymphatic system by opacifying them with radio-opaque contrast medium. It is of two types – direct and indirect.

Direct lymphangiography is done by injecting the contrast (ultrafluid lipiodol) into a lymphatic of first web space of foot identified by injecting methylene blue or patent blue violet. The contrast is injected into the lymphatic with the help of a special injector, and then serial radiography is done. It may take 12–24 h to visualize the inguinal and retroperitoneal lymphatics. It is a "gold standard" investigation for detecting the structural defects of lymphatics and lymph nodes, especially larger lymphatics.

Indirect lymphangiography is done by intradermal injection of water soluble nonionic contrast (Iotasul, Schering) into the first web space from where it is absorbed into the lymphatics when they can be radiographed (initial lymphatics, precollectors, and subcutaneous collectors). It shows only the distal lymphatics and not proximal lymphatics and lymph nodes (Bergan 1995).

The lymphangiography is the ideal investigation to see the anatomy of lymphatic system. However, the disadvantages of this procedure are as follows:

1. It is technically difficult and time consuming.
2. It is unpleasant to the patient.
3. It may cause further damage to lymphatics.

Hence, it is not done as a routine but done only for preoperative evaluation in a patient with megalymphatics where bypass or fistula ligation is being planned.

Lymphoscintigraphy It is radioisotopic visualization of the lymphatic system, which has nearly completely substituted lymphangiography (Barrett et al. 2006; Szuba et al. 2003). It is done by injection of technetium-99m-labeled human albumin or sulfur colloid particles into interdigital web space of foot. The limb is exercised intermittently, and the images are taken with a whole-body gamma camera. It provides more information about the function than about the structure of lymphatics. It is minimally invasive and can be done as an outdoor procedure. It has a low exposure of radiation (~5 mCi).

In normal persons, the tracer activity may be detected in the inguinal lymph nodes within 15–60 min. The isotope should be present in the pelvic and retroperitoneal lymph nodes a little later.

In lymphedema, there may be absent or delayed transport, abnormal accumulation of isotope in the collaterals, and obstruction at the level of regional lymph nodes. It cannot differentiate between primary and secondary lymphedemas, but

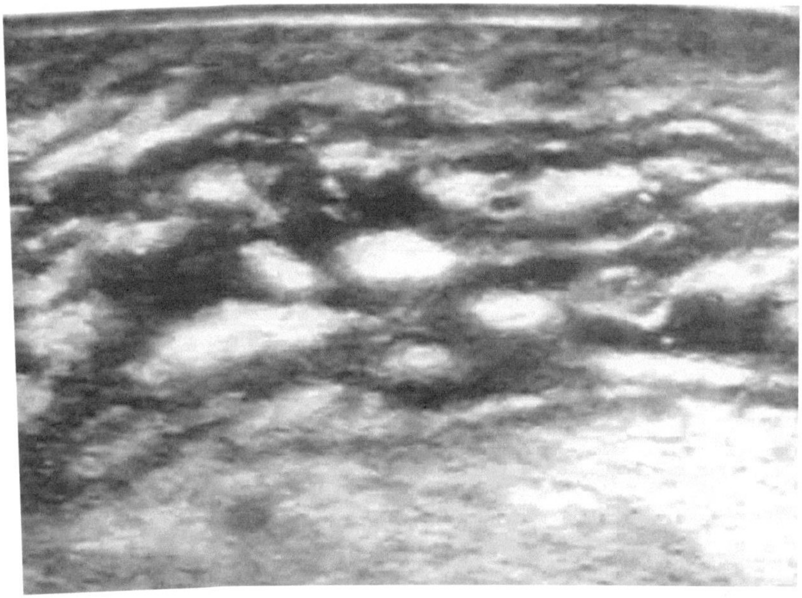

Fig. 21.10 Ultrasonography of chronic lymphedematous leg showing accumulation of lymph in subcutaneous tissue

it has a sensitivity of 70–90 % and a specificity of almost 100 % in differentiating lymphedema from other causes of a swollen extremity (Pipinos and Baxter 2012).

Contrast Magnetic Resonance Lymphangiography It is a new diagnostic test which is performed after intracutaneous injection of gadobenate dimeglumine into the interdigital webs of dorsal foot (Liu et al. 2009). It visualizes the anatomy and function including the lymph flow in lymphatics and lymph nodes.

Further, *MRI* may help in the diagnosis of lymphatic hyperplasia. It may help in differentiating between venous and lymphatic causes of swollen extremity, and also in the diagnosis of tumors of pelvis causing lymphedema due to extrinsic pressure.

Ultrasonography The lymphedema can be imaged by ultrasound (Figs. 21.10 and 21.11). If an abscess has formed it can also be imaged. It also provides useful information about the local veins.

Many patients of lymphedema show venous reflux on duplex ultrasound, which may lead to the wrong diagnosis of chronic venous disease and subsequent surgery on veins, i.e., saphenofemoral or saphenopopliteal junction ligation together with saphenous stripping. It will further damage the lymphatics as the subcutaneous lymph bundles run along the major superficial veins.

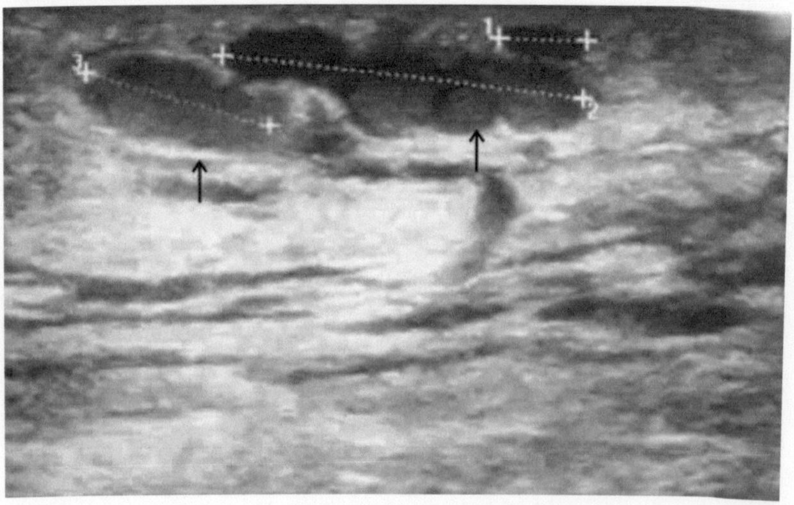

Fig. 21.11 Ultrasonography of chronic lymphedema–elephantiasis of lower leg showing abscess cavities in subcutaneous tissue

CT Scan It can be done to confirm the diagnosis of lymphedema for which a single axial CT slice is taken through the midcalf. It shows a coarse, nonenhancing reticular "honeycomb" pattern in the enlarged subcutaneous compartment. On the contrary, in phlebedema, it reveals increased volume of muscular compartment and in lipedema increased thickness of subcutaneous fat. It may help in differentiating filarial lymphedema from primary lymphedema as the primary lymphedema is characterized by lack or absence of lymph nodes draining the area involved. In filarial lymphedema, the lymph nodes are usually enlarged (Jenkins 2005).

These two investigations, i.e., CT scan and MRI, are essential for the exclusion of underlying oncologic states as the cause of lymphedema (Barrett et al 2006).

Biopsy If a tumor is suspected as the cause or effect of chronic lymphedema FNA, core biopsy or open biopsy may be done. Enlarged inguinal lymph nodes may also be studied by FNA or biopsy.

Near Infrared (NIR) Fluorescence Imaging It is a new technique of imaging lymph vessels by injecting indocyanine green (ICG) into the skin followed immediately by imaging with a dynamic (real time) infrared fluorescence camera. With this method even very small lymphatic vessels can be seen. This study is dynamic as the actual function of the lymphatic vessels can be analyzed. The diseased lymphatics that do not contract (or pulsate) normally can be seen. It is a safe dye that is used in very small amounts to image the lymphatics.

This technique can diagnose lymphedema and may find lymphatic abnormalities at an early stage.

This technique is currently available at a very few centers and most of them are involved in research (Unno et al. 2010, Rasmussen et al. 2009, Damstra 2008).

Measurement of Volume The volume measurements are used to quantify the fluid accumulation and to follow the response of treatment. The limb volume can be measured by three methods:

1. *Tape measurement* – Tape measurements are taken at defined intervals and the total volume of the limb is calculated using geometric formulas. This technique is accurate if it is done in the same way each time by the same person.
2. *Perometry* – It uses an infrared optical electronic scanner and computer to calculate the volume of the body part. It is accurate if the limb is positioned exactly the same way each time and the machine is calibrated for accuracy.
3. *Water displacement* – It is a long used "gold standard" for measurement of limb volume, but it is rarely used these days due to its inconvenience. The limb is inserted in a large cylinder containing water and the volume of water pushed out or displaced is measured.

The measurement of volume does not diagnose the cause of lymphedema and cannot differentiate the lymphedema from other types of swollen limb (NLN 2011).

Bioimpedance Spectroscopy (BIS) This method measures the interstitial fluid in patients of lymphedema. It is done by passing a small painless electrical current through the extremity and the resistance to the current (impedance) is measured, and it is compared with the resistance to current in the opposite limb. The higher the water content in the interstitial space, the lower is the resistance (impedance) to the electronic flow. It is not accurate in advanced lymphedema or fibredema and does not differentiate between various types of edemas (Moseley et al. 2002; Ward 2006).

All the investigations described above are not needed in every patient of lymphedema–elephantiasis. The treating team should use its own judgment in selecting the appropriate investigations.

21.10 Treatment

This problem is difficult to treat and should be treated by a multiprofessional team. Although the surgery has very little role, the surgeons usually supervise the treatment of these patients. Early diagnosis and treatment is very important because at this stage the removal of the cause and very simple therapeutic measures are very effective and may give nearly complete relief to the patient. In late lymphedema, i.e., elephantiasis, only palliative measures are available, which provide partial relief. The components of treatment include removal of the cause, relief of pain, prevention of complications, and reduction of the swelling.

21.10.1 Treatment of the Cause

A course of diethylcarbamazine (DEC) 100 mg three times a day orally after meals is given for 3–4 weeks. It kills the parasite but does not reverse the pathologic changes caused by infection. To prevent further attacks, a single annual dose of DEC (6 mg/kg orally) alone or in combination with ivermectin (400 mcg/kg orally) may be used. Further mosquito bite is prevented by reduction of mosquito breeding and by use of protective clothing, mosquito netting and mosquito repellants.

Weight loss – The lymphedema risk increases with obesity. Hence, weight loss should be a part of lymphedema treatment in obese patients.

21.10.2 Pain Relief

There may be significant pain at the onset and in between due to attacks of acute infection. It is relieved by treatment of the cause and use of analgesics as required.

21.10.3 Prevention of Complications

The lymphedematous part is more prone for infection which may be mild or severe. It causes further lymphatic injury. It must be prevented by careful inspection of affected part daily and good skin care, which consists of the following:

1. Washing the part gently daily with special attention to folds and grooves, drying it (use of hair dryer on low heat is the best hygienic method), and application of a bland emollient (aqueous cream) to keep it hydrated. If the skin is dry, a bland ointment (made of equal parts of white soft paraffin and liquid paraffin) should be applied twice daily.
2. Hyperkeratosis is treated by local use of 5 % salicylic acid ointment. It has keratolytic properties.
3. Fungal infections are common at entry point but the fungi do not invade the tissues; hence, antifungal drugs are applied locally. Prolonged use of an antifungal cream may cause maceration of skin. Hence, antifungal powders are used in socks and foot wears. Athlete's foot is prevented by 3 % benzoic acid, which can be used for prolonged periods without any ill effects.
4. Acute infections (cellulitis, lymphangitis) are mostly streptococcal or staphylococcal in origin. They are treated with benzyl (intravenous) or phenoxymethyl (oral) penicillin and flucloxacillin (or clindamycin or a cephalosporin) for 2 weeks. Co-amoxiclav is a good alternative. If the attacks are frequent (3 or more episodes per year), long-term prophylactic antibiotic therapy may be considered (Cooper et al. 2009; Al Niaimi et al. 2009, Schook et al. 2014).

21.10.4 Reduction of Swelling

Most patients with chronic lymphedema have some residual lymph vessels although they may be less efficient than normal ones. By making the best use of the residual lymphatics and helping them to drain lymph from the tissues, the swelling may be reduced or checked (Kinmonth 1982).

The methods of reduction of swelling include bed rest, elevation of swollen limb, centripetal massage, pressure bandaging, compression garments, exercise, and surgical methods. The current term used for the treatment of lymphedema is decongestive lymphedema therapy (DLT), which has two phases – the first phase of short intensive period of therapist-led care (3–8 weeks) and the second phase of a long duration in which the patient looks after himself with intermittent professional intervention (Ko 1998; Mayrovitz 2009). The surgery may be used as a last weapon to reduce the swelling in a failed case. It reduces the swelling mostly by excision of lymphedema and fibredema.

Patient Education Since lymphedema–elephantiasis is a life-long problem, the patient education in self-management is very important (Fu et al. 2008). Hence, all the patients of lymphedema or at risk for lymphedema should be instructed in essential self-care, including skin care, recognition of skin infection, care of lymphedema garments, nutrition, exercise, and weight control.

The methods of reducing the swelling of lymphedema–elephantiasis are described as follows:

1. *Elevation of part* – When the patient is at rest, the swollen part should be kept above the level of heart by putting 6 in. thick blocks under the foot end of the bed.
2. *Manual lymphatic drainage* (*MLD*) – It evacuates fluid and protein from the interstitial space of the affected limb and stimulates lymphangion contraction. MLD is a light skin technique designed to improve fluid removal from congested areas with not properly working lymphatics into the lymph vessels and lymph nodes that are functioning (McNeely 2004). It is done daily by the therapist who trains the patient at the same time to do a simple massage himself which causes simple lymphatic drainage (SLD).
3. *Pneumatic compression devices, e.g., Lymphapress* (Zelikovski and Urca 1981) – They may be used to reduce the swelling quickly. These methods reduces the swelling by sequential inflation of multiple chambers with the swollen limb kept inside with a pressure of up to 100 mmHg with distal to proximal compression (Richmand et al. 1985). Computer-controlled pumping devices are also available (Bergan 1995).

   There are smaller machines available such a Flowtron with a single large bag, which is intermittently inflated and deflated (Kinmonth 1982).

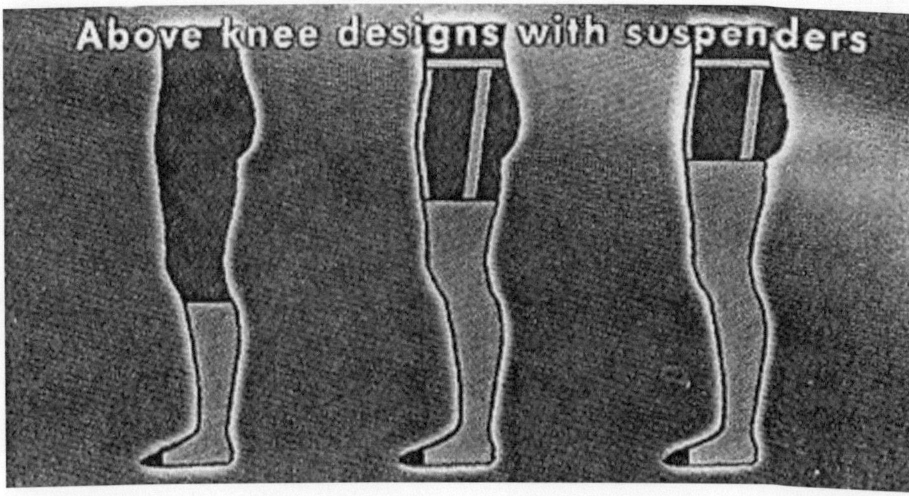

Fig. 21.12 Compression garments of different size for chronic lymphedema of lower extremity

4. *Multilayer lymphedema bandaging* (*MLLB*) – Elastic compression bandaging produces sustained high resting pressure and continued compression ("follow in") as the edema reduces. This effect is lost when there is muscular activity. Nonelastic pressure bandaging is better during the intensive phase of DLT when there is severe swelling. The pressure exerted by bandaging must be graduated to 100 % at ankle and foot, 70 % at knee, 50 % at mid thigh, and 40 % at groin maintaining the arterial circulation, but it is impossible to decide it by arterial palpation in the swollen limb. Hence, the noninvasive assessment of the ankle-brachial pressure index (ABPI) using a handheld Doppler ultrasound probe is performed. MLLB is a very effective and safe method of reducing lymphedema if applied by a trained therapist (Badger et al. 2000).
5. *Compression garments* – Use of compression garments (hosiery, sleeves) is recommended in mild lymphedema and during the maintenance phase of therapy after the edema has been reduced significantly by therapist-led intensive phase of treatment (Fig. 21.12). The patient should have a pair of garments, one to wear and one to wash and dry so that he/she has not to wear a dirty or wet garment. It is to prevent infection. Properly fitting garments are essential for long-term control of lymphedema (Yasuhara et al. 1996; Badger et al. 2000). Ready-made garments come in a variety of sizes and can be fitted to many patients. Otherwise, custom-made garments are used that are specifically made for the patients who cannot fit a ready-made garment. They are more expensive and may be required for patients with irregularly shaped extremity. Most of the garments must be replaced every 4–6 months to maintain compression pressure. The patient wears it in the morning before getting out of bed and removes it at night before going to sleep. The typical pressures used are 30–40 mmHg in the arm and 40–60 mmHg in the leg

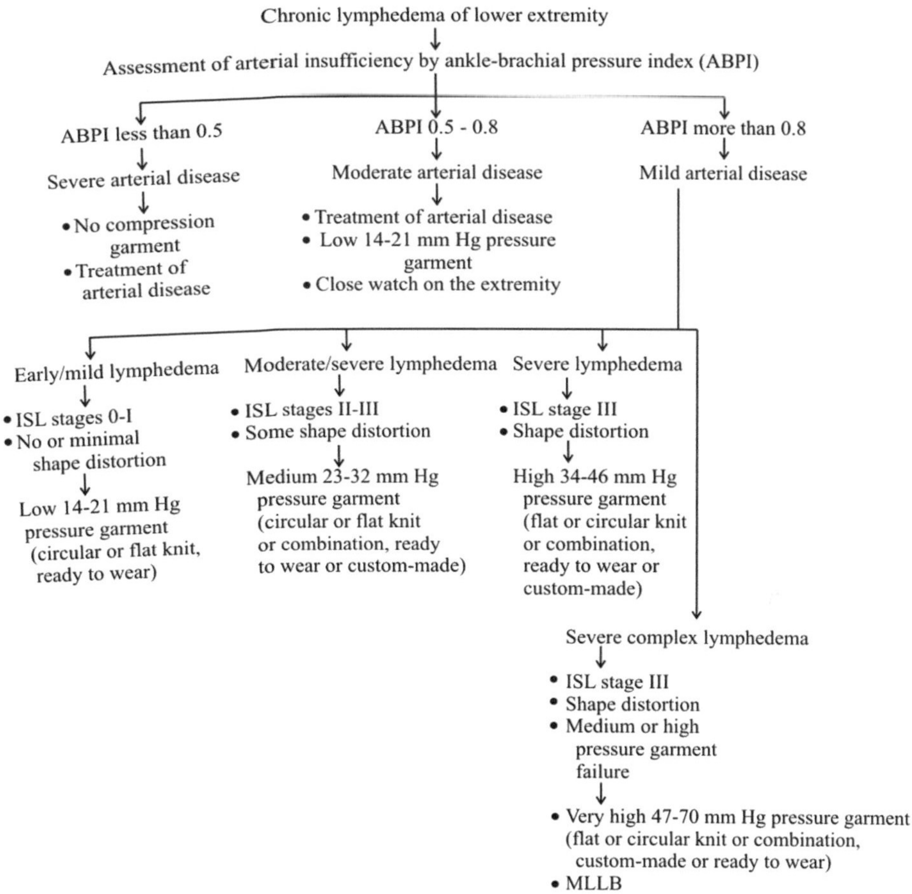

Flow Chart 21.1 Use of compression garments in lymphedema of lower extremity

(Yasuhara et al. 1996). They may be reduced in patients with arterial insufficiency (see the Flow Chart 21.1). The disadvantages of pressure garments include the following:

1. The putting on and taking off the compression garment is difficult and cumbersome.
2. The wearing it in warm climate is uncomfortable.

6. *Exercise* – 40 % of the lymph is formed in the skeletal muscles and the formation is directly proportionate to the arterial inflow. Hence, the patient should avoid vigorous exercise, especially anaerobic and isometric and prolonged static activities such as prolonged standing. The slow rhythmic isotonic movements, e.g., swimming increase lymphatic and venous return, hence are useful. The exercise also helps in maintaining the joint mobility. If the patient cannot do active exercise, passive exercise is recommended.

7. *Drugs* – So far there is no drug available which can reduce or control lymphedema (Casley-Smith et al. 1993). Benzopyrones is a big group of naturally occurring substances of which the flavinoids have been used but their beneficial effect remains unproven. They are thought to reduce the capillary permeability, improve microcirculatory perfusion, stimulate interstitial macrophage proteolysis, reduce erythrocyte and platelet aggregation, engulf free radicals, and exert an anti-inflammatory effect. Oxerutins (Paroven) are the drugs of this group used to treat venous disease. Diuretics do not have any beneficial role.
8. *Molecular lymphangiogenesis* – This treatment is based on the activation of VEGFR-3 pathways by administration of cognate ligands VEGF-C and VEGF-D using a variety of methods (Nakamura and Rockson 2008). This treatment is under study, but the danger in this treatment is the possibility of stimulation of dormant tumor cells due to increased angiogenesis (Tervala et al. 2008).
9. *Alternate heating and cooling* – The Chinese have devised a new method of treatment of chronic lymphedema by heating and cooling the swollen limb alternately. A microwave oven is used for heating. This method is reported to be very effective though cumbersome (Chandy et al. 2011).

   Zhang et al. (1984) treated 1017 patients of filarial lymphedema of lower extremity by putting the limb in electrocontrolled heating chamber at 80–90 °C for 1 h. One course consisted of 20 such treatments with the interval between courses of about 7–10 days. There to five of such courses are needed. Following treatment, elastic bandage was tied during the day. The overall effectiveness of this treatment was 68.3 %. It is a safe, simple, and easy to perform method of treatment. Following treatment hair regrowth was frequently noticed over the legs.
10. *Surgical treatment* – The swelling of lymphedema is adequately controlled in about 95 % of patients by the conservative measures described above (Pipinos and Baxter 2012). Hence, the surgical treatment is required in a very few patients. It gives quick relief by reducing the swelling but does not treat its cause. A large number of operations have been described which have been used as given in the following table (Kinmonth 1982, Goel 1985; Pipinos and Baxter 2012) -

21.11 Operations for Chronic Lymphedema–Elephantiasis of Lower Extremity

- *Drainage or bypass or physiological operations (lymphangioplasties)*
  (a) *Use of nonliving conduits or material*
    1. Insertion of silk threads (Handley 1908)
    2. Buried rubber tubes (Walther 1919)
    3. Insertion of nylon sutures (Ransohoff 1945; Mohan Rao 1958)
    4. Insertion of polythene tubes (Hogeman 1955)
    5. Insertion of fine bore nylon or portex tubes (Jantet et al. 1961)
    6. Strands of Teflon threaded into tissues (Silver and Puckett 1976)

(b) *Use of living tissues*
   1. Pedicled deep fascial strips inturned into muscle layer or bone marrow (Lanz 1911)
   2. Strips of deep fascia (Lexer 1962)
   3. Grafting a flap of full thickness skin from lower abdomen and buttock into the thigh (Kimura 1925)
   4. Swinging a broad pedicle skin flap from the flank into the leg (Gillies and Fraser 1935)
   5. Insertion of aponeurotic strips (Martorell 1958)
   6. Nodo-venous anastomosis (Nielubowicz and Olszewski 1966, 1968)
   7. Mesenteric bridge (Pugnaire 1968) – implantation of a flap of mesentery of ileum under inguinal ligament
   8. Mircovascular lymphovenous anastomosis (Sedlacek 1969; Cordeiro 1969; Yamada 1969)
   9. Enteromesenteric bridge (Kinmonth et al. 1971; Hurst et al. 1978, 1985)
   10. Microlymphatic bypass (Ho et al. 1983)

- *Excisional operations*
  1. Excision of skin and subcutaneous tissue followed by split-thickness grafting (Charles 1912)
  2. Excision of subcutaneous tissue including deep fascia – in two stages (Sistrunk 1918) and in four stages (Homans 1936)
  3. Macey's excision (1948) of skin and subcutaneous tissue with split-thickness grafting in stages
  4. Excision of subcutaneous tissue with covering of raw area with Wolfe graft obtained from the affected limb (Mansoor 1968)
- *Combined operations*
  1. Rosanow's (1913) modification of Lanz (1911) operation – inturning of cellulo-aponeurotic flaps into muscle layer with excision of overlying cutaneous rhomboid
  2. Creation of a window in deep fascia by excision of long strips of subcutaneous tissue with deep fascia of whole limb (Kondoleon 1912)
  3. Matas modification (1913) of Kondoleon's operation – Creation of a medial and a lateral window in leg by excising strips of elephantoid tissue with deep fascia
  4. Excision of subcutaneous tissue with buried shaved skin flap (Thompson 1962)
  5. Omental transposition (Goldsmith and Santos 1966, Goel and Misra 1973)
- *Reduction of fluid supply to limb* – Femoral artery ligation (Carnochan 1852; Jaju 1975)

21.12 Comments on the Surgical Procedures for Chronic Lymphedema–Elephantiasis

- *Drainage or bypass operations*
  (a) *Use of nonliving conduits or material*
    1. Subcutaneous insertion of threads and sutures work temporarily for some time. Subsequently they do not work as they are enclosed in scar tissue.

2. The subcutaneous insertion of a variety of fine tubes also does not work. They do not have pumping mechanism and valves to propel the fluid against gravity. They are also walled off by scar tissue and often contain old clotted lymph or blood in the lumen (Kinmonth 1982).

(b) *Use of living tissue to improve drainage* (*reconstructive surgery*) – In these operations, an alternative route is created for the drainage of static lymph. They are indicated in ilio-inguinal obstruction with patent (dilated) distal lymphatics and megalymphatics (Campisi and Boccardo 2002). Five modern drainage procedures are described as follows:

1. *Mesenteric bridge* – It is implantation of a flap of mesentery of small bowel brought below the inguinal ligament. Pugnaire (1968) did it in a case of chronic lymphedema of right lower limb where the swelling disappeared completely and remained so for some 10 years.
2. *Enteromesenteric bridge* (Kinmonth et al. 1971) – A vascularized segment of ileum is disconnected from the rest of the bowel opened at the antimesenteric border and stripped off its mucosa. It is put over the cut ends of lymph vessels and lymph nodes of inguinal region to drain the lymph into the mesenteric lymphatics (Fig. 21.13). It has given some promising results in some patients (Hurst et al. 1985).
3. *Nodo-venous shunt* (Nielubowicz and Olszewski 1966, 1968) – It is the anastomosis of cut raw surface of an enlarged dilated lymph node (lymphadenovarix) with most of the lymphatic attachments to the side of a vein in the vicinity, e.g., long saphenous or femoral vein (Fig. 21.14). The results of this procedure are not predictable.
   There may be 5–10 afferent lymphatics draining into one lymph node. Hence, if two nodes are implanted, the possible number of shunted lymphatics may be considerable (Kinmonth 1982).
4. *Lymphatico-venular anastomosis* (Sedlacek 1969; Yamada 1969; Koshima 2000) – It is a recent addition to drainage procedures. In this operation, anastomosis is done between the dilated lymphatic channels

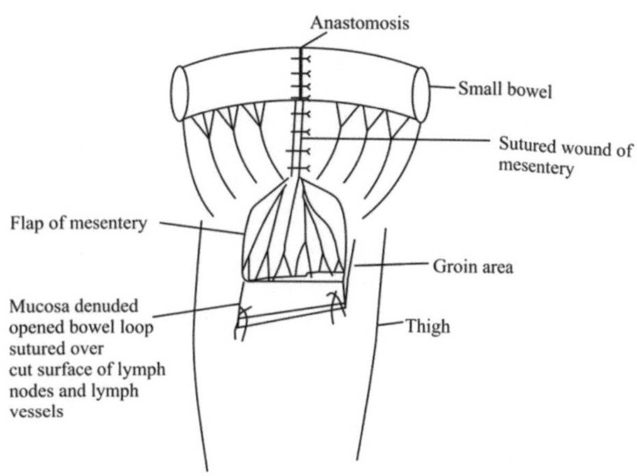

Fig. 21.13 Enteromesenteric bridge

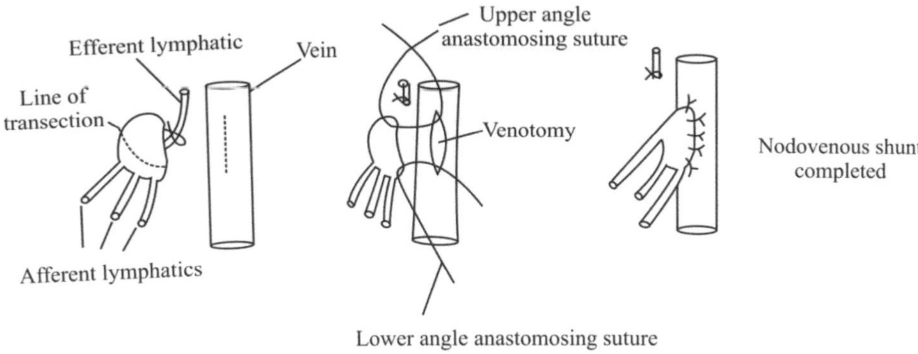

Fig. 21.14 Nodo-venous shunt – anastomosis of raw surface of a hemisectioned lymph node in situ (with tissue connections) with the side of a vein in the vicinity

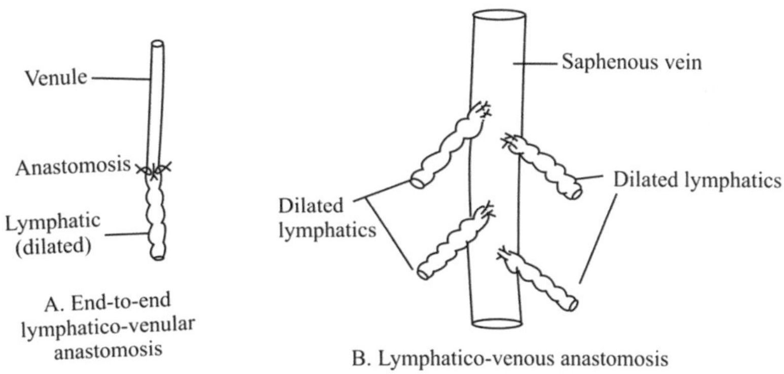

Fig. 21.15 Microvascular lymphatico-venular and lymphatico-venous anastomosis

distal to the obstruction identified by lymphangiography and venules of 0.3–0.8 mm in diameter using supermicrovascular technique. Three to four of such anastomoses are done (Fig. 21.15A). This procedure is difficult and time consuming and does not give the desired results especially in filarial lymphedema because of multiple level lymphatic obstruction. In selected patients of lymphedema, this procedure resulted in objective improvement in 30–60 % of patients with initial reduction of excess limb volume by 40–50 % (Damstra et al. 2009).

The lymphatico-venous anastomosis includes anastomosis of dilated lymphatics in the vicinity of saphenous vein to it by end-to-side method (Fig. 21.15B) (Shenoy and Shenoy 2010).

O'Brien and Shafiroff (1979) made four lymphatic to vein anastomoses with clinical improvement.

5. *Omental transposition* – The greater omentum is lengthened maintaining its vascularity and brought in the leg through a subcutaneous tunnel in the

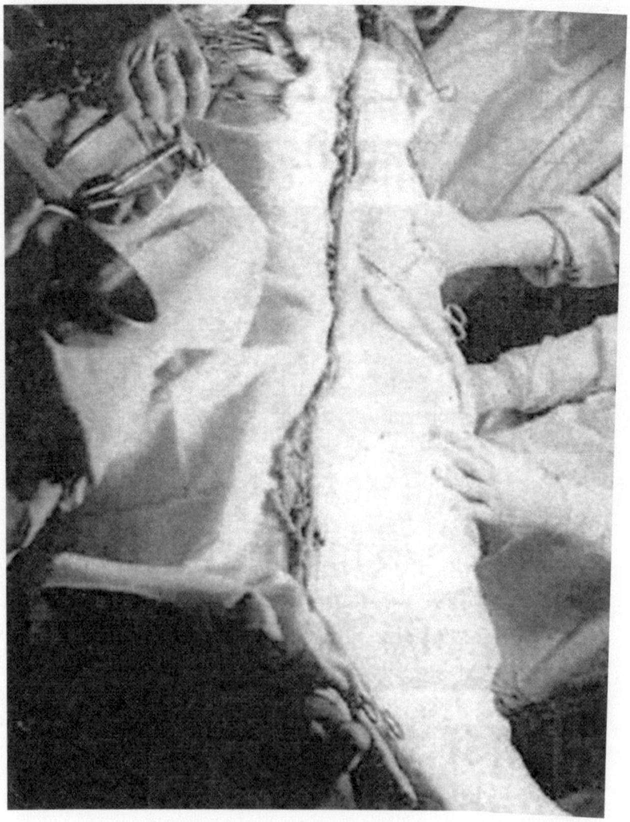

Fig. 21.16 Omental transposition in chronic lymphedema

thigh and spread in the subcutaneous plane after excision of elephantoid tissue (Fig. 21.16) (Goldsmith and De Los Santos 1966; Goldsmith 1974; Goel and Misra 1973). The results of this procedure are not better than pure excision of elephantoid tissue.

- *Limb reduction or debulking operations* – These operations are indicated when there is marked swelling and disability or severe deformity. They reduce the bulk but the shape of the limb is never restored to normal, and they cause significant scarring. They are the only option in patients without optimum residual lymphatics for reconstructive procedures. There are many operations in this group of which four are being described as follows:

1. *Sistrunk* (1918) – The subcutaneous tissue, including the overlying skin of the extremity, is excised by two long semi-elliptical incisions on lateral and medial aspects of the limb in two stages.
2. *Homans* (1936) – Kondoleon in 1918 did "staged subcutaneous excision underneath flaps," which was later popularized by Homans, who did excision of elephantoid tissue in four stages. In the first stage, the elephantoid tissue of anteromedial surface of leg is removed down to muscles (subcutaneous tissue

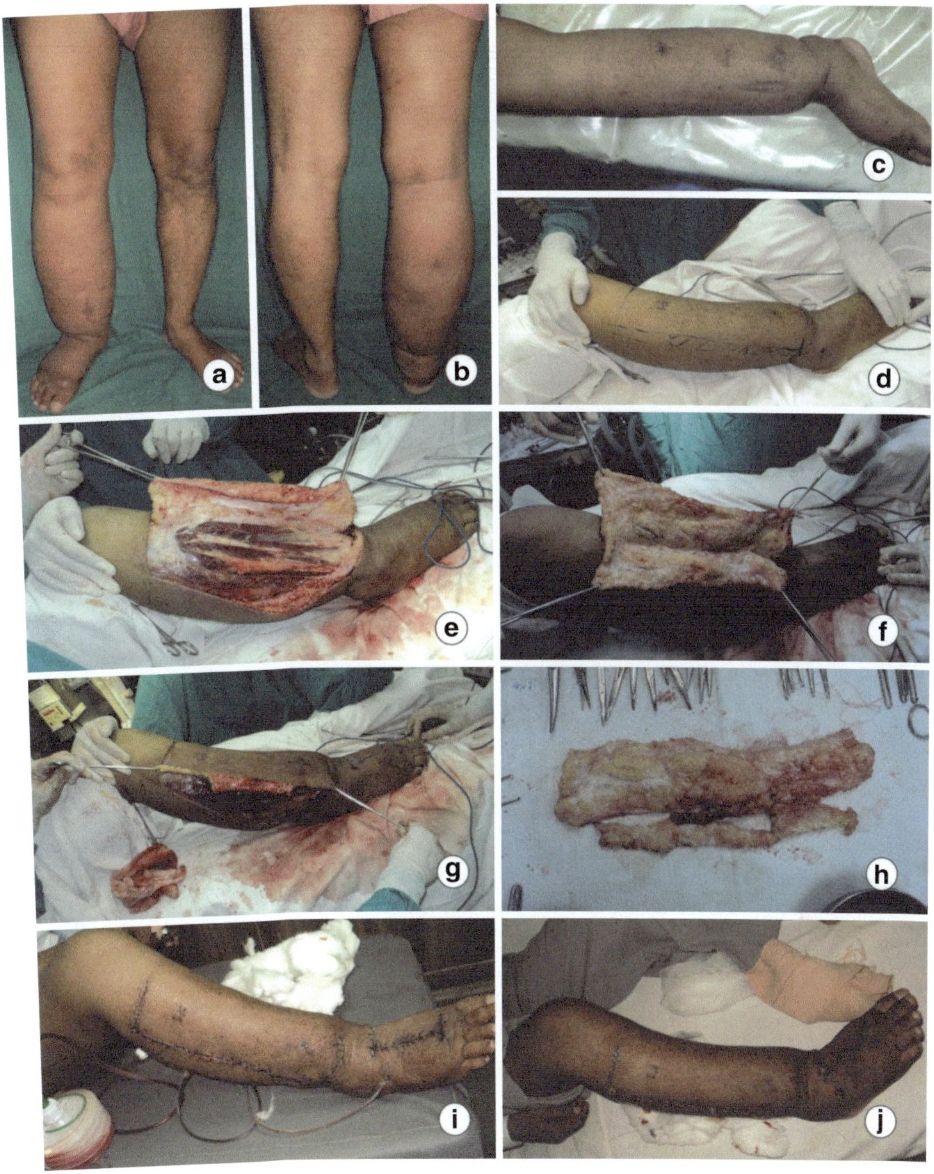

Fig. 21.17 Excision of elephantoid tissue of leg and foot: (**a–c**) Preoperative images; (**d**) Flaps worked; (**e–g**) Operative steps; (**h**): excised tissue; (**i, j**) Postoperative images (Courtesy or Dr. Brijesh Mishra)

and deep fascia). After sometime (ideally 6 months), the posterolateral aspect of the leg is cleared (Figs. 21.17 and 21.18). The remaining surfaces are debulked subsequently. The swelling of the thigh reduces spontaneously after excision of elephantoid tissue of leg. It gives good results. The skin flap necrosis is the main complication. Hence, during dissection, the flap elevation must not pass the midline.

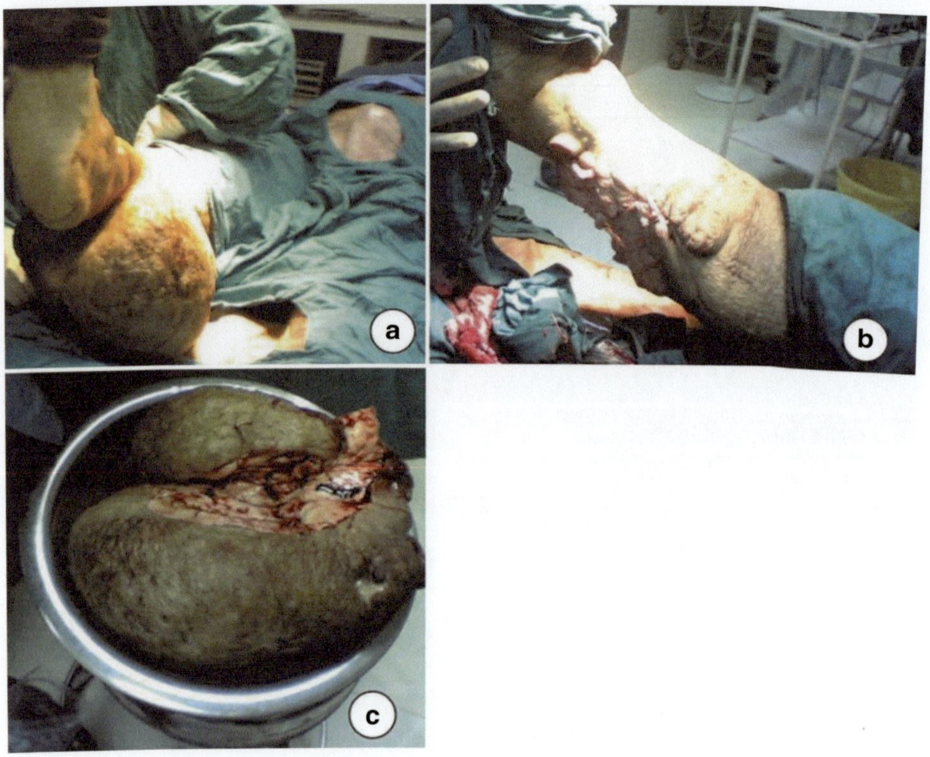

Fig. 21.18 (**a–c**): Intraoperative pictures of pendulous filarial elephantiasis of leg. (**a**) Preoperative appearance. (**b**) After excision. (**c**) Excised specimen in the bucket (Courtesy – Dr. A. C. Dwivedi)

3. *Thompson's buried dermis flap operation* (1962) – Following excision of elephantoid subcutaneous tissue including the deep fascia of a segment of limb, the epidermis of the extra width of one flap is shaved from the edge, and its cut edge is stitched to the cut edge of the deep fascia of opposite side close to the main vascular bundle of the limb and buried beneath the second flap (Swiss-roll operation) (Fig. 21.19). It is hoped that the superficial lymphatics of the dermis of buried flap, which are never involved in filarial elephantiasis (Shenoy and Shenoy 2010), will establish communication with the deep lymphatics situated along the main vessels of the extremity. However, there is no evidence of such occurrence. The local skin must be healthy for this operation (Kinmonth 1982). The long-term results of this operation are no better than Homan's operation. The occurrence of a pilonidal sinus is a common complication. Hence, this operation is not popular.
4. *Charles' operation* (1912) – In this operation, all elephantoid tissue of the involved leg and dorsum of foot including the skin and deep fascia is excised

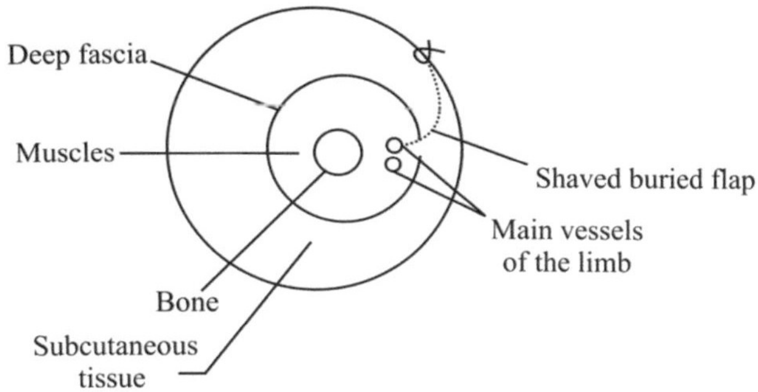

Fig. 21.19 Thompson buried shaved skin flap operation (Swiss roll operation)

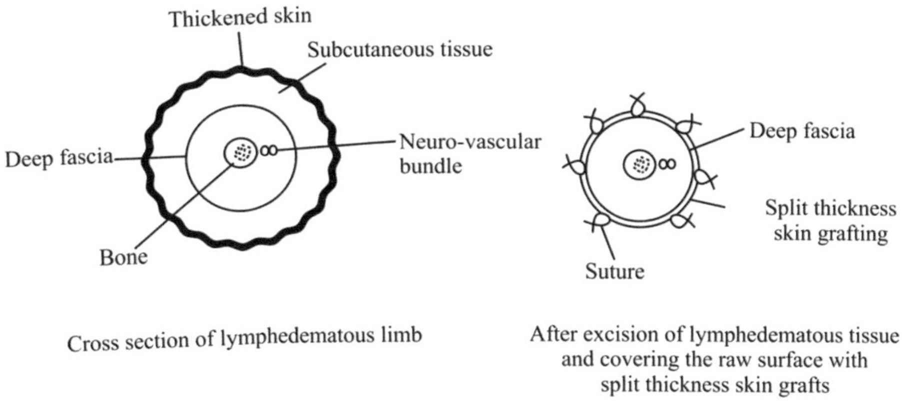

Fig. 21.20 Charles' operation

(Dellon and Hoopes 1977) followed by split-thickness skin grafting taken from the healthy donor areas of the body (Figs. 21.20, 21.21, 21.22, and 21.23). This operation is indicated when the lymphedema is pronounced and the overlying skin is unhealthy and infected. The grafts take very well (88 %). The advantages of this operation are as follows:

1. It immediately provides normal contour to the limb.
2. Recurrence does not occur as there is no subcutaneous tissue and space.

However, the disadvantages of this procedure are –

1. Patchwork appearance of skin (may be masked by skin color stockings)
2. Inflexibility of joints, especially ankle joint if the total skin of ankle is excised (better to leave a strip of relatively healthy skin around ankle)
3. Step deformity of upper limit of excision
4. Unpredictable healing of skin grafts
5. Hyperkeratosis and verrucae on toes or on the grafts (Kinmonth 1982) (Fig. 21.24)

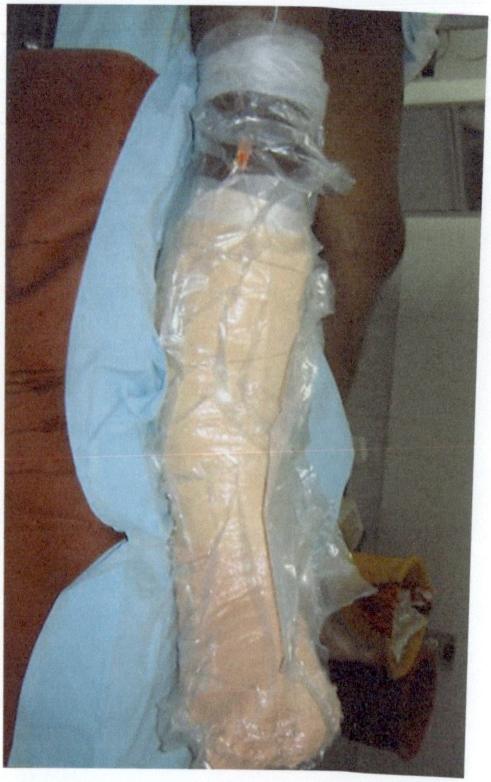

Fig. 21.21 Vacuum-assisted closure of the wound after excision of filarial elephantoid tissue to make it fit for subsequent skin grafting (Courtesy of Dr. Surajit Bhattacharya)

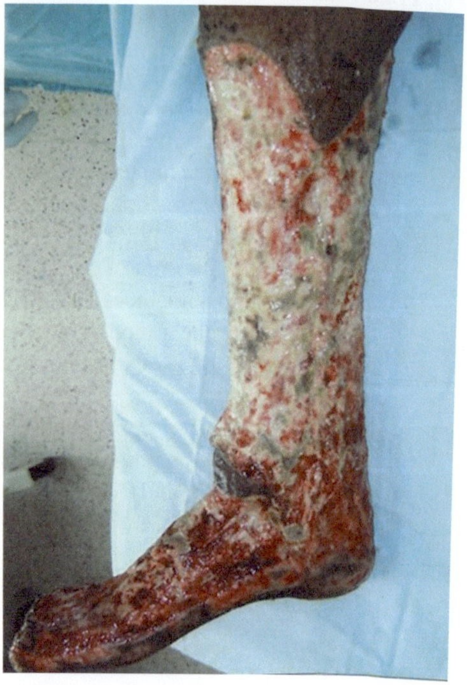

Fig. 21.22 Raw area of leg a few days after excision of elephantoid tissue being prepared for partial thickness skin grafting

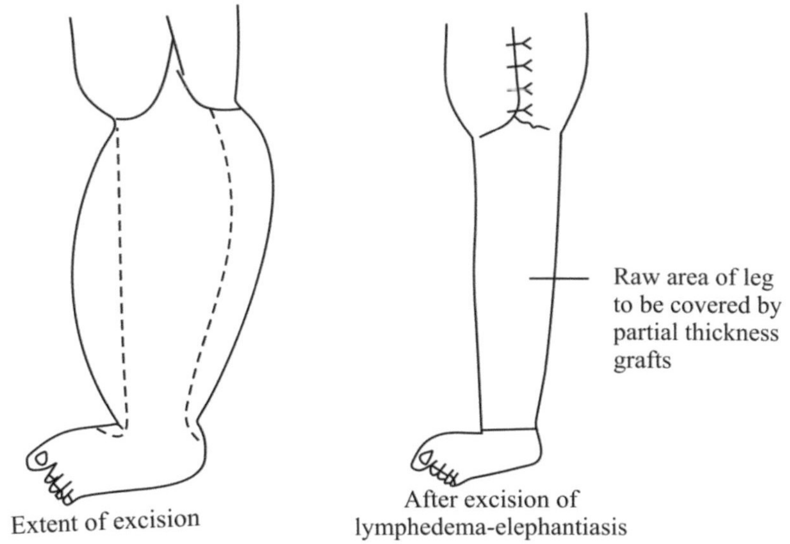

Fig. 21.23 Charles' operation

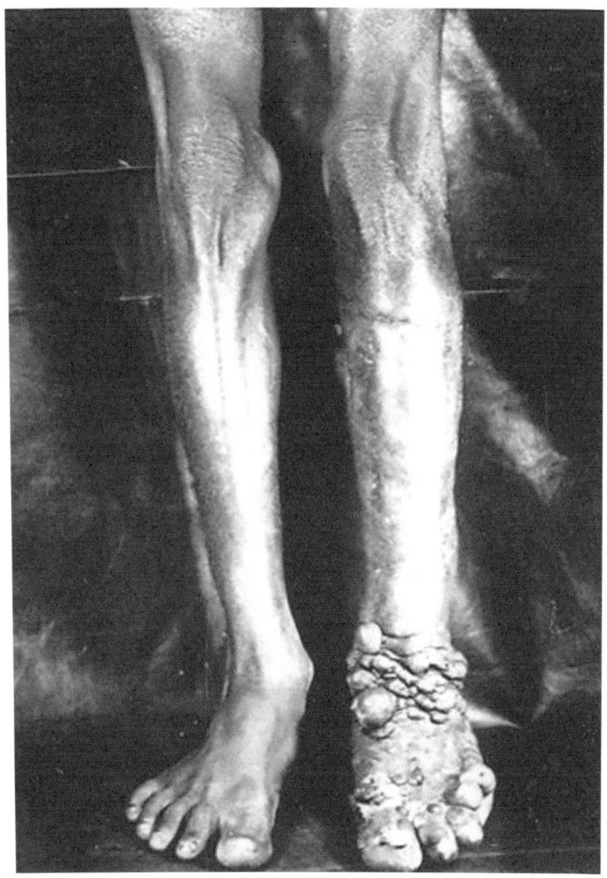

Fig. 21.24 Multiple fibrous nodules on the dorsum of left foot and around ankle in a patient of filarial elephantiasis of left lower extremity in whom Charles' operation was done several years ago. The girth of the leg looks normal

21.13 Femoral Artery Ligation

Carnochan (1852) ligated the femoral and external iliac arteries with the view of reducing the arterial supply to reduce lymph production, stasis, and edema. It is based on the assumption that the blood supply to the elephantoid limb is increased (Feder and McDonald 1967; Jacobsson 1967; Pelug and Calnan 1971). Jaju (1975) have reported some good results following this procedure. The arterial supply of the limb must be carefully studied before this operation is done. After due reduction is achieved, the excess skin is excised with thickened and fibrosed deep fascia. This artery is ligated just below the origin of profunda femoris artery. We have found this operation to be useful in patients with massive lymphedema of short duration with lymphorrhea

Varma and Dwivedi (1988) did this operation in five patients of massive elephantiasis of relatively short duration with good results except in one patient who had some recurrence of edema 6 months after operation.

21.14 Liposuction

A procedure similar to liposuction is now being done at some centers where the blubbery subcutaneous tissue is sucked by subcutaneous cannulas inserted at multiple points. It would not help in fibredema (Brorson et al. 2008; Espinosa-de-Los-Monteros et al. 2009). It may be combined with intermittent pneumatic compression for better results. The risks of liposuction include bleeding, infection, skin loss, and abnormal sensation such as numbness, tingling, and "pins and needles" (NLN 2011).

21.15 Debulking of Foot

Foot is a less favorable site for excisional operations than other common sites. It should always be done as an independent procedure separate to that of leg debulking (Kinmonth 1982).

Homans procedure is the recommended operation. It is done by a midline incision extending from the front of ankle joint to a finger's breadth above the base of the toes. Postoperative minor necrosis of corners of the flaps is a common complication.

The chronic lymphedema–elephantiasis of lower limb is a crippling complication which does not kill but causes life-long disability. Hence, it should be prevented as far as possible.

The operations for chronic lymphedema–elephantiasis are given in Flow Chart 21.2

The pathogenesis, diagnosis and treatment of chronic lymphedema–elephantiasis of lower extremity are described in Flow Chart 21.3.

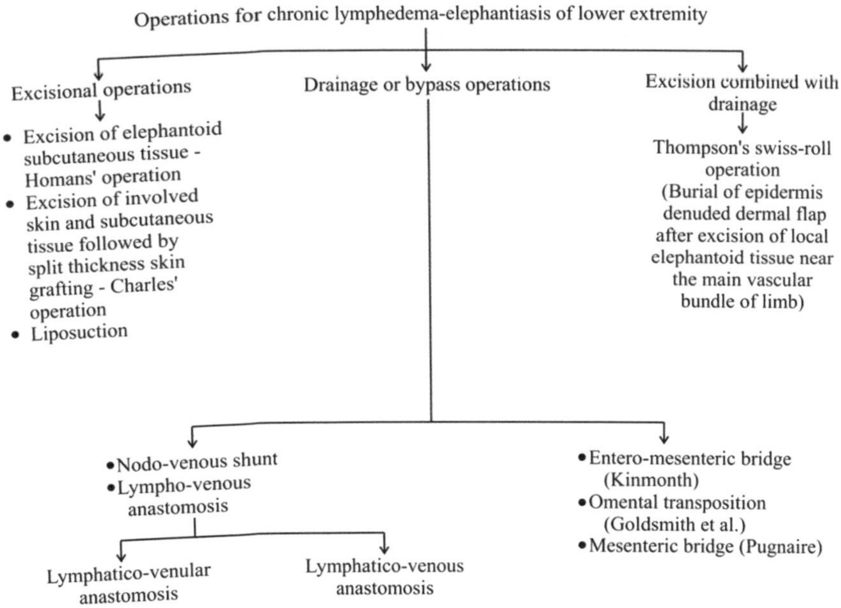

Flow Chart 21.2 Various operations for the treatment of chronic lymphedema–elephantiasis of lower extremity

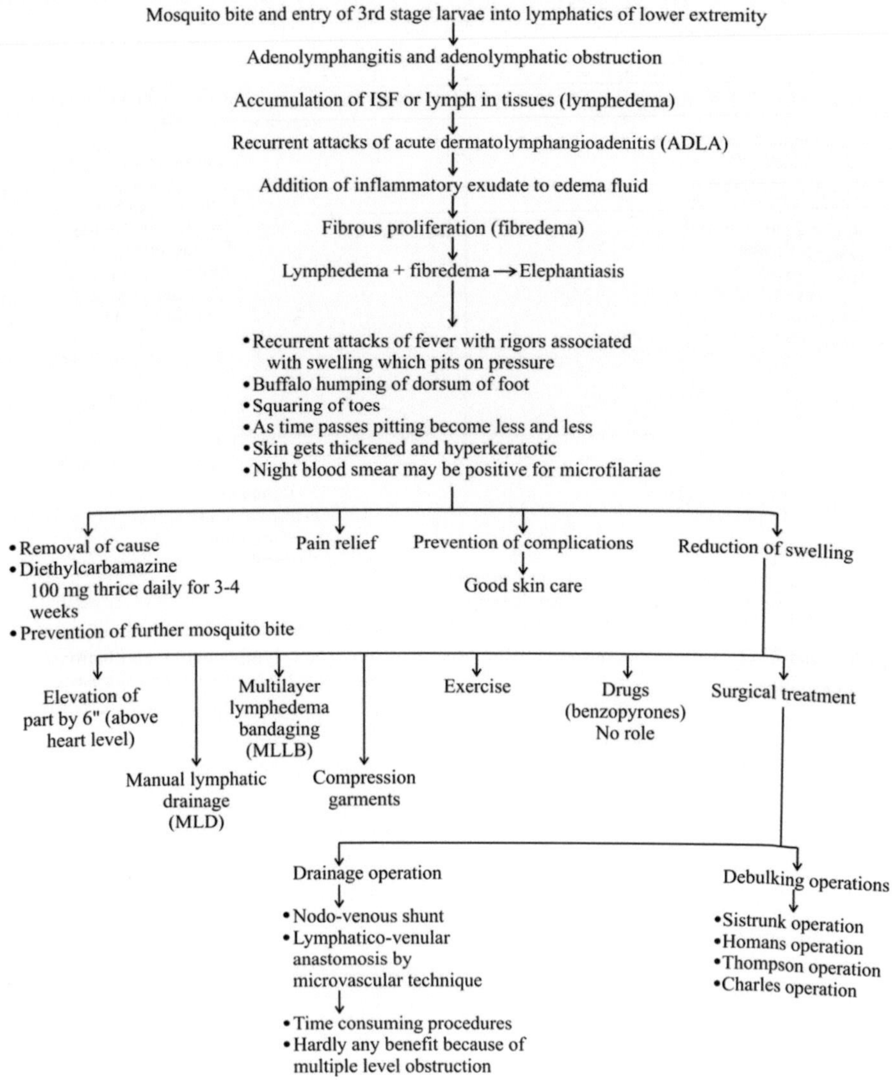

Flow Chart 21.3 Management of filarial lymphedema–elephantiasis of lower extremity

References

Al Niaimi F, Cox N. Cellulitis and lymphedema:a vicious cycle. J Lymphoedema. 2009;4:38–42. http://www.overtherainbow.ie/Over_the_Rainbow/Price_list_files/Cellulitis%20and%20Lymphoedema.pdf.

Badger CM, Peacock JL, Mortimer PS. A randomized controlled parallel-group clinical trial comparing multilayer bandaging followed by hosiery versus hosiery alone in the treatment of patients with lymphedema of the limb. Cancer. 2000;88:2832–367.

Barrett T, Choyke PL, Kabayashi H. Imaging of the lymphatic system: New horizons. Contrast Media Mol Imaging. 2006;1:230–45.

Bergan JJ. Venous and lymphatic surgery. In: Cuschieri A, Giles GR, Moossa AR, editors. Essential surgical practice. 3rd ed. Oxford: Butterworth Heinemann; 1995. p. 948–50.

Bhishagratna KKL. An English translation of Shusruta Samhita based on the original Sanskrit text. Vol 2. Varanasi: Chowkamba Sanskrit Series Office; 1963. p. 439–49.

Brorson H, Ohlin K, Olsson G, et al. Controlled compression and liposuction treatment for lower extremity lymphedema. Lymphology. 2008;41:52–63.

Burri H, Loutan L, Kumaraswami V, Vijayasekaran V. Skin changes in chronic lymphatic filariasis. Tran R Soc Trop Med Hyg. 1996;90:671–4.

Campisi C, Boccardo F. Lymphedema and microsurgery. Microsurgery. 2002;22:74–80.

Carnochan JM. Elephantiasis arabum of the right inferior extremity successfully treated by ligature of femoral artery, part I. NY J Med. 1852;9:162.

Casley-Smith JR, Morgan RG, Piller NB. Treatment of lymphedema of the arms and legs with 5, 6-benzo-α-pyrone. N Engl J Med. 1993;329:1158–63.

Chandy A, Thakur AS, Singh MP, Manigauha A. A review of neglected tropical diseases: filariasis. Asia Pac J Trop Med. 2011;4(7):581–6.

Charles H. Elephantiasis scroti. In: Latham A, English TC, editors. A system of treatment, vol. 3. Calcutta: Butterworth & Co (India) Ltd; 1912. p. 511–6.

Cho S, Atwood JE. Peripheral edema. Am J Med. 2002;113:580–6.

Cooper R, White R. Cutaneous infections in lymphedema. J Lymphedema. 2009;4:44–8. http://www.woundsinternational.com/media/issues/831/files/content_11153.pdf.

Cordeiro AK. Lynfoedema primario, anstomose linfo-venosa 16th Brazilian Congress for Angiology, Nov 1969.

Damstra RJ. Diagnosis and therapy in children with lymphedema. Phlebology. 2008;23:276–86.

Damstra RJ, Vocsten HG, et al. Lymphatic venous anastomosis (LVA) for treatment of secondary arm lymphedema with breast cancer-related lymphedema and a critical review of literature. Breast Cancer Res Treat. 2009;113:199–206.

Dellon AL, Hoopes JE. The Charles procedure for primary lymphedema. Long-term clinical results. Plast Reconstr Surg. 1977;60:589–95.

Devi L, Bahuleyan CK. Lymphangiosarcoma of lower extremity associated with chronic lymphedema of filarial origin. Indian J Cancer. 1977;14:176–8.

Espinosa-de-Los-Monteros A, Hinojosa CA, Abarca L, et al. Compression therapy and liposuction of lower leg for bilateral hereditary primary lymphedema praecox. J Vasc Surg. 2009;49:222–4.

Feder FP, McDonald D. Changes in renal function produced by lymphatic obstruction. J Urol. 1967;97:432–8.

Fu MR, Axelrod D, Haber J. Breast-cancer-related lymphedema: information, symptoms and risk reduction behaviors. J Nurs Scholarsh. 2008;40:341–8.

Gillies HD, Fraser FR. Treatment of lymphedema by plastic operation. Br Med J. 1935;1:96.

Goel TC. Filarial elephantiasis of lower extremity: a review. Indian J Plast Surg. 1985;18:22–34.

Goel TC, Misra SC. Omental transposition in the treatment of tropical elephantiasis of lower limb. Indian J Surg. 1973;35:381–5.

Goldsmith HS, De Los Santos R. Omental transposition for the treatment of chronic lymphedema. Rev Surg. 1966;23:303.

Goldsmith HS. Long-term results of omental transposition for chronic lymphedema. Ann Surg. 1974;180:847–9.

Handley WS. Lymphangioplasty: a new method for the relief of the brawny edema of breast cancer and for similar conditions of lymphatic oedema: preliminary note. Lancet. 1908;1:783.

Jenkins MP. Venous and lymphatic disorders. In: Henry MM, Thompson JN, editors. Clinical surgery. 2nd ed. Edinburgh: Elsevier Saunders; 2005. p. 540–1.

Ho LC, Lai MF, Kennedy PJ. Microlymphatic bypass in the treatment of obstructive lymphedema of the arm: a case report of new technique. Br J Plast Surg. 1983;36:350–57.

Hogeman KE. Artificial subcutaneous channels in draining lymphedema. Acta Chir Scandinav. 1955;110:154.

Homans J. Treatment of elephantiasis of leg. N Engl J Med. 1936;215:1099.
Hurst PA, Kinmonth JB. Ruth DL.A gut and mesentery pedicle for bridging lymphatic obstruction. Experimental studies. J Cardiovasc Surg. 1978;19:589–96.
Hurst PA, Stewart G, Kinmonth JB, et al. Long-term results of enteromesenteric bridge operation in the treatment of primary lymphedema. Br J Surg. 1985;72:272–4.
Jacobsson S. Studies in blood circulation in lymphedematous limb. Scand J Plast Recons Surg Suppl. 1967;3:1-81. Quoted In: Kinmonth JB. The lymphatics. London: Edward Arnold; 1982. p. 135.
Jaju JR. Elephantiasis–lymphoedema. A new concept in management based on physiologic observations. Transactions of the sixth International Congress of Plastic & Reconstructive Surgery. Paris: Masson. 1975. p. 616.
Jantet GA, Taylor GW, Kinmonth JB. Operations for the primary lymphoedema of lower limb. J Cardiovasc Surg. 1961;2:27.
Kimura H. On the treatment of elephantiasis. Japan Med World. 1925;5:201.
Kinmonth JB, Hurst PA, Edwards JM, Butt DL. Relief of chronic lymph obstruction by the use of bridge of mesentery of ileum. Br J Surg. 1971;65:829.
Kinmonth JB. The lymphatics. 2nd ed. London: Edward Arnold; 1982. p. 105–44.
Ko D. Effective treatment of lymphedema of the extremities. Arch Surg. 1998;133:452–8.
Kondoleon E. Die Chirurgische Behandlung der elephantiastichen Oedeme. Munch Med Wschr. 1912;59:525 and 2726.
Koshima I. Supermicrosurgical lymphaticovenular anastomosis for the treatment of lymphedema in the upper extremities. J Reconstr Microsurg. 2000;16:437–42.
Lanz O. Erofnung neuer Abfurhwege bei straunung in Bauch and unteren Extremia ten. Zentralbl Chir. 1911;38:153.
Lexer E. Erworbenes Elephantiasis. Munchen, Mee. Wchnschr 1919; Quoted by Thompson N. Surgical treatment of chronic lymphoedema of the lower limb. With preliminary report of new operation. Br Med J. 1962;2(5319):1566–73.
Liu NF, Lu Q, Jaing JH, et al. Anatomic and functional evaluation of the lymphatics and lymph nodes in diagnosis of lymphatic circulation disorders with contrast magnetic resonance lymphangiography. J Vasc Surg. 2009;49:980–7.
Macey HB. A surgical procedure for lymphedema of extremities. A follow-up report. J Bone Joint Surg. 1948;30:339.
Mansoor A. Elephantisis – amethod of treatment. Br J Plast Surg. 1968;21:378–57.
Martorell F. A new therapyof lymphedema: pedicled lymphangioplasty. Angiologia. 1958;10:151–7.
Matas R. Surgical treatment of elephantoid states dependent upon chronic obstruction of lymphatic and venous channels. Am J Trop Dis. 1913;1:60.
Mohan Rao U. Lymphangioplasty for filarial lymphedema. Indian J Surg. 1958;20:40.
McNeely M. The addition of manual lymphatic drainage to compression therapy for breast cancer-related lymphedema: a randomized controlled trial. Breast Cancer Res Treat. 2004;86:95–106.
Moseley A, Piller N, Carati C. Combined opto-electronic perometry and bioimpedance to measure objectively the effectiveness of a new treatment intervention for chronic secondary leg lymphedema. Lymphology. 2002;35:136–43.
Muller R, Hajdu SI, Brennan MF. Lymphangiosarcoma associated with chronic filarial lymphedema. Cancer. 1987;59:179–83.
Mayrovitz HN. The standard of care for lymphedema: current concepts and physiological considerations. Lymphat Res Biol. 2009;7:101–8.
Nakamura K, Rockson SG. Molecular targets for therapeutic lymphangiogenesis in lymphatic dysfunction and disease. Lymphat Res Biol. 2008;6:181–9.
Nielubowicz J, Olszewski W. Special issue for XVth Congress of European Society of Cardiovascular Surgery. J Cardiovasc Surg. 1966;384.
Nielubowicz J, Olszewski W. Surgical lymphatico-venous shunts. Br J Surg. 1968;55:440.
NLN Position Statement of National Lymphedema Network. The diagnosis and treatment of lymphedema. 2011;1–16. www.lymphnet.org.

O'Brien BM, Shafiroff BB. Microlymphatico-venous and resectional surgery in obstructive lymphedema. World J Surg. 1979;3:3–15.
Pelng JJ, Calnan JS. The experimental production of chronic lymphedema. Br J Plast Surg. 1971;24:1–9.
Pipinos II, Baxter BT. The lymphatics. In: Townsend Jr CM, Beauchamp RD, Evers BM, Mattox KL, editors. Sabiston textbook of surgery, vol. 2. 19th ed. Philadelphia: Elsevier Saunders; 2012. p. 1819.
de Pugnaire M. R. Linfangioplastia mesenterica en al tratamiento de las elefantiasis de los membros inferiores. Angiologia. 1968;20:146–52.
Ransohoff JL. Surgical treatment of lymphedema. Arch Surg. 1945;50:209.
Rasmussen J, Tan IC, Marshall MV, Fife CE, Sevick-Muraca EM. Lymphatic imaging in humans with near-infrared fluorescence. Curr Opin Biotechnol. 2009;20:74–82.
Richmand DM, O'Donnell Jr TF, Zelikovski A. Sequential pneumatic compression for lymphedema. A controlled trial. Arch Surg. 1985;120:1116–9.
Rosanow WM. Zentralbl. f. chir. 1913;2:59.
Schook CC, Kulungowski AM, Greene AK, Fishman SJ. Male genital lymphedema: clinical features and management of 25 pediatric patients. J Pediatr Surg. 2014;49:1647–951.
Sedlacek J. Lympho-venous shunt as supplementary treatment of elephantiasis of lower limb. Acta Chirurgica Plastica. 1969;11:157–62.
Shenoy KR, Shenoy A. Manipal manual of surgery. 4th ed. New Delhi: CBS; 2010. p. 110–8.
Silver D, Puckett CL. Lymphangioplasty: a ten-year evaluation. Surgery. 1976;80:748–55.
Sistrunk WE. Modifications of the operation for elephantiasis. JAMA. 1918;71:800.
Sordillo EM, Sordillo PP, Hajdu SI, Good RA. Lymphangiosarcoma after filarial infection. J Dermatol Surg Oncol. 1981;7:236–9.
Szuba A, Shin WS, Strauss HW, et al. The third circulation: radionuclide lymphoscintigraphy in the evaluation of lymphedema. J Nucl Med. 2003;44:43–57.
Tervala T, Souminen E, Saaristo A. Targeted treatment for lymphedema and lymphatic metastasis. Ann N Y Acad Sci. 2008;1131:215–24.
Thompson N. Surgical treatment of chronic lymphoedema of lower limb. Br Med J. 1962;2:1566–73.
Unno N, Nishiyama M, Suzuki M, Tanaka H, Yamamoto N, Sagara D, Mano Y, Konno H. A novel method of measuring human lymphatic pumping using indocyanine green fluorescence lymphography. J Vasc Surg. 2010;52:946–52.
Venkata Phani Deepthi B, Govinda Rajan R, Gopal PNV. Review on elephantiasis – a long-term disability. Int J Res Pharm Biomed Sci. 2011;2(2):375–81.
Varma KD, Dwivedi B. Evaluation of various surgical procedures in chronic lymphedema of inferior extremities. Surgery. 1988;1:20–30.
Walther C. Buried tube drainage of elephantiasis. Bull Acad Nat Med. 1919;80:262.
Ward L. Bioelectrical impedance analysis: proven utility in lymphedema risk assessment and therapeutic monitoring. Lymphat Res Biol. 2006;4:51–6.
Yamada Y. The studies of lymphatic venous anastomosis in lymphoedema. Nagoya J Med Sc. 1969;1:32.
Yasuhara H, Shigematsu H, Muto T. A study of the advantages of elastic stockings for leg lymphedema. Int Angiol. 1996;15:272–7.
Yimer M, Hailu T, Mulu W, Abera B. Epidemiology of elephantiasis with special emphasis on podoconiosis in Ethiopia: a literature review. J Vector Borne Dis. 2015;52:111–5.
Zhang T-s, Huang W-y, Han L-y, Liu W-y. Heat and bandage treatment of chronic lymphedema of extremities: report of 1045 patients. Chinese Med J. 1984;97:567–57. Quoted in SGO 162: 30, 1986.
Zelikovski A, Urca I. Progress in lymphology. Prague: Avicenum, Czechoslovak Medical Press; 1981.

22 Chronic Lymphedema–Elephantiasis of Scrotum

After the chronic lymphedema of lower extremity, the chronic lymphedema–elephantiasis of scrotum is the next common chronic manifestation of lymphatic filariasis (Figs. 22.1, 22.2, and 22.4). It is mostly associated with chronic lymphedema–elephantiasis of penis. In tropical countries, about 20 % of male population has elephantiasis of external genitals (De Greef 1938). It produces a very ugly deformity which is a source of extreme mental anguish (Dandapat et al. 1985).

Khanna (1970) reported his experience of managing 28 cases of filarial elephantiasis of external genitalia in whom 25 patients had penoscrotal lymphedema and 3 had lymphedema of penis only.

Dandapat et al. (1985) described their experience of dealing with 350 patients of filarial elephantiasis of scrotum, including 282 patients of scrotal elephantiasis with buried penis and 68 patients with elephantiasis of both scrotum and penis without penis being buried.

Singh et al. (2011) reported 48 patients of filarial male genital lymphedema, including 34 patients of penoscrotal disease and 14 patients with isolated penile involvement.

22.1 Etiology

There are many causes of chronic lymphedema of scrotum as described below Kinmonth (1982):

1. *Lymphatic filariasis*—It is the commonest cause of scrotal lymphedema–elephantiasis in tropical and subtropical countries. It is caused by adenolymphatic obstruction of inguinal lymphatics.

   Other causes of inguinal lymphatic obstruction that can cause scrotal lymphedema include tuberculosis, lymphogranuloma venereum (LGV), and metastatic disease of inguinal lymph nodes including its treatment with node dissection, and/or radiotherapy.

T.C. Goel, A. Goel, *Lymphatic Filariasis*, DOI 10.1007/978-981-10-2257-9_22

Infections involving inguinal lymph nodes are the commonest cause of chronic lymphedema of scrotum in tropical and underdeveloped countries, while malignancy involving these lymph nodes is the commonest cause in advanced western countries.

2. *Obesity*—massive obesity may cause scrotal lymphedema due to pressure on lymphatics. Lee et al. (2014) reported 6 cases of massive lymphedema of scrotum associated with obesity. Machol et al. (2014) reported 4 patients of massive localized lymphedema (MLL) in obese persons. This condition may be confused with liposarcoma and lymphangiosarcoma, hence described as pseudosarcoma.
3. *Primary lymphedema*—This type of lymphedema of scrotum is attributed to hypoplasia of lymphatics (developmental defect).
4. *Idiopathic*—It is usually seen in small children where scrotum and penis swell up fairly rapidly without any known cause. It can occur in adults.

   Many authors have reported patients of idiopathic chronic scrotal lymphedema–elephantiasis (Paradysz et al. 2010; Singh and Sandhu 2011; Schook et al. 2014). Brotherhood et al. (2014) reported 2 patients of idiopathic scrotal elephantiasis in Canadian men.
5. *As a part of general anasarca*—The edema of scrotum is a part of general anasarca seen in patients of congestive cardiac failure, cirrhosis of liver, chronic renal failure, and hypoproteinemia. This problem is managed with the help of a physician.

22.2 Pathology

It may be associated with chronic lymphedema of penis and lower extremity. However, it may occur alone without involving the extremity and/or penis indicating that the lymph nodes draining the scrotum are distinct from those of penis and lower extremity.

The whole scrotum is enlarged, i.e., 4–9 kg is common (Manson-Bahr and Apted 1982), but 20–25 kg is by no means unknown. It may hang down up to the knees or more. The swelling is maximum at the fundus giving the scrotum a pyriform shape.

The skin of the scrotum is grossly thickened and may become 2–4 cm thick. The rugosity is increased, and it may be covered by wart-like or nodular excrescences. Usually, the whole of rugose skin is affected. It is thickest toward the lower part and gradually thins out as it merges around into the normal skin of pubis, perineum, and thighs. The posterior and posterolateral skin, which is nonrugose, is much less affected.

Burial of penis As the anterior wall of enlarging scrotum advances forward, the skin of the penis, which is normal, flares out from the root of penis and gradually becomes flush with the skin of scrotum. As time passes, the penis is totally buried in the anterior wall of scrotum (Figs. 22.1 and 22.2).

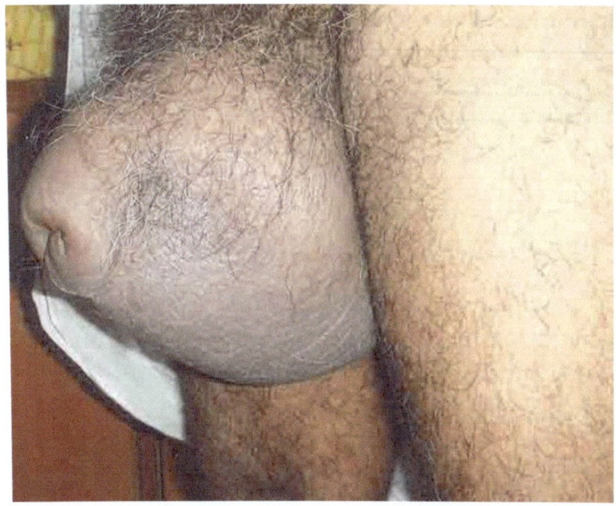

Fig. 22.1 Filarial chronic lymphedema–elephantiasis of scrotum with embedding of the penis in its anterior wall

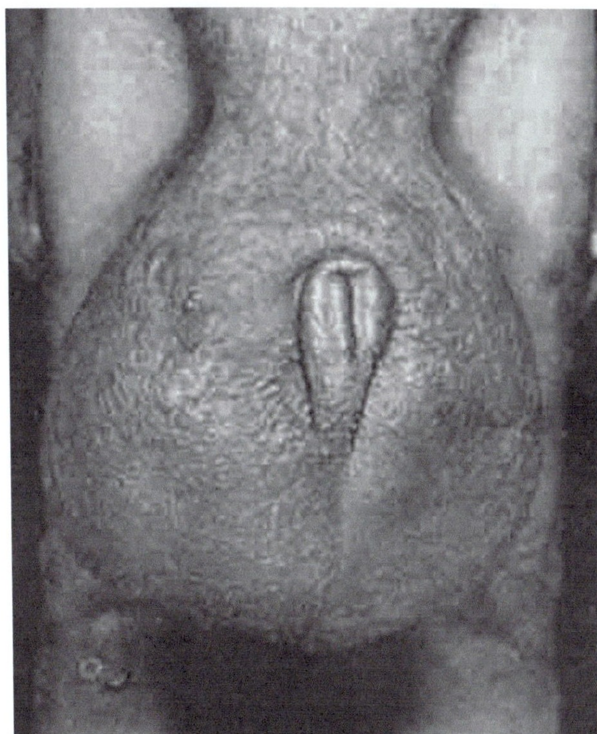

Fig. 22.2 Filarial chronic lymphedema–elephantiasis with penis buried in the anterior wall of scrotum

Further advancement of scrotal swelling elongates the prepucial tube resulting in downward displacement of the prepucial orifice. This skin also becomes elephantoid, but the inner layer of the prepuce remains normal.

Posterior advancement The posterior enlargement of the scrotum lifts the skin of the perineum, which becomes the skin of posterior wall of scrotum. However, this skin remains nearly normal. As time passes, most of the skin of the perineum may be lifted up, but it stops at the anus. There is no distortion of anal orifice no matter how massive the elephantiasis of the scrotum grows.

The inner surface of Colles' fascia in the perineum and the inner surface of the dartos muscle are continuous, and it is most likely that the elephantoid tissue of the scrotum does not extend beyond this continuous surface.

This disease process involves the skin and subcutaneous tissue of the scrotum. In patients where the subcutaneous tissue is predominantly involved, the scrotum goes on enlarging and may attain a huge size (mega-scrotum) as the skin is stretchable. If the skin is predominantly involved due to recurrent attacks of lymphangitis or cellulitis (acute dermatolymphangioadenitis, ADLA), it loses its stretchability due to early fibrosis. Hence, it prevents unlimited enlargement of scrotum when the scrotal swelling is not massive.

Cut surface External to external spermatic fascia of scrotum there is a layer of loose areolar tissue. This layer is normal even in advanced disease. The great bulk of elephantoid tissue forms in the dartos muscle layer of scrotum (Fig. 22.3).

In a fully developed disease, there are two clearly differentiated zones surrounding the central hydrocele. The outer zone consists of a dense rind of the thickened edematous dermis consisting of a lot of fibrous connective tissue and thick inner zone of soft myxomatous blubbery tissue. Bilateral scrotal hydrocele is invariably present and contributes to the scrotal swelling. It is associated with thickened tunica vaginalis. The testes are pushed posteriorly and attached firmly by the

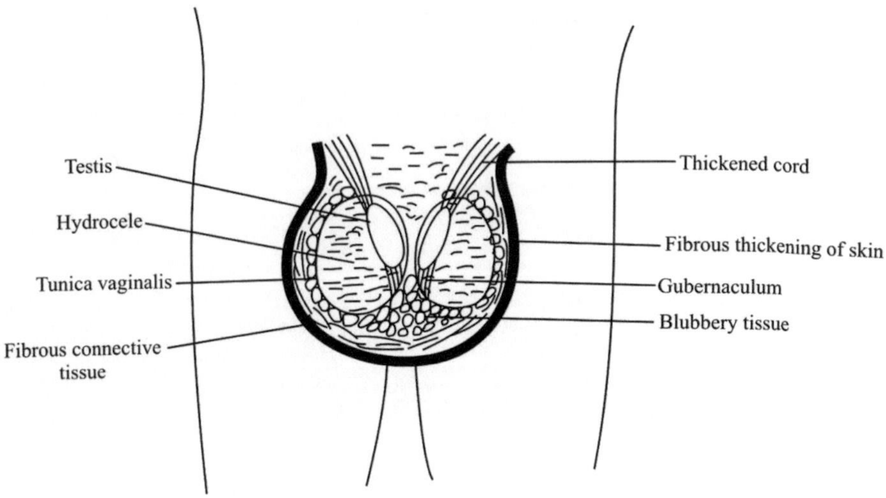

Fig. 22.3 Pathology of chronic lymphedema–elephantiasis of scrotum

hypertrophied remains of gubernaculum testis. The structure and function of the testes are usually normal (Manson-Bahr and Apted 1982).

The testes may be atrophic due to persistent pressure and loss of temperature regulation mechanism (Khanna 1970).

Micropathology Microscopically, the scrotal lesion shows stromal fibrosis with marked edema, perivascular chronic inflammation, eosinophilic infiltration, and lymphangiectasia. Varying degrees of hyperplasia and hypertrophy of the dartos muscle is usually seen (Lee et al. 2014).

22.3 Clinical Features

The patient is usually a middle-aged person who presents with a gradually enlarging swelling of the scrotum, which may attain a huge size and may hang up to the knees or even more (mega-scrotum). The commonly recorded weight of scrotum has been 4–9 kg and the highest recorded weight has been 102 kg (Manson-Bahr and Apted 1982). It may result in some discomfort and difficulty in walking.

A history of recurrent attacks of fever with rigor and increase of the swelling with every attack is usually present. The patient may have difficulty in maintaining local hygiene, voiding in standing position and sexual intercourse (Modolin et al. 2006). The erection is inhibited (Prpic 1966). There may be difficulty in finding clothes that fit the patient comfortably.

The swelling commences at the most dependent part of the scrotum (fundus) and grows uniformly upward. Initially the scrotum is swollen due to edema that pits on pressure. Gradually it becomes solid when the skin looks thick and rugose like that of a bitter gourd. Bilateral nontranslucent hydrocele is usually present.

The penis is usually buried in the anterior wall of the scrotum with stretched out prepuce on the surface of lower part of scrotum (Figs. 22.1 and 22.2). The patient urinates without any hindrance, but it makes the scrotum wet every time he urinates. The penis can be manipulated out of the scrotum, but it returns into buried position as soon as it is left. The prepucial sac contains offensive and blackish dirty smegma.

The penis may not be buried when it may be elephantoid and looks like a ram horn (Figs. 22.4 and 22.5). Rarely, it may be normal. The spermatic cords are thickened and the cremaster is hypertrophied.

Hai et al. (1987) reported 195 patients of male external genital chronic lymphedema with 135 patients of scrotal elephantiasis, 45 patients of scrotal elephantiasis with partially or completely buried penis, and 10 patients is penile elephantiasis.

It may be associated with other manifestations of lymphatic filariasis, and may be physically, mentally, and socially disturbed (Machol et al. 2014).

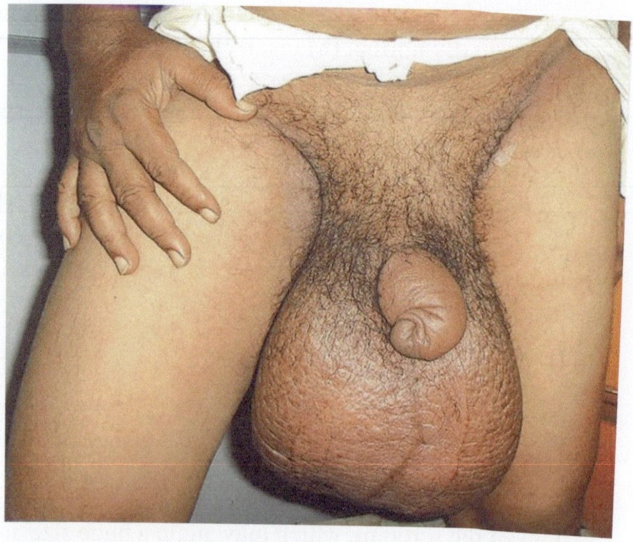

Fig. 22.4 Filarial chronic lymphedema of scrotum and bilateral hydrocele with early ram-horn penis

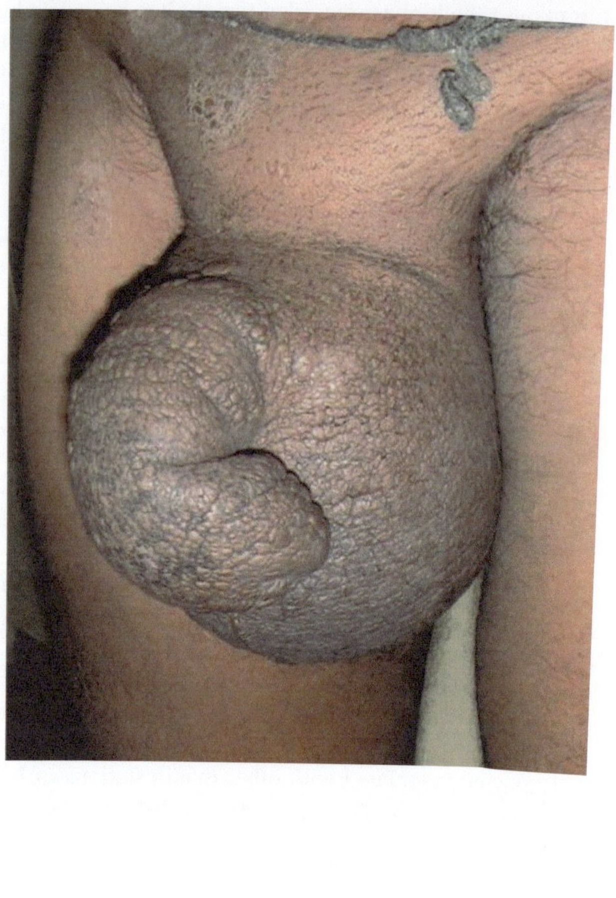

Fig. 22.5 Filarial elephantiasis of scrotum and penis with a ram-horn penis

22.4 Extent of Chronic Lymphedema of Scrotum

Justine Whitaker method of measuring scrotal lymphedema (Fig. 22.6) consists of taking following three measurements in standing position (Reddick 2012)—

1. Girth in the middle of scrotum
2. Girth at the neck of scrotum
3. Length of scrotum

However, as there are no normal standard dimensions there is difficulty in assessing the degree or extent of swelling. Hence, these figures are used to assess the benefits of conservative treatment.

22.5 Complications

The complications of chronic lymphedema–elephantiasis of the scrotum include skin papillomatosis, hyperkeratosis, recurrent cellulitis, intertrigo, ulceration, and lymphatic fistulae (Schook et al. 2014).

22.6 Investigations

- *Blood*—It may show eosinophilia, and microfilariae in the night blood smear, especially during an acute attack of filariasis.
- *Imaging*—The pathology of this disease can be imaged by ultrasonography, CT scan, or MRI.

The pathological changes in the lymphatic drainage of the scrotum can be seen by lymphography or lymphoscintigraphy. This investigation is usually not required.

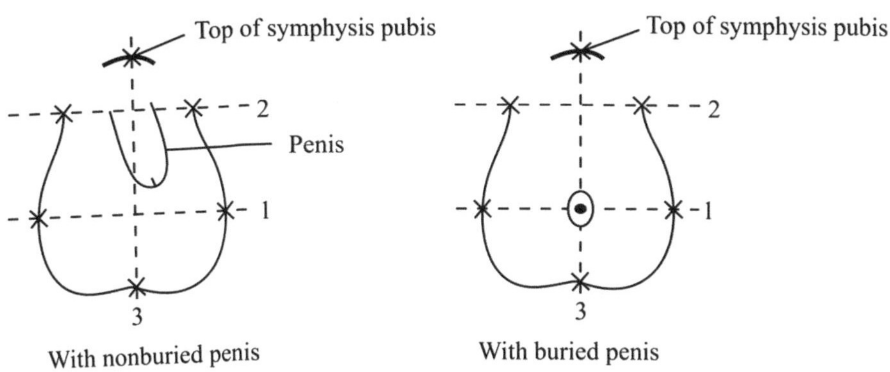

Fig. 22.6 Justine Whitaker method of measuring scrotal lymphedema

22.7 Glasgow Benefit Inventory (GBI)

Glasgow Benefit Inventory (GBI) is an established tool that assesses how a procedure has altered the quality of life of the patient. It is based on the answers to 18 questions given by the patient. It not only allows the calculation of "total" quality of life as influenced by the intervention but also permits a break-down of results into "general subscale," "social support subscale," and "physical health subscale."

The score is calculated as described here—the sum of the responses is first divided by the number of questions in the respective subscale to get an average response score. From the average response score, 3 is subtracted and the result is multiplied by 50. It gives a score between −100 and 100 with −100 being the worst possible change, 0 no change and 100 the best possible change. (Torio-Padron, et al. 2015).

22.8 Treatment

There is no known drug which can reverse the elephantoid process. The cause of the problem is treated, e.g., in filarial elephantiasis a course of diethylcarbamazine is given and further mosquito bite is prevented. Al-Sindi et al. (2008) reported first case of elephantiasis of scrotum from Bahrain which was suspected to be filarial. Hence, he was given a 8-week course of doxycycline to eradicate potential filarial infection. It acts on adult filarial worms by killing the endosymbiont, Wolbachia. The patient was subsequently treated by scrotectomy and scrotoplasty.

Complex Decongestive Physiotherapy (CDP) Complex decongestive physiotherapy was first described by Foldi (1998) and consists of skin hygiene, manual lymphatic drainage, compression bandages and therapeutic exercises. All these measures are not applicable to the lymphedema of external genitalia because of the anatomical peculiarities. However, if they are given by an experienced therapist they may reduce the swelling significantly (de Godoy et al. 2014; Torio-Padron et al. 2015).

Skin hygiene of scrotum External genitalia is washed daily with soap and water and dried (ideally with a hair dryer) followed by application of a bland emollient.

Acute infections such as lymphangitis and cellulitis are mostly streptococcal or staphylococcal. They are controlled with appropriate antibiotics, e.g., oral penicillin, flucloxacillin or co-amoxiclav. If the attacks are more frequent, i.e., 3 or more per year (Schook et al. 2014) long-term prophylactic antibiotic therapy may be indicated.

Manual lymph drainage (MLD) It may be done by a therapist, but it is not readily accepted by the patient. Hence, the patient can be provided with a video for instructions on self-manual lymphatic massage (Reddick 2012).

Elevation of the part may be done by putting a wedge under the pelvis during the night (Schook et al. 2014).

Compression bandaging The bandaging protocol is effective but difficult to practice. It is done with Coban 2 short stretch compression bandaging maintained with class 2 Whitaker pouch (Reddick 2012).

Surgical treatment The benefits of conservative treatment stop as soon as this therapy is stopped. Hence, surgical intervention in required to give proper size and shape to the genitalia for the rest of life (Charles, 1912). Two types of surgical procedures may be used:

1. *Procedures to improve lymphatic drainage*—These procedures aim at improving the lymphatic drainage of the external genitalia. Historically, it has been done by implantation of silk threads, metal tubes or polythene tubes, and permanent suture of scrotum to adjacent thigh (Dandapat et al. 1985). Some other methods to improve the lymphatic drainage are—
   (a) Use of skin flap between the scrotum and inguinal area (Orr 1962)
   (b) Suturing the scrotum permanently to upper medial thigh as done in the Keetley–Torek operation for incompletely descended testis (Nesbit cited by Bulkley 1962)
   (c) Bilateral inguinal nodo-venous shunt (Nielubowicz and Olszewski 1966)—The scrotum-draining lymph node is identified by subcutaneous isosulfan injection into the scrotum by color as done for sentinel lymph node biopsy. The raw surface of hemisectioned lymph node is anatomized to the side of long saphenous vein in the vicinity. The afferent lymphatics of this lymph node are protected from injury.
   (d) Lymphatico-venular anastomosis—Yamamoto et al. (2011) successfully treated 2 patients of genital lymphedema by multiple lymphatico-venular anastomoses.

   These procedures are more theoretical than practical as they do not give satisfactory results. Hence, they have been abandoned.
2. *Excisional operations*—Complete excision of elephantoid tissue is the definitive curative treatment of this problem (Gelbke 1954; Farina et al. 1958).

Larry (1803)) is credited with describing the scrotal reduction surgery, Delpech (1832) for minute details of surgery, and Gibson (1956) for its entertaining and informative reflection. Depending upon the size of the scrotum a partial, subtotal and total scrotectomy may be done, the last being required very rarely. After taking informed consent, general or spinal anesthesia is given and a no 14 Foley's self-retaining catheter is passed in the urinary bladder. As the tissues are quite vascular, there may be significant intraoperative bleeding and lymphorrhea. Therefore arrangements may be made for blood transfusion and fluid replacement (Ollapallil and Watters 1995). There are two types of scrotal excision depending upon the extent of resection—

Partial or subtotal excision (reduction scrotoplasty) Charles reduction (1912) includes excision of diseased skin and defect coverage with adjacent healthy skin with midline suturing simulating median raphe (Modolin et al. 2006; Parmar 2013) or split thickness skin grafting (Martinez et al. 1988).

In elephantiasis of scrotum it is mainly the rugose (anterior) skin that is diseased. It needs removal. The skin of the sides and posterior aspect of scrotum is healthy and normal. It is saved and utilized to reconstruct a new scrotum. Dog ears must be avoided during closure of the wound. The scrotal skin has a great capacity to stretch out which betters the reconstruction as the time passes.

The associated bilateral hydrocele is treated by eversion of sac if sac wall is thin (Singh et al. 2011), or excision (hydrocelectomy) if it is thick. This step reduces the scrotal size markedly.

The testes are put back into the scrotum avoiding torsion (Ndoye et al. 1999).

This operation can be done with a midline elliptical incision enclosing the diseased skin to be excised or two curved transverse incisions enclosing the diseased skin and subcutaneous tissue to be excised (Figs. 22.7, 22.8, 22.9, and 22.10).

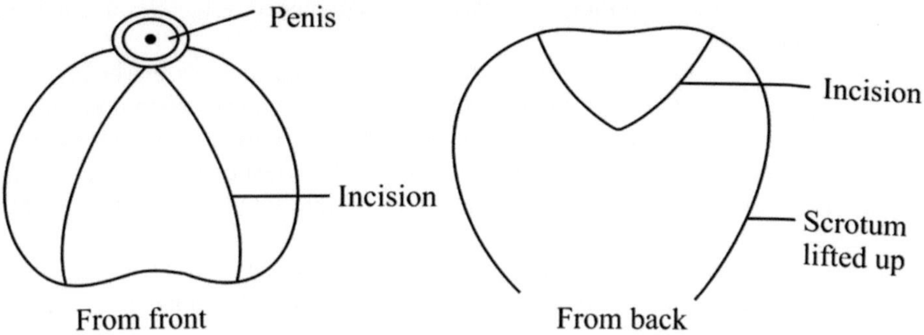

Fig. 22.7 Midline elliptical incision for partial or subtotal scrotectomy

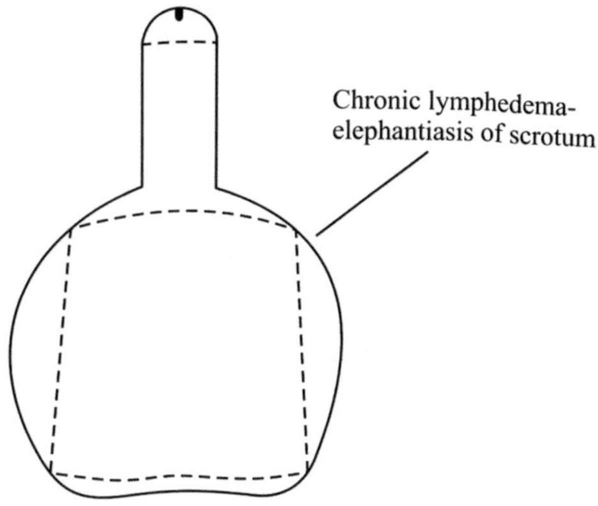

Fig. 22.8 Transverse incisions with vertical side incisions for reduction scrotoplasty for chronic lymphedema–elephantiasis of scrotum without involvement of penis aimed at excising the rugose skin

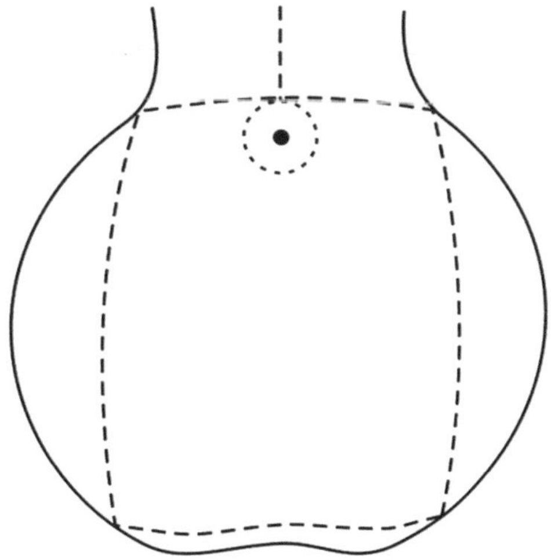

Fig. 22.9 Transvere incisions with vertical side incisions for reduction scrotectomy and scrotoplasty (reduction scrotoplasty) in chronic lymphedema–elephantiasis of scrotum with embedded penis (Ndoye et al. 1999)

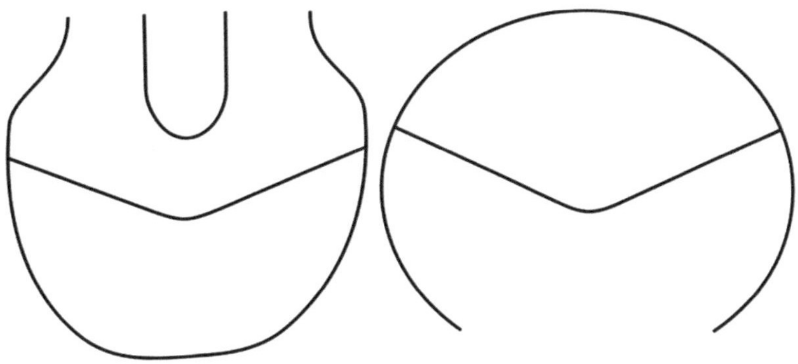

Fig. 22.10 Incision for partial or subtotal scrotectomy for chronic lymphedema–elephantiasis of scrotum with normal penis

A vertically located (midline) incision in the scrotum may result in regrowth of lymphedematous tissue on either side of the scar giving a labia majora-like appearance. (Schook et al. 2014). Hence, other incisions described above may be employed.

The steps of partial scrotectomy for elephantiasis of scrotum are shown in the following pictures (Fig. 22.11):

Total scrotectomy Total excision of the scrotum is required in extensive involvement of scrotum which is rare. Hence, this operation is rarely indicated. The scrotum is excised with a transverse elliptical incision near the neck of scrotum (Fig. 22.12). During operation, the injury to the testes and spermatic cords on either

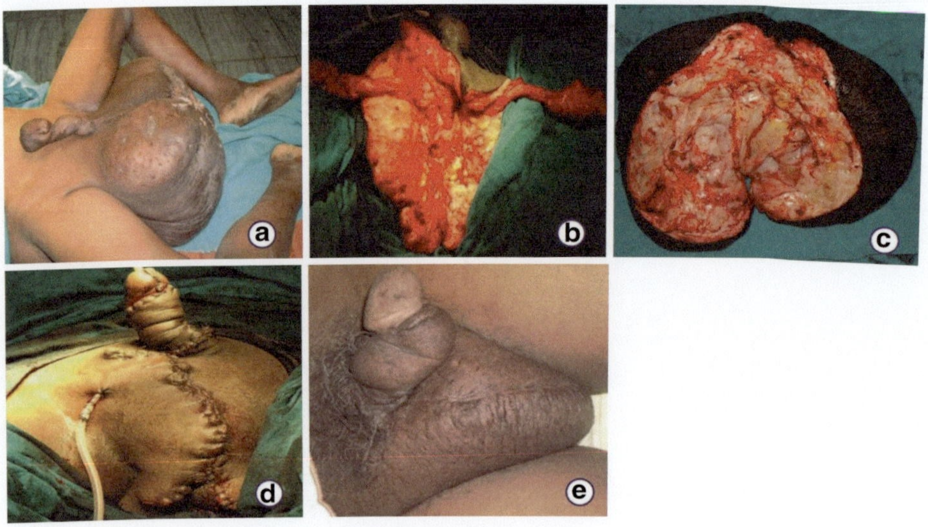

Fig. 22.11 Steps of the surgical treatment in a patient of elephantiasis of scrotum and penis with postoperative picture (Courtesy or Professor Brijesh Mishra.)

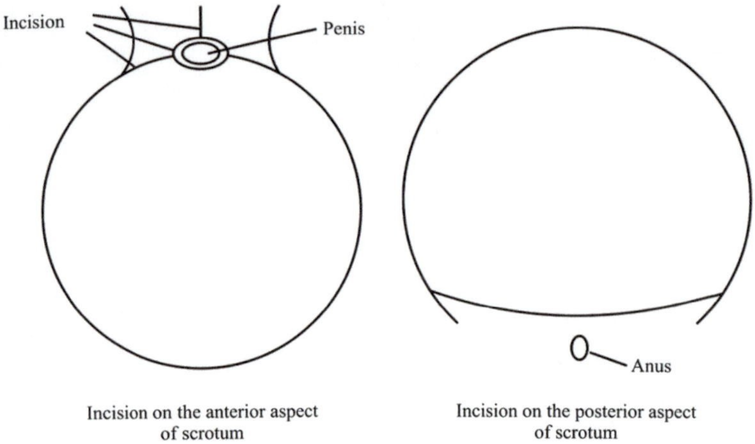

Fig. 22.12 Curved transverse incision at the neck of scrotum with an ellipse in the middle to enclose penis to save it for total scrotectomy (Dandapat et al. 1985)

side and the penis and urethra in the midline must be prevented. The methods of dealing with the exposed testes are described below (Khanna 1970):

(a) *Implantation of the testes into the thighs*—The testes may be put in a subcutaneous pocket on either side into the corresponding thighs as done in some cases of scrotal avulsion injury (Owens 1842).

There are some conflicting reports about the function of these testes in future. Huffman (1956) studied the temperature of abdominal cavity, inguinal canal, scrotum and thigh pockets and found that temperature in the scrotum and superficial thigh pockets is the same. Hence, the temperature of thigh pocket is no problem. However, there seems to be some unknown factors in the scrotum favoring normal spermatogenesis.

Apart from the functional aspect, the implantation of testes into the thighs does not satisfy the cosmetic, psychological, and the emotional aspects of the problem. The proper place for the testes to lie is where the nature intended them to be, i.e., in a separate bag outside the abdomen hanging just below the root of penis in the midline (Khanna 1970). However, the only indication for implantation of testes in the thigh is an old enfeebled patient where the scrotal reconstruction will add to the operation time thereby the operative risk.

(b) *Reconstruction of a new scrotum*—After excision of diseased scrotum and complete hemostasis, both the testes are sutured together and to the Colles' fascia with fine interrupted absorbable sutures and then to the saved skin of the posterior wall of scrotum to from a stable mass for skin grafting. The raw area is then covered with partial thickness skin grafts. The take of these grafts is excellent resulting in a scrotum of reasonable look (Khanna 1970).

A new scrotum can also be reconstructed by rotating the skin flaps from the lower abdomen or thighs. McDougal (1983) described reconstruction of scrotum with superior and laterally based thigh flaps in 3 patients of massive traumatic loss of scrotal skin with acceptable cosmetic results.

Hodjati and Khezri (1996) did reduction scrotoplasty in a case of marked penoscrotal lymphedema where a neoscrotum was made by combining the anterior suprapubic and posterior U-shaped scrotal flaps.

Prica et al. (2008) mentions scrotal coverage with a gracilis myocutaneous flap to establish a channel for lymph flow.

The scrotoplasty is completed by insertion of a closed suction drain in the scrotal sac. It is removed when the drain output is reduced to <15 mL per day (Singh, 2011). The Foley's catheter is removed about 2 weeks after operation.

The complications of excision of elephantoid scrotum include bleeding, hematoma and injury to testes, spermatic cords, penis and urethra; wound infection, painful erection, wound dehiscence, lymphorrhea, flap necrosis and loss of skin grafts, delayed healing and recurrence (Khanna 1970; Nasehi and Azadi 2004; Singh et al. 2011; Torio-Padron et al. 2015).

Chatterjee (1965) reported that excision of median septum of scrotum may result in adhesions between the two testes which may cause postoperative discomfort or pain. However, no other author has mentioned about this problem.

The excised tissue must be sent for histopathological examination as rarely sarcomatous changes may be found in it (Machol et al. 2014).

Compression therapy after operation must continue to prevent reacumulation and deposition of adipose tissue into the newly formed scrotum (Schook et al. 2014).

Recurrence—Despite the care and precautions the problem may recur. Hence, multiple-staged serial excision procedures may be necessary over the life-time of the patient to treat recurrence and re-recurrence (Schook et al. 2014).

The management of chronic lymphedema–elephantiasis of scrotum is summarized in the following Flow Chart 22.1.

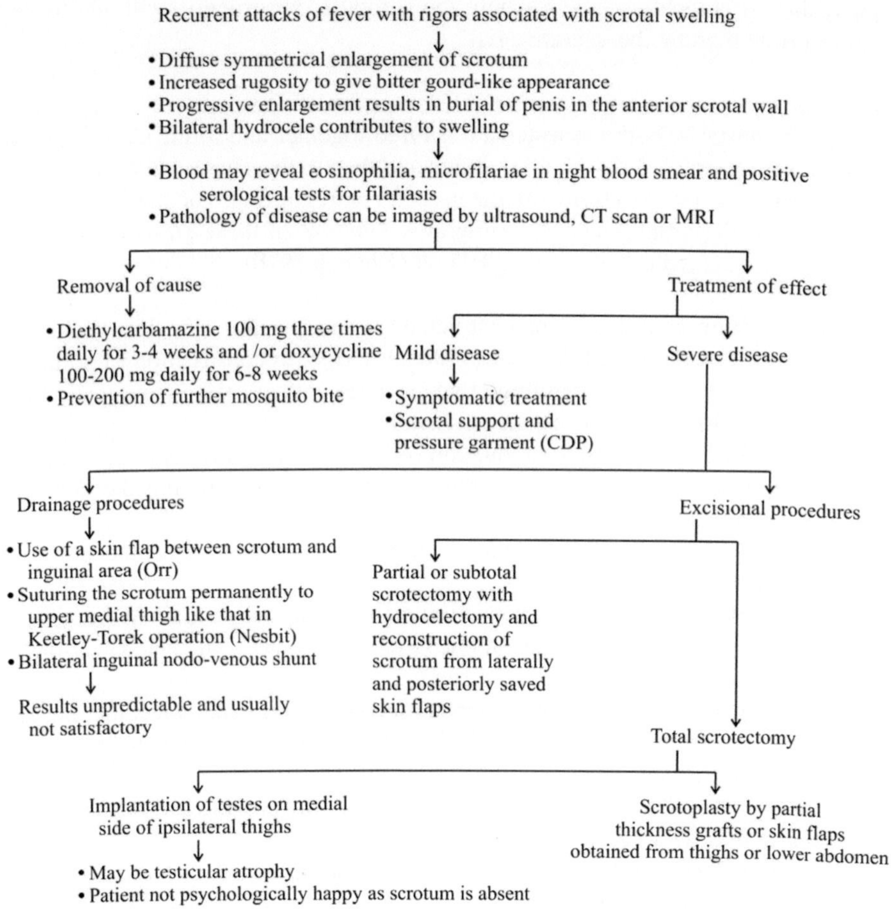

Flow Chart 22.1 Management of chronic lymphedema–elephantiasis of scrotum

References

Al-Sindi K, Golbahar J, Al Moosa D, Nagraj V, Essam W. Scrotal elephantiasis: a first case report from Bahrain. Bahrain Med Bull. 2008;30(3).

Brotherhood HL, Metcalfe M, Goldenberg L, Pommerville P, Bowman C, Naysmith D. A surgical challenge: idiopathic scrotal elephantiasis. Can Urol Asso J. 2014;8:1500–4.

Charles H. Elephantiasis scroti. In: Latham A, English TC, editors. A system of treatment. Vol 3. Calcutta: Butterworth & Co (India) Ltd; 1912. p. 511–6.

Chatterjee P. Filariasis. In; Clinical Surgery (Tropical) edited by Robs C & Smith R. 1st ed. London. Butterworths 1965:99–100.

Dandapat MC, Mahapatro SK, Patro SK. Elephantiasis of the penis and scrotum: a review of 350 cases. Am J Surg. 1985;149:686–90.

de Godoy JMP, Facio Jr FN, de Carvalho EC M, de Godoy Mde FG. New compression mechanism in penile-lymphedema and sexual rehabilitation. Urol Ann. 2014;6(1):88–90.

De Greef R. Ann Soc Belg Med Trop. 1938;87:422. Quoted by Prpic I. Severe elephantiasis of penis and scrotum. Brit J Plast Surg. 1996;19:173–78.

Delpech JM. Chirurgic Clinique de Montpellier. Paris and Montpellier. 1832. Quoted by Torio-Padron N, Bjorn Stark G, Foldi E,Simunovic F. Treatment of male genital lymphedema: an integrated concept. J Plast Reconstr Aesth Surg. 2015;68:262–8.

Farina R, De Freire GC, Macedo A. Elephantiasis of the male genitalia; phallus-oscheo-plasty. Urol Int (Basel). 1958;6:50–60.

Foldi E. The treatment of lymphedema. Cancer. 1998;83:2831–4.

Gelbke H. Penisskin transplantation. Zentralbl Chir. 1954;79(22):935–42.

Gibson T. Delpech: his contributions to plastic surgery and the astonishing case of scrotal elephantiasis: case report. Brit J Plast Surg. 1956;6:4–10.

Hai AA, et al. Filarial lymphoedema of male genitalia. Second international conference on surgery in tropics, Bombay Hospital Institute of Medical Sciences. 22–27 Feb 1987.

Hodjati H, Khezri AA. A new modified surgical approach in lymphedema of the penis and scrotum. Medical J Islamic Rep Iran. 1996;10(2):113–5.

Huffman WC, Gulp DA. Greenleef JS et al. Injuries to male genitalia. Plast Reconstr Surg. 1956;18:344–53.

Khanna NN. Surgical treatment of elephantiasis of male genitalia. Plast Reconstr Surg. 1970;46(5):481.

Kinmonth JB. The lymphatics. 2nd ed. London: Edward Arnold; 1982. p. 193.

Larry DJ, 1803. Quoted by Bulkley GJ: Scrotal and penile lymphedema. J Urol. 1962;87:422–9.

Lee S, Han JS, Ross HM, et al. Massive localized lymphedema of the male external genitalia: a clinicopathologic study of 6 cases. Hum Pathol. 2014;44:277–81.

Machol JA, Langenstroer P, Sanger JR. Surgical reduction of scrotal massive localized lymphedema (MLL) in obesity. J Plast Reconstr Aesth Surg. 2014;67:1719–25.

McDougal WS. Scrotal reconstruction using thigh pedicle flaps. J Urol. 1983;129:757–9.

Manson-Bahr PEC, Apted FIC. Filariases. In: Manson's tropical diseases. 18th ed. London: Bailliere Tindal; 1982. p. 148–80.

Martinez RE, Couchell SH, Raffel B, Swartz WM. Primary lymphedema of scrotum: surgical treatment and reconstruction. Ann Plast Surg. 1988;21:354–7.

Modolin M, Mitre AI, et al. Surgical treatment of lymphedema of the penis and scrotum. Clinics (Sao Paulo, Brazil). 2006;61:289–94.

Nasehi A, Azadi SH. Elephantiasis of penis and scrotum. Urol J. 2004;2:55–7.

Ndoye A, Sylla C, Gueye MBASM, Diagne BA. Management of penile and scrotal elephantiasis. BJU Int. 1999;94:362–4.

Nesbit RM. Quoted by Bulkley GJ: Scrotal and penile lymphedema. J Urol. 1962;87:422–9.

Nielubowicz J, Olszewski W. Special issue for XVth congress of European society of cardiovascular surgery. J Cardiovasc Surg. 1966;384.

Ollapallil JJ, Watters DAK. Surgical management of elephantiasis of male genitalia. Br J Urol. 1995;76:213–315.

Orr TG. Quoted by Bulkley GJ: Scrotal and penile lymphedema. J Urol. 1962;87:422–9.
Owens N. Reconstruction for traumatic denudation of the penis and scrotum. Surgery. 1842;12:88.
Paradysz A, Prokopowicz G, Pindycka-Piaszczynska M, Bryniarski P, Zyczkowski M. Idiopathic scrotal, penile and perineal elephantiasis – Successful surgical treatment. Centr Eur J Urol. 2010;63:51–3.
Parmar HD. The surgical approach in huge scrotal lymphedema. Int J Med Sc Pub Hlth. 2013;2(1):153–5.
Prica S, Donati OF, Schaefer DJ, Peltzer J. Genital elephantiasis; reconstructive treatment of peno-scrotal lymphedema with myocutaneous M gracilis flap: experience from a district hospital in Ethiopia. Handchir Mikroch Chir. 2008;40(4):272–8.
Prpic I. Severe elephantiasis of penis and scrotum. Br J Plast Surg. 1966;19:173–8.
Reddick M. Scrotal lymphedema: Compression solutions for a challenging condition. Lymphedema pathways 2012; Ca 22. http://canadalymph.ca/wp-content/uploads/2015/04/Scrotal-Lymphedema-compression-solutions-for-a-challenging-condition.pdf.
Schook CC, Kulungowski AM, Greene AK, Fishman SJ. Male genital lymphedema: clinical features and management of 25 pediatric patients. J Pedia Surg. 2014;49:1647–951.
Singh G, Sandhu AS. Gaint peno-scrotal elephantiasis. Int J Clin Cases Invest. 2011;3(1).http://ijcci.info/component/content/article/149-giant-peno-scrotal-elephantiasis?showall=1.
Singh V, Sinha RJ, Sankhwar SN, Kumar V. Reconstructive surgery for penoscrotal filarial lymphedema : a decade of experience and follow up. Urology. 2011;77:1228–31.
Torio-Padron N, Bjorn Stark G, Foldi E, Simunovic F. Treatment of male genital lymphedema : an integrated concept. J Plast Reconstr Aesthet Surg. 2015;68:262–8.
Yamamoto T, Koshima I, Yoshimatsu H, Narushima M, Miahara M, Iida T. Simultaneous multisite lymphatiovenular anastomoses for primary lower extremity and genital lymphedema complicated with severe lymphorrhea. J Plast Reconstr Aesthet Surg. 2011;64:812–5.

Chronic Lymphedema–Elephantiasis of Penis

23

After the chronic lymphedema–elephantiasis of lower extremity and that of scrotum, it is the next common type of chronic lymphedema–elephantiasis (Fig. 23.1). It is a disease of integuments of penis as the erectile tissue of the glans and shaft cannot be affected as there are no lymphatics in these parts of penis.

The chronic lymphedema–elephantiasis of penis commonly occurs in association with lymphedema of scrotum (Fig. 23.2) but it can occur alone indicating that the penile lymphatic drainage may be distinct from scrotal lymphatic drainage.

De Greef (1938), Manson-Bahr and Apted (1982), Kinmonth (1982), Dandapat et al. (1985), Paradysz et al. (2010), Lee et al. (2014), and Schook et al (2014) have described about peno-scrotal lymphedema-elephantiasis.

Khanna (1970) reported his experience of treating 20 patients of chronic lymphedema–elephantiasis of male external genitals in whom three patients has lymphedema of penis only. Others had lymphedema of scrotum with lymphedema of penis of varying degrees.

Singh et al. (2011) reported 48 patients of filarial male genital lymphedema which included 14 patients of isolated penile and 34 patients of penoscrotal lymphedema.

23.1 Etiology

The etiology of chronic lymphedema of penis is nearly the same as that of chronic lymphedema of scrotum, as described below (Kinmonth, 1902):

1. *Infection* – In this group the lymphatic filariasis is the commonest cause in tropical and subtropical countries. It causes lymphedema due to adenolymphatic obstruction of inguinal lymphatics. Other infections which can cause inguinal lymphatic obstruction include tuberculosis and lymphogranuloma venereum (LGV).
2. *Malignancy* – The metastatic disease of inguinal lymph nodes and its treatment with node dissection or radiotherapy may also cause penile lymphedema–

T.C. Goel, A. Goel, *Lymphatic Filariasis*, DOI 10.1007/978-981-10-2257-9_23

elephantiasis. The infections involving the inguinal lymph nodes are the commonest cause in tropical and underdeveloped countries while malignancy involving these lymph nodes is the commonest cause in advanced western nations.

3. *Primary lymphedema* – This type of lymphedema of penis is attributed to developmental defect of lymphatics, i.e., hypoplasia. Sandeepa et al. (2015) described a patient of primary isolated penile lymphedema which was treated by excision.
4. *Idiopathic* – Edema of penis and of scrotum can occur without a known cause.

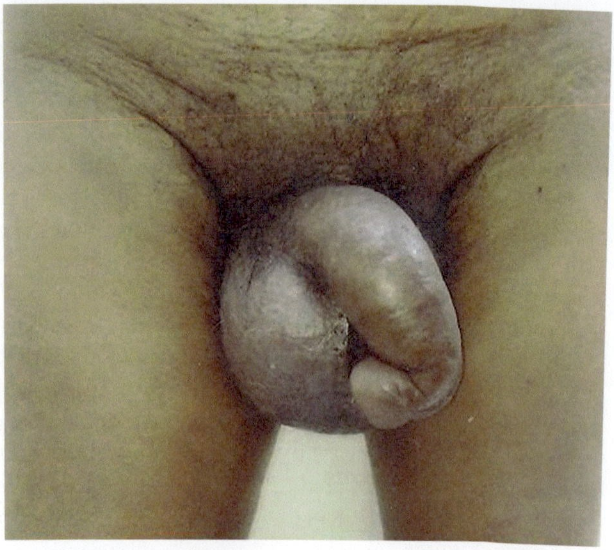

Fig. 23.1 Ram-horn penis of filariasis. The scrotum is also affected and there is right-sided hydrocele (Courtesy – Dr. SK Vaish)

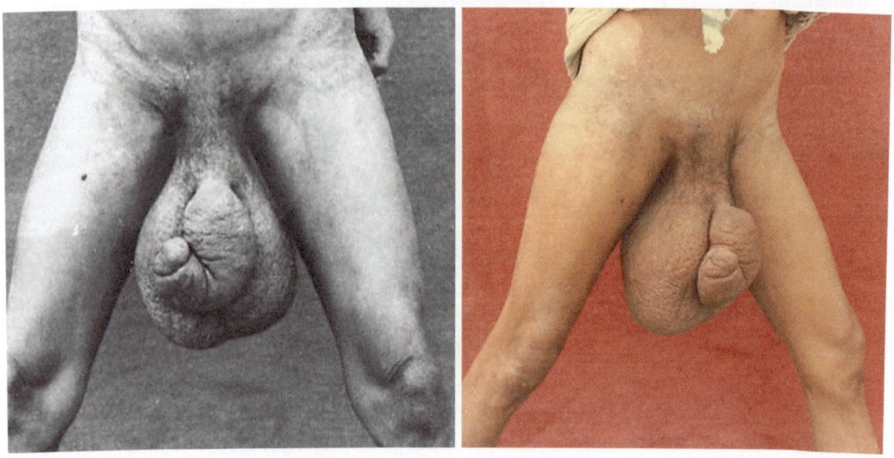

Fig. 23.2 Chronic filarial lymphedema–elephantiasis of scrotum and penis in which the penis is curved like a snail or angulated like ram horn

5. *As a part of general anasarca* – Swollen penis may be a part of general anasarca that occurs in congestive heart failure, cirrhosis of liver, chronic renal disease, and hypoproteinemia. This swelling disappears following successful treatment of the cause.
6. *Other causes* – de Godoy et al. (2014) described a case of lymphedema of penis and scrotum following surgery of pancreas.

23.2 Pathology

The loose cellular tissue under the skin of penis is a zone which is continuous with the loose cellular tissue within the scrotal wall. Just external to this there is a plane where the lymph of chronic lymphedema accumulates. The inner layer of prepuce is fixed intimately with the fascial sheath of penis for some distance in the post-coronal area. In this area the lymphedema does not occur.

The chronic lymphedema–elephantiasis involves the skin of the penis and the outer layer of prepuce which may become markedly thickened, rough and dry and may be warty or nodular (Fig. 23.3). It can be easily dissected and separated from the body of penis and inner layer of prepuce by separation through the plane of loose cellular tissue (Fig. 23.12). The inner layer of prepuce is normal.

The length of prepuce is increased. Due to lymphedema and subsequent fibrosis the prepuce may lose its retractile property to expose the glans ("filarial phimosis"). Dirty blackish smegma may accumulate in the prepucial sac mainly in post-coronal sulcus. Rarely the prepuce may become nodular (Figs. 23.4 and 23.5):

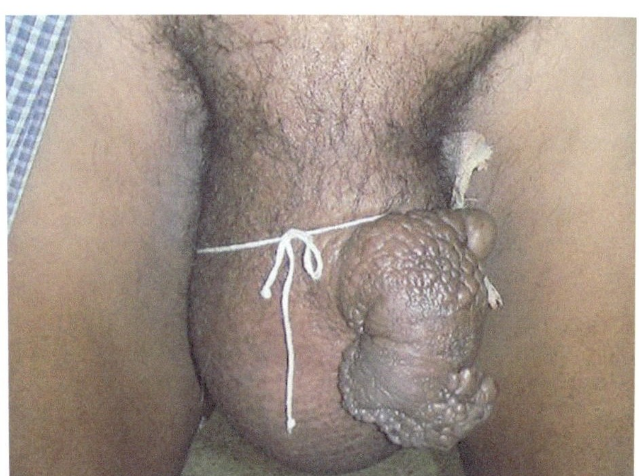

Fig. 23.3 Filarial elephantiasis of penis and scrotum. The penis has thickened and warty skin and it is curved anteroposteriorly

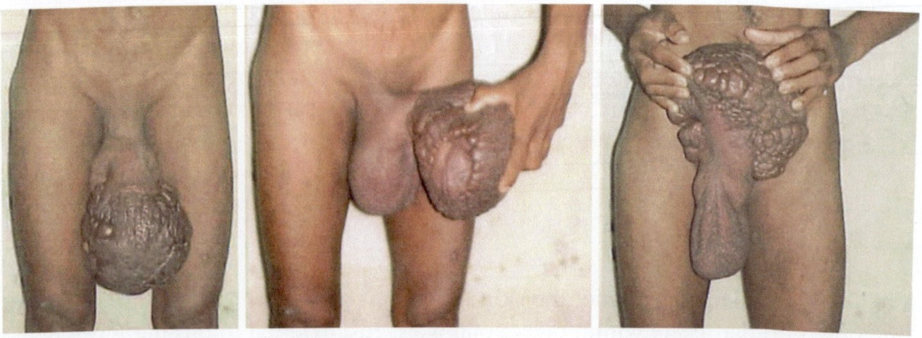

Fig. 23.4 Filarial elephantiasis of penis with markedly enlarged and nodulated prepuce (Courtesy – Professor Sandeep Kumar)

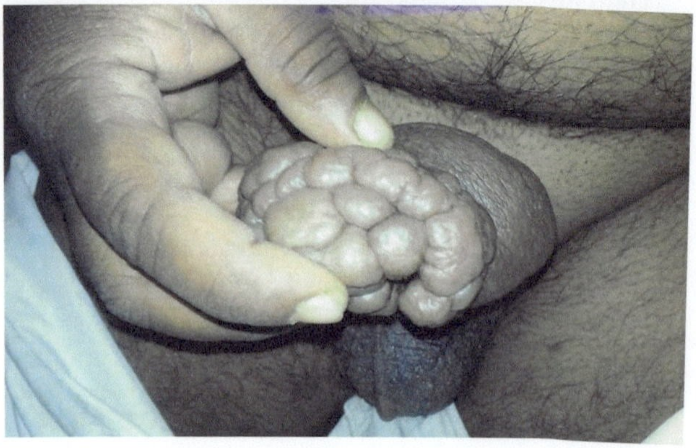

Fig. 23.5 Nodular elephantiasis of prepuce due to filariasis (Courtesy – Dr Ravi Mishra)

23.3 Clinical Features

The patient is usually a middle-aged person who presents with swelling of penis of gradual onset. There is usually a history of recurrent attacks of fever with rigors increasing the swelling with every attack (recurrent progressive swelling). The prepuce is markedly swollen due to edema which pits on pressure. Subsequently the skin gets thickened, roughened and dry and the shape of distal penis becomes crooked (Prpic 1966) or coiled due to irregular fibrosis (ram-horn or snail-like penis) (Figs. 23.6, 23.7, and 23.8).

The micturition is normal, and it may not be possible to retract the prepuce. The patient may not be able to do sexual intercourse which may lead to severe psychosocial problems.

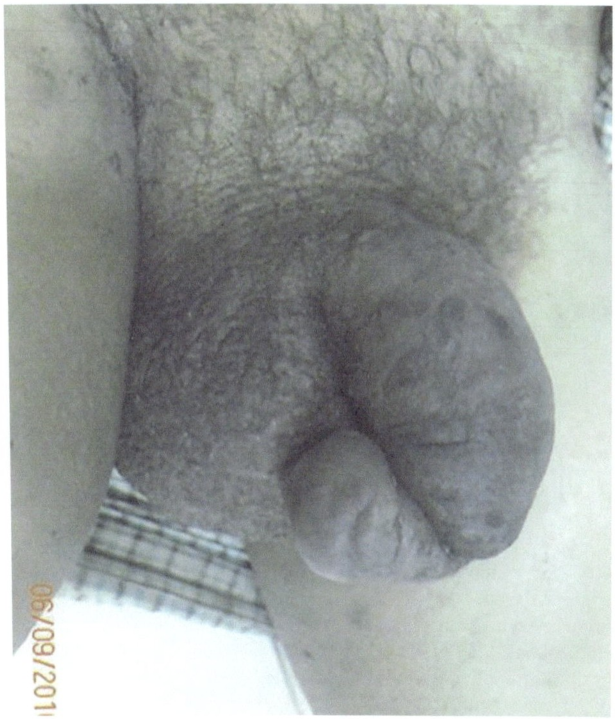

Fig. 23.6 Ram-horn penis of filariasis

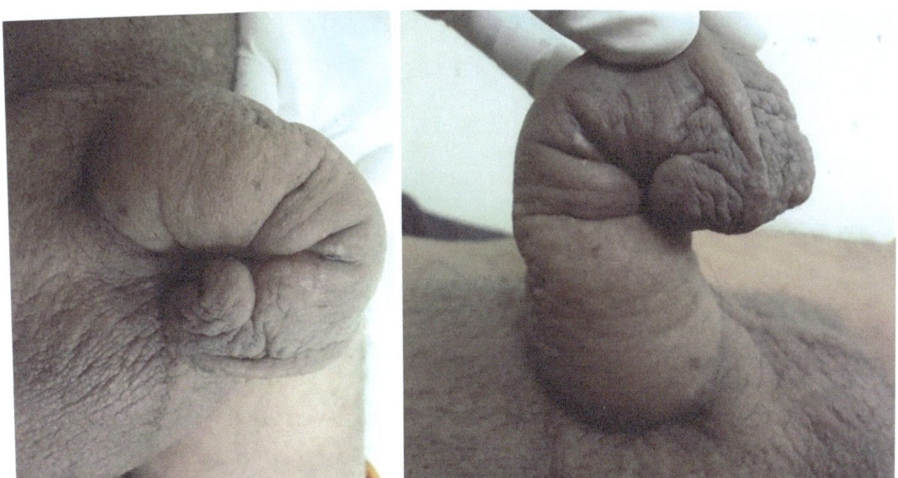

Fig. 23.7 Ram-horn penis of elephantiasis (Courtesy – Professor D Dalela)

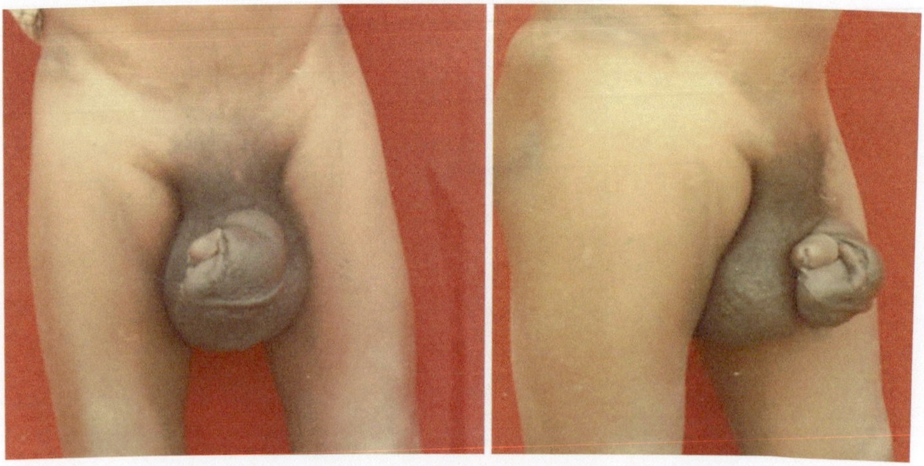

Fig. 23.8 Elephantiasis of penis and scrotum. The penis is curved like a snail

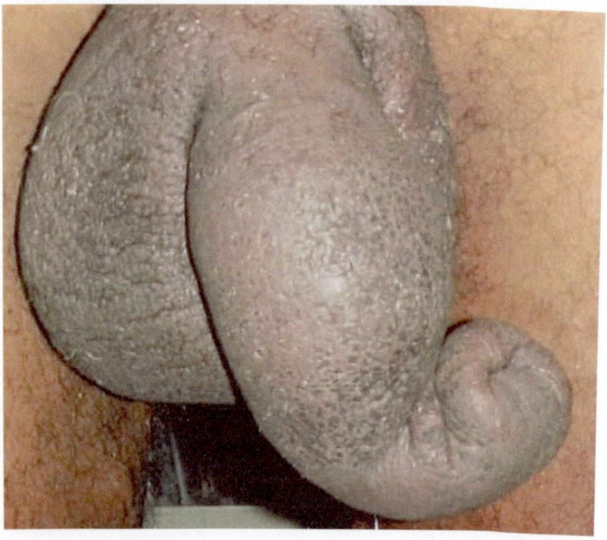

Fig. 23.9 Elephantiasis of penis with ram-horn penis or penis bent like trunk of an elephant. The scrotum has mild lymphedema (Courtesy – Professor Sandeep Kumar)

23.4 Types of Chronic Lymphedema–Elephantiasis of Penis

Ahmed (1941) has described three types of penile involvement in chronic filarial lymphedema:

1. *Ram-horn penis* – The lymph accumulates more in the distal part of penis than in its proximal part. With passage of time fibrosis sets in this fluid due to increasing protein levels. Due to unequal fibrosis and contraction of the scar tissue the swollen prepuce becomes distorted and angulated giving it a ram-horn shape or like that of a snail (Figs. 23.6, 23.7, 23.8, and 23.9). It is the commonest type of elephantiasis of penis.

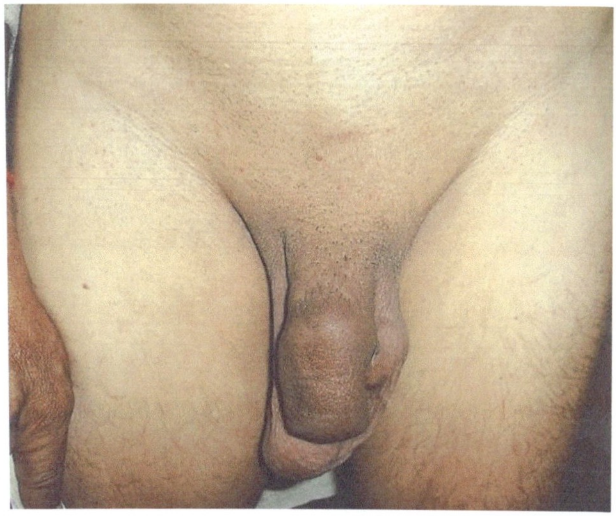

Fig. 23.10 Filarial lymphedema of penis with swelling of distal half of penis with straight penis

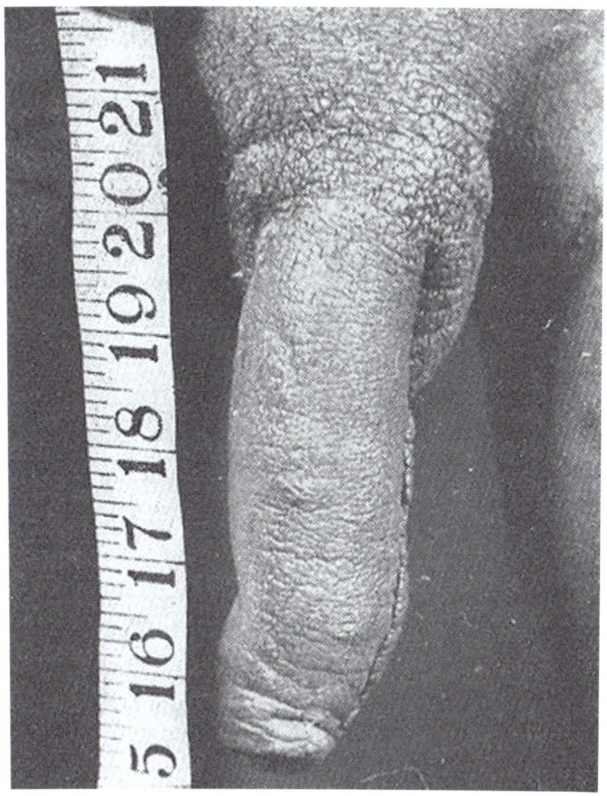

Fig. 23.11 Elephantiasis of penis – straight hypertrophied penis

2. *Straight hypertrophied penis* – This type is chronic lymphedema of penis is characterized by lymphedema and elephantiasis of distal penile skin without distortion (Figs. 23.10 and 23.11). It is relatively uncommon type and may be a stage earlier than ram-horn penis.
3. *Buried penis* – It is truly speaking not the disease of penis. Here the penis is gradually buried in the anterior wall of progressively enlarging scrotum due to chronic filarial lymphedema–elephantiasis. It is usually possible to deliver the penis on the surface by manipulation and pressure, but it returns to its buried position as soon as the manipulating hand is lifted up (Khanna 1970). It is the commonest clinical presentation of chronic filarial penoscrotal lymphedema–elephantiasis.

In the first two types of elephantiasis the penis cannot be buried into the scrotum as the penile skin has lost its elasticity and stretchability and cannot be pulled into it by the enlarging scrotum. Hai et al. (1987) described 195 cases of filarial lymphedema of male external genitals consisting of 15 patients of penile lymphedema and 45 cases of buried penis in elephantoid scrotum. Ollapallil and Watters (1995) described 12 patients of elephantiasis of male genitalia in whom four patients had buried penis.

23.5 Investigations

- *Blood* – It may show eosinophilia and microfilaremia during an acute attack of filariasis. The immunological tests for filariasis are usually positive.
- *Imaging* – The pathology of the disease can be imaged by ultrasonography, CT scan, or MRI. The adenolymphatic obstruction can be imaged by lymphography.

23.6 Treatment

The patient is given a course of diethylcarbamazine 100 mg three times daily for 3–4 weeks and further attacks of filariasis are prevented by prevention of mosquito bite.

The swelling may be reduced by doing self-massage of swollen penis and with continuous use of a cotton–polyester compression garment (Godoy & Godoy technique quoted by de Godoy et al. 2014).

Nodo-venous shunt (Nielubowicz and Olszewski 1966, 1968) – It is a drainage operation which may help in mild to moderate lymphedema without fibrous proliferation. In this procedure bilateral inguinal nodo-venous shunt is combined with circumcision.

Excision of elephantoid tissue – The operation is done under general or spinal anesthesia and a Foley's catheter is passed in the bladder and kept in situ for 10–15 days.

The buried type of penis is brought out of the swollen scrotum during surgical treatment of chronic lymphedema–elephantiasis of scrotum.

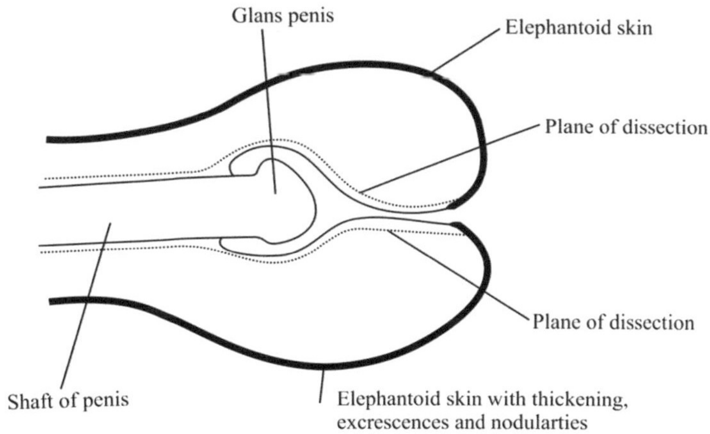

Fig. 23.12 Excision of elephantoid tissue in penile elephantiasis

The other two types of penile elephantiasis are treated by excision of all elephantoid tissue including the outer layer of prepuce by a racket incision at the root of penis and a circumferential incision around the prepucial orifice with both the incision joined together by a longitudinal dorsal midline incision. There is a good plane of cleavage between the normal and elephantoid tissue which is quite avascular (Fig. 23.12). Hence, the excision is not difficult. The distal limit of the excision is the distal junction of external and inner layers of prepuce. The whole elephantoid tissue is excised to give proper shape to the penis preventing injury to its vessels and nerves.

Resurfacing of the penis is required after excision of elephantoid tissue of penis. There are many methods of doing it:

1. DeSavitsch (1941) left the raw penis to spontaneous epithelialization. It is not acceptable as it takes a lot of time in healing and causes scarring of penis.
2. Use of excised skin of the penis (after debulking) as a full thickness graft, but this skin should not be used as it is not healthy (Farina et al. 1958).
3. Use of inner layer of prepure (Bowesman 1960) – The raw area of the penis is commonly covered by inner layer of prepuce which is turned back on the penis to cover it like a pillow cover and its edge is stitched to the cut edge of the skin around the root of penis. To prevent seroma formation under the skin envelope the prepucial tube is punctured at many places before suturing. Also to prevent a circumferential scar at the root of penis a Z-plasty is usually required. If there is deficiency of the skin near the root of penis, it is made good by partial thickness skin grafts.
4. Use of skin flaps from suprapubic, inguinal, or femoral region and even scrotum (Ross 1941–1942), but they make the penis bulky while this operation is being done to debulk the penis. Also it requires staging of the procedure.

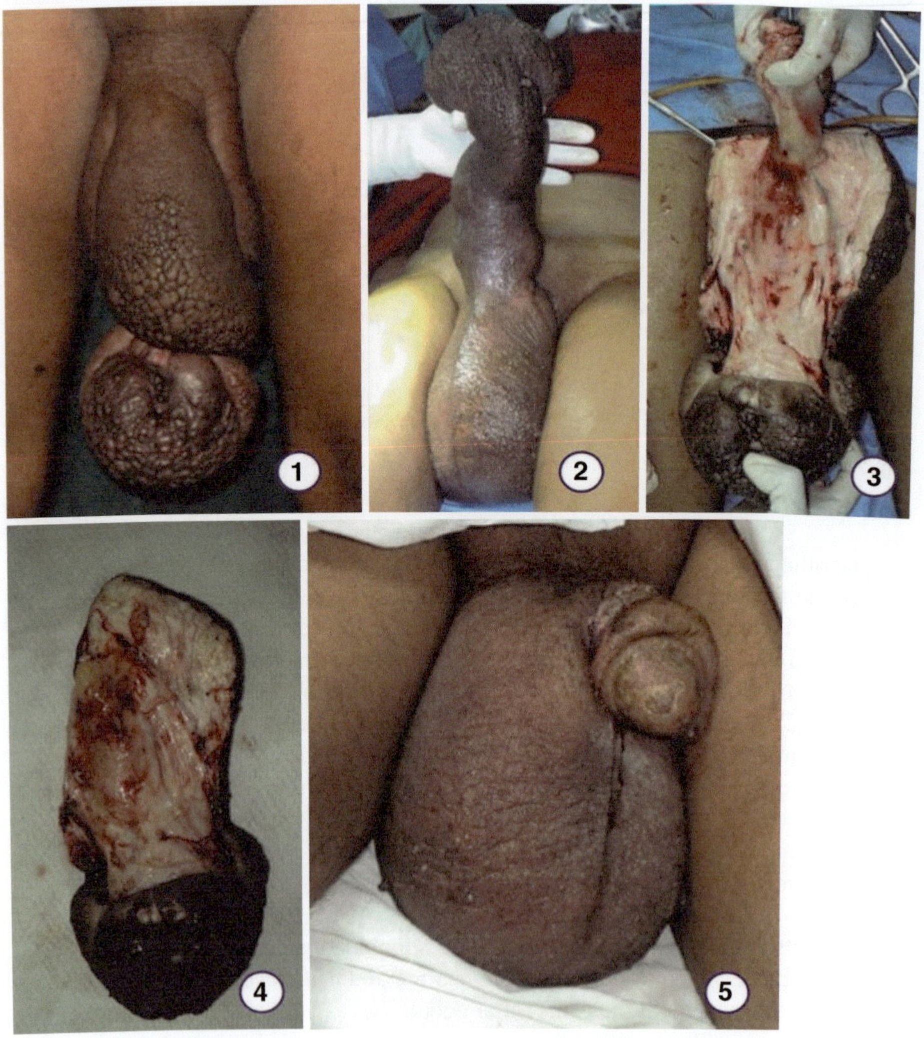

Fig. 23.13 Steps of the surgical treatment of elephantiasis of penis with postoperative result (Courtesy – Professor Brijesh Mishra)

5. Use of partial thickness skin grafts 0.7–0.8 mm thick (Gelbke 1954; Morales et al. 1954). The graft is stitched at the root of penis in a zigzag manner to avoid a circular scar and on the ventral surface also in a zigzag manner to prevent scar contracture. Kubacek (1957) also sutures the graft on the ventral side of penis. Ferris (1949) stitches the graft on the dorsal surface and Paletta (1952) on the lateral side. However the contracture of any scar can occur but the scar contracture on the dorsal surface is not troublesome. Hence, Khanna (1970) used dorsal suturing.

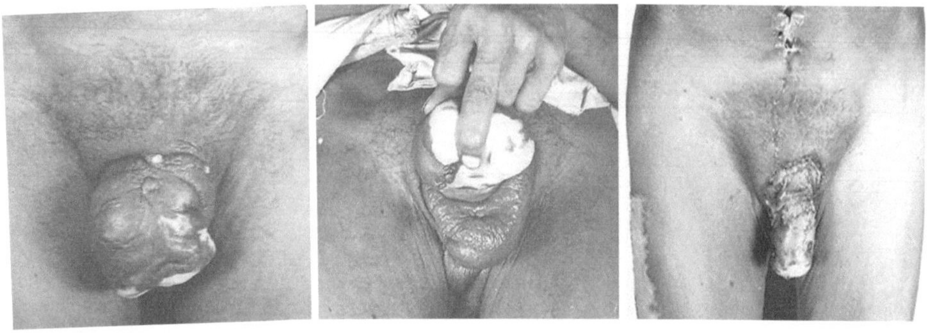

Fig. 23.14 Elephantiasis of penis with marked scarring, nodularity and curvature of penis. The third picture is taken 11 days after excision of elephantoid tissue

The patients whose penile shaft was covered with prepucial skin (Fig. 23.13) had better penile sensation than those whose shaft was covered with split thickness skin grafts (Khanna 1970; Feins 1980; Modolin et al. 2006; Singh et al. 2011).

Some authors recommend interdigitation of the suture lime (Ferris 1949) or suture of the grafts in a spiral fashion (Cullen 1966).

For grafting the penis is pulled to elongate it to its maximum and then grafts are put and sutured (Khanna 1970).

To avoid formation of a hematoma under the grafts the grafts are fenestrated, and penis is covered with Etheron sponge dressing (Rowan and Howley 1965).

Immobilization of penis is a must for healing of the grafts. Streli (1958) immobilizes the penis in a vertical position, while Boeminghaus (1950) recommends a wire stirrup. Russe (1955) used a bandage and spiral Elastoplast bands. Prpic (1966) immobilized the penis in the groove of the rubber tube. The results of excision are good (Fig. 23.14).

The *complications* of operation of chronic lymphedema–elephantiasis of penis include bleeding, wound infection and painful erections of penis which can cause partial necrosis of the grafts. Hence, stilbesterol (Morales et al. 1954) or lupulin and bromide (Prpic 1966) may be given in the postoperative period.

The *delayed complications* include mild pain during erection (Singh et al. 2011), scarring, and recurrence. Prasad (1976) reported a patient age 58 years who had recurrence 17 years after excision of penile and scrotal elephantiasis with left orchiectomy. The mass looked like scrotum 20 cm in diameter. It covered the glans penis with urinary opening at the bottom.

As both penis and scrotum are affected together in this disease, both are operated in one operation. The operative steps of one such patient are given below (Fig. 23.15).

The management of chronic lymphedema–elephantiasis of penis is described in brief in the following Flow Chart 23.1:

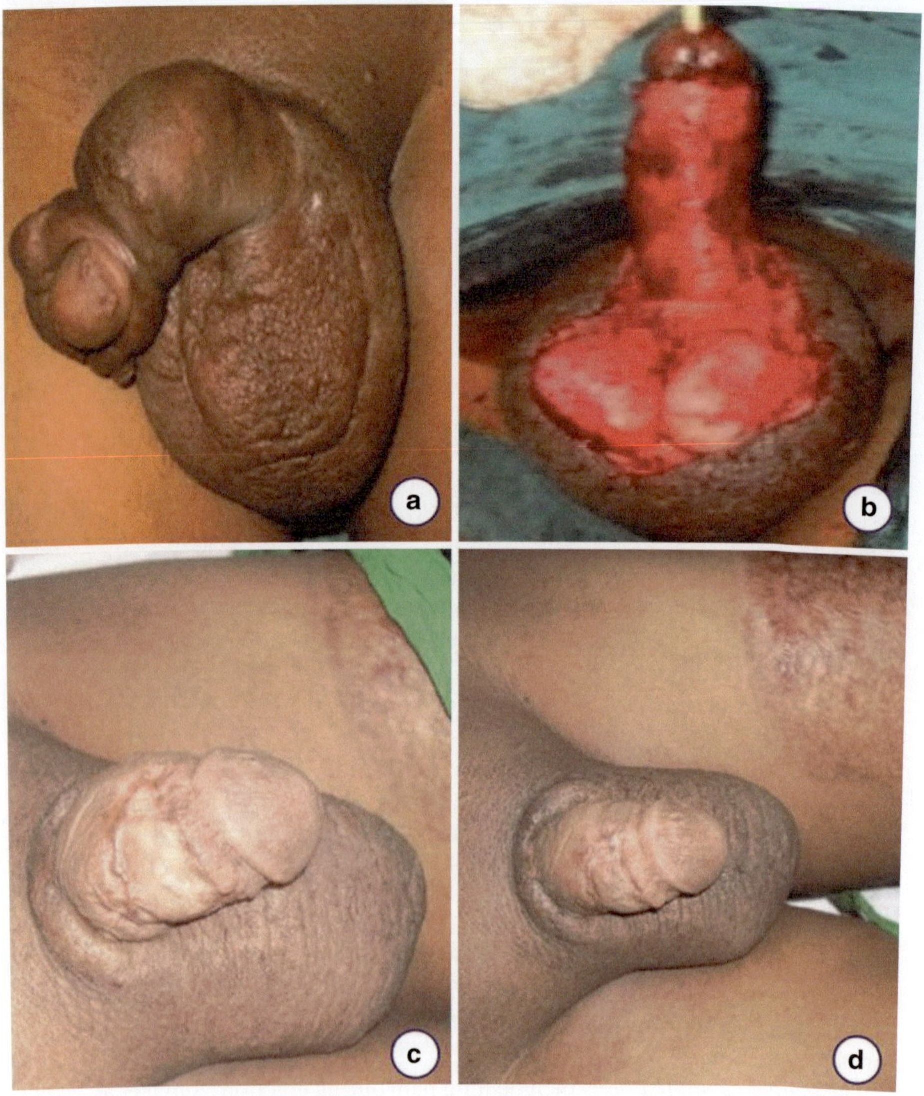

Fig. 23.15 Steps of surgical treatment of elephantiasis of penis and scrotum (Courtesy – Professor Brijesh Mishra)

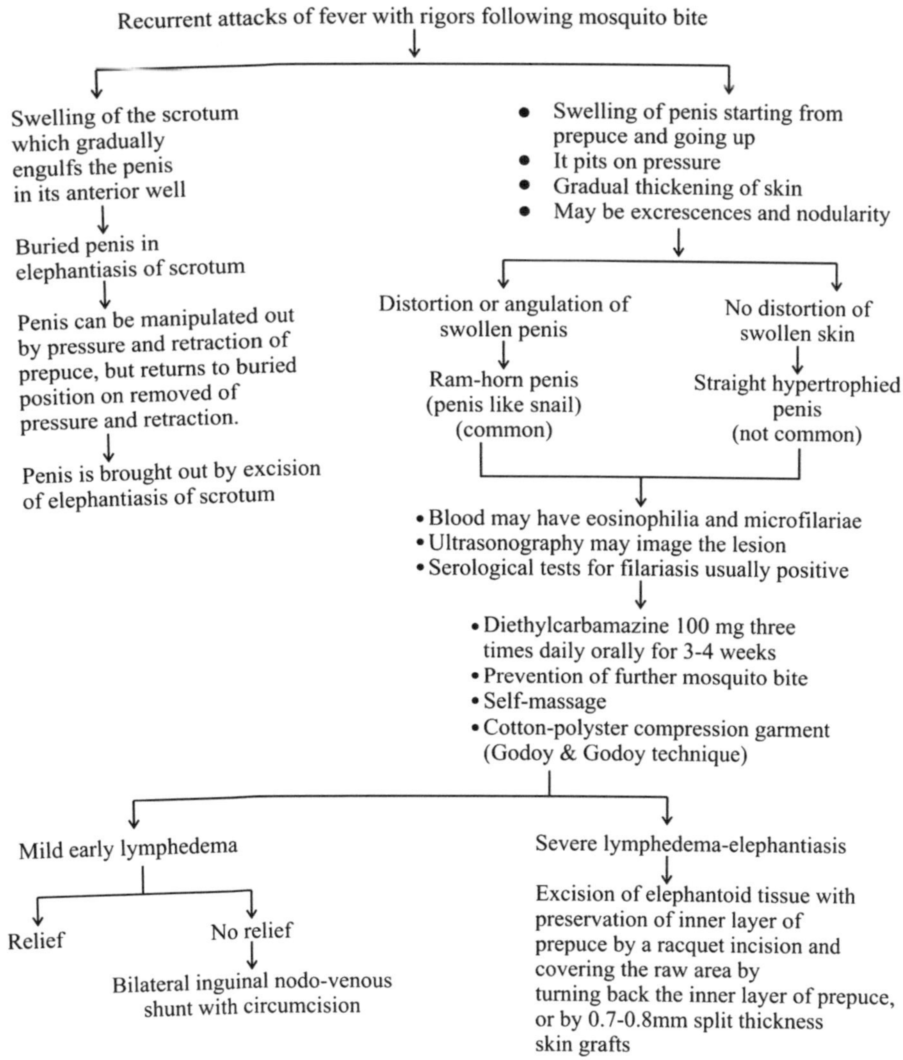

Flow Chart 23.1 Management of chronic lymphedema–elephantiasis of penis

References

Ahmed N. Filarial penis – Its variations and treatment. Indian J Surg. 1941;3:16–22.

Boeminghaus H. Chirurgie der Urogenitalorgane. Bad Worishofen: Banaschewski. 1950. Quoted by Prpic, 1966.

Bowesman C. Surgery and clinicel pathology in the topics Edinburgh & London: E&S Livingstone 1960; p 1036.

Cullen TH. Avulsion of skin of penis and scrotum. Br J Urol. 1966;38:99.

Dandapat MC, Mahapatro SK, Patro SK. Elephantiasis of the penis and scrotum: a review of 350 cases. Am J Surg. 1985;149:686–90.

de Godoy JMP, Facio Jr FN, Matias dc Carvalho EC, de Godoy Mde FG. New compression mechanism in penilelymphedema and sexual rehabilitation. Urol Ann. 2014;6(1):88–90.
De Greef R. Ann Soc Belges Med Trop Parasitol Mycol. 1938;18:5.
DeSavitsch 1941. Quoted by Morales PA, O'Connor JJ, Gordon SG. Surgical treatment of severe lymphedema of penis. J Urol. 1954;72:880.
Farina R, De Freire GC, Macedo A. Elephantiasis of the male genitalia; phallus-oscheo-plasty. Urol Int (Basel). 1958;6:50–60.
Feins NR. A new surgical technique for lymphedema of penis and scrotum. J Pediatr Surg. 1980;15:787–9.
Ferris DO. Traumatic avulsion of the skin of penis and scrotum. J Urol. 1949;62:523–7.
Gelbke H. [Penisskin transplantation]. Zentralbl Chir. 1954;79(22):935–42.
Hai AA, et al. Filarial lymphoedema of male genitalia. Second international conference on surgery in tropics, Bombay Hospital Institute of Medical Sciences. 1987. p. 22–27.
Khanna NN. Surgical treatment of elephantiasis of male genitalia. Plast Reconstr Surg. 1970;46(5):481–7.
Kinmonth JB. The lymphatics. 2nd ed. London: Edward Arnold; 1982. p. 193.
Kubacek V. Brit J Plast Surg 1957;10:25. Quoted by Prpic I. Severe elephantiasis of penis and scrotum. Brit J Plast Surg. 1966;19:173–8.
Lee S, Han JS, Ross HM, et al. Massive localized lymphedema of the male external genitalia: a clinicopathologic study of 6 cases. Hum Pathol. 2014;44:277–81.
Manson-Bahr PEC, Apted FIC. Filariases. In: Manson's tropical diseases. 18th ed. London: Bailliere Tindal; 1982. p. 148–80.
Modolin M, Mitre AI, et al. Surgical treatment of lymphedema of the penis and scrotum. Clinics (Sao Paulo). 2006;61:289–94.
Morales PA, O'Connor JJ, Gordon SG. Surgical treatment of severe lymphedema of penis. J Urol. 1954;72:880–5.
Nielubowicz J, Olszewski W. Surgical lymphatico-venous shunts. Br J Surg. 1968;55:440–2.
Nielubowicz J, Olszewski W. J Cardiovasc Surg. Special issue for XVth Congress of European Society of Cardiovascular Surgery. 1966;384.
Ollapallil JJ, Watters DAK. Surgical management of elephantiasis of male genitalia. Br J Urol. 1995;76:213–315.
Paletta FX. Reconstructive surgical problems of penis. Plast Reconstr Surg. 1952;10:191–203.
Paradysz A, Prokopowicz G, Pindycka-Piaszczynska M, Bryniarski P, Zyczkowski M. Idiopathic scrotal, penile and perineal elephantiasis – successful surgical treatment. Cent European J Urol. 2010;63:51–3.
Prasad S. Filariasis penis. Br J Urol. 1976;48:426.
Prpic I. Severe elephantiasis of penis and scrotum. Br J Plast Surg. 1966;19:173–8.
Ross JC. Brit J Surg. 1941–1942;29:194. Quoted by Prpic I. Severe elephantiasis of penis and scrotum. Brit J Plast Surg. 1966;19:173–8.
Rowan RL, Howley TF. Etheron sponge dressing for skin grafting. J Urol. 1965;93:709–10.
Russe O. [Dermatome plastic surgery of the penis]. Chirurg. 1955;26(5):228–9.
Sandeepa S, Rao K, Hemalatha AN, Shenoy V. A rare case of isolated primary penile lymphedema. Indian J Appl Res. 2015;5(3):449–50.
Schook CC, Kulungowski AM, Greene AK, Fishman SJ. Male genital lymphedema: clinical features and management of 25 pediatric patients. J Pediatr Surg. 2014;49:1647–951.
Singh V, Sinha RJ, Sankhwar SN, Kumar V. Reconstructive surgery for penoscrotal filarial lymphedema: a decade of experience and follow up. Urology. 2011;77:1228–31.
Streli R. Traumatic avulsion of skin of penis and scrotum (with amputation of both testes). Chirurg. 1958;29:467–70.

Chronic Lymphedema–Elephantiasis of Upper Extremity

24

The lymphatic filariasis is an uncommon cause of chronic lymphedema–elephantiasis of upper extremity but filarial lymphedema–elephantiasis of upper limb is still seen in tropical and subtropical countries.

24.1 Etiology

The causes of chronic lymphedema of upper extremity are given below.

1. Post-mastectomy lymphedema – It is the most common cause of upper limb lymphedema that occurs following radical mastectomy. A combination of excision of axillary lymphatics and postoperative radiotherapy is most likely to cause lymphatic obstruction (Kinmonth 1982). Another etiological factor is destruction of lymphatics by tumor invasion.
2. Lymphatic filariasis causing adenolymphatic obstruction following mosquito bite in the upper extremity – Gooneratne (1969) has shown that the site of mosquito bite and inoculation of third stage larvae determines the site of development of future adult worms in the regional lymphatics and lymph nodes, hence the probable future site of lymphedema.

   Babu et al. (2001) have reported two patients of elephantiasis of arm in males and five patients in females from Khurda district of Orissa (India).
3. Tuberculosis of axillary lymph nodes with destruction of lymph nodes.
4. Chronic eczema and recurrent bacterial infection of the upper extremity – Multiple repeated bacterial infections by streptococci or staphylococci damage the lymphatics permanently causing lymphedema. The lymphedema itself with its stagnant protein-rich fluid is more prone to infections and inflammation. Hence, the condition becomes self-perpetuating (Kinmonth 1982).
5. Wounds with extensive or circumferential skin loss and scar formation (Kinmonth 1982) – Such a wound should be repaired with flaps or pedicle grafts supplying normal lymphatics in the defect as early as possible before the occurrence of irreversible damage to the distal normal lymphatics.

T.C. Goel, A. Goel, *Lymphatic Filariasis*, DOI 10.1007/978-981-10-2257-9_24

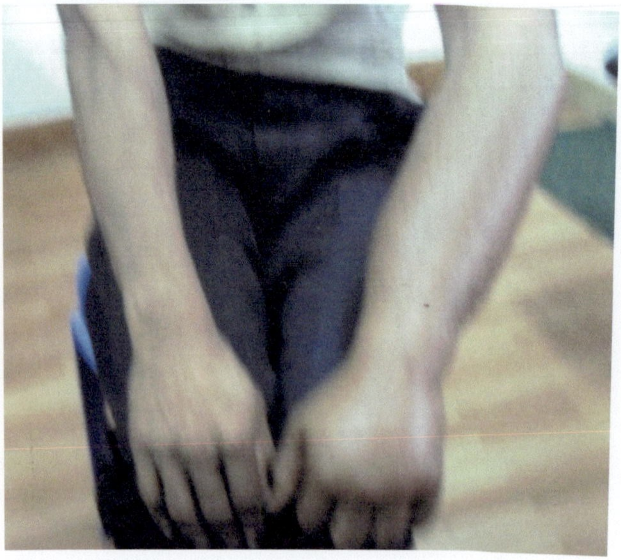

Fig. 24.1 Lymphedema of left upper extremity

6. Rheumatoid arthritis of distal upper extremity, i.e., hand and forearm.
7. Extrinsic pressure of lymphatics (and veins) (Fig. 24.1).

The risk factors include obesity, congenital predisposition, venipuncture and injection in upper extremity, measuring blood pressure, insertion of pacemaker leads, arterio-venous shunt for dialysis, and air travel (Homer-Vanniasinkam and Russell 2013).

The complications, investigations, and treatment are nearly the same as described for chronic lymphedema–elephantiasis of the lower extremity.

References

Babu BV, Acharya AS, Mallick G, et al. Lymphatic filariasis in Khurda district of Orrisa, India: An epidemiological study. SE Asian J Trop Med Public Health. 2001;32(2):240–3.

Gooneratne BWM. Lymphography of filarial infections. Lecture at St Thomas's Hospital, London, 1969. Quoted by Kinmonth, 1982.

Homer-Vanniasinkam S, Russell DA. Lymphatic disorders. In: Williams NS, Bulstrode CJK, O'Connell PR, editors. Bailey & love's short practice of surgery. 26th ed. London: CRC Press; 2013. p. 923–40.

Kinmonth JB. The lymphatics. 2nd ed. London: Edward Arnold; 1982. p. 145–58.

25 Filarial Manifestations of Female Breast

The breast is not commonly affected by lymphatic filarial infection. When it is involved, it is usually bancroftian filarial infection.

The adult filarial worms may reside in the lymphatics of the breast. The containing lymphatic is dilated and tortuous (varicose) due to the action of certain "toxins" produced by the live worms, though Kinmonth (1982) does not agree with this hypothesis. Here, they can be detected by finding "filarial dance sign" of actively moving worms with the use of Doppler probe with ultrasonography (Fig. 25.1).

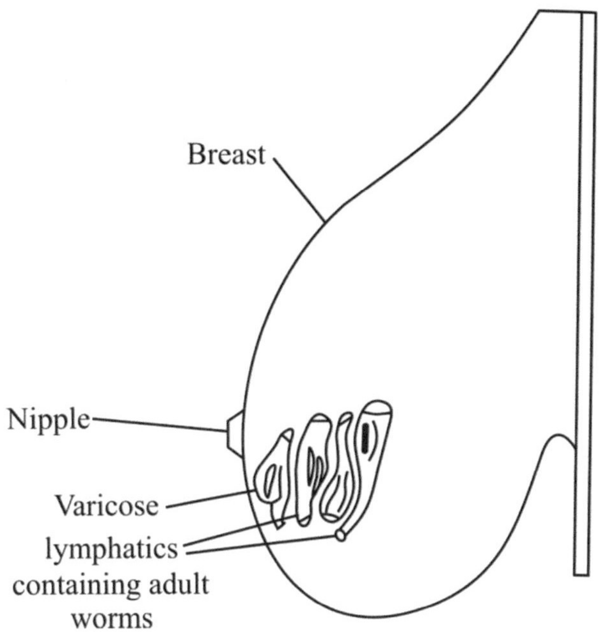

Fig. 25.1 Lump of varicose lymphatics with "filarial dance sign" due to presence of live and active worms

T.C. Goel, A. Goel, *Lymphatic Filariasis*, DOI 10.1007/978-981-10-2257-9_25

25.1 Classification of Filarial Manifestations of Breast

- Acute manifestations – lymphangitis, cellulitis, abscess
- Chronic manifestations
  1. Chronic lymphedema–elephantiasis
  2. Filarial lump or nodules
  3. Filarial lymph varix

25.1.1 Acute Manifestations

When the adult worm residing in the dilated lymphatics die either spontaneously or following the use of filaricidal drugs, there is an acute reaction leading to acute inflammation of the containing lymphatics (lymphangitis) and diffuse inflammation of the surrounding tissue (cellulitis).

Acute lymphangitis is characterized by the presence of linear red streaks in an ill-defined red area radiating from a central nodule. Cellulitis is characterized by a diffuse red patch of acute inflammation with an indistinct edge or border. As time passes, one or more abscesses may appear which contain dead or decaying worms as a whole or its segments.

The treatment is symptomatic and supportive. The ideal antibiotic is doxycycline 100–200 mg daily for 4–6 weeks because of its cidal action on Wolbachia, an intracellular endosymboint of adult filarial worms.

25.1.2 Chronic Lymphedema–Elephantiasis of Breast

It is an uncommon manifestation of lymphatic filariasis occurring in female breast in filaria-infested regions (Fig. 25.2).

This manifestation is characterized by chronic lymphedema of skin and the underlying subcutaneous tissue of the breast due to adenolymphatic obstruction in the axilla. The glandular tissue of the breast remains unaffected. The edema and subsequent elephantoid change starts in the most dependent part of the breast (fundus) and progresses slowly upwards.

25.1.2.1 Clinical Features

The patient is about 30–40 years of age and presents with recurrent attacks of fever with rigors associated with severe pain and lymphangitis. Every attack leaves behind some swelling of the breast which grows in size with every fresh attack of filariasis. Due to increasing weight, the breast becomes pendulous and may hang down up to the thigh or even knee of that side.

The edema starts in the lowermost part of the breast and then grows upwards as the disease progresses. Initially, the skin is edematous but is otherwise normal, Later on, it becomes thick, rough and dry due to fibrosis in the lymphedematous

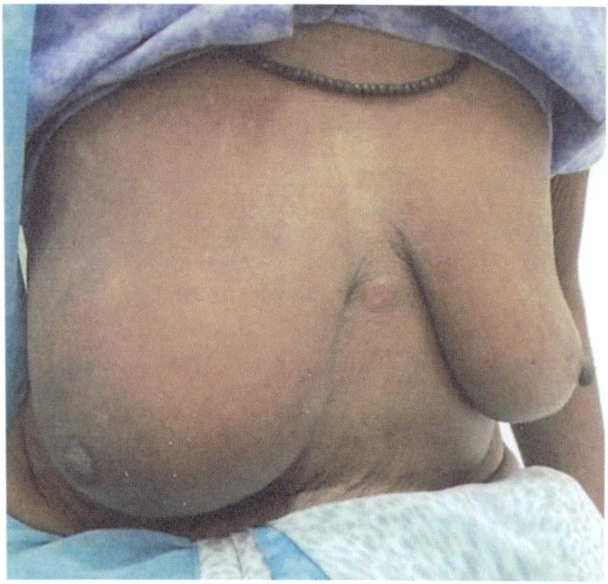

Fig. 25.2 Chronic filarial lymphedema–elephantiasis of female breast with swollen and hanging down breast

tissue. With further progress, the skin may have wart-like projections, excoriations and ulceration.

The areola may have similar changes. The nipple may be retracted with fissures in the areola. The veins of the skin may stand out prominently under the skin. The ipsilateral axillary lymph nodes may be enlarged, discrete and rubbery.

25.1.2.2 Investigations

The blood may show eosinophilia and microfilariae in the night blood smear, especially during the acute attacks. The serological tests for filariasis may be positive.

The chronic lymphedema–elephantiasis can be imaged by ultrasonography, especially to rule out a malignant lesion by FNAC done at the same time. Live motile adult worms may be found in the dilated and tortuous lymphatics in the breast ("filarial dance sign"; Amaral et al. 1994).

25.1.2.3 Treatment

A course of diethylcarbamazine 100 mg three times daily orally is given for 3–4 weeks together with symptomatic treatment, elevation of breast and breast support. It may be enough in early disease.

The late disease is treated by excision of elephantoid tissue, i.e. the diseased skin and subcutaneous tissue is excised and the hanging breast is lifted up (reduction mammoplasty). The reconstruction of nipple and areola may be required. The treated breast must match with the opposite breast. The management of chronic lymphedema–elephantiasis of the breast is described in the following Flow Chart 25.1:

- Recurrent attacks of fever with rigors with increasing swelling of one breast
- Maximum in the lower-most part or fundus of breast
- Initially it pits on pressure which gradually becomes less and less
- Breast hangs lower down and may reach up to thigh or knee

↓

- Blood may show eosinophilia and microfilariae
- Ultrasonography images the lesion and may show live adult worms in a dilated lymphatic ('filarial dance sign')

↓

Chronic filarial lymphedema-elephantiasis of breast

↓ Early disease

↓

- Diethylcarbamazine 100 mg three times daily orally for 3-4 weeks
- Breast support, compression and elevation
- Prevention of further mosquito bite

↓ Late or advanced disease

↓

Excision of elephantoid tissue with reconstruction to match with the opposite breast (reduction mammoplasty)

Flow Chart 25.1 Management of chronic lymphedema–elephantiasis of female breast

25.1.3 Filarial Lump or Nodules

Sometimes the patient presents with a lump or nodule in the breast which is a mass of granulation tissue formed around a dead adult worm or its decaying segments. It is a unilateral, painless and nontender mass of insidious onset. The most common sites are the upper and lower outer quadrants. Hyperemia of the overlying skin with peau de orange and axillary lymph node enlargement may be present (Lahiri 1975; Lang et al. 1987).

Mukerjee et al. (1977) reported a patient who had a stationary lump in the breast due to filariasis.

Upadhyaya et al. (2006) reported a case of an ill-defined lump in the central part of left breast due to filariasis in a female 55 years of age.

The blood may show eosinophilia and microfilaremia. The serological tests for filariasis are usually positive. Lahiri (1975) found microfilariae in the nipple secretion of a patient with a filarial breast mass.

Mammography Upadhyaya et al. (2006) did mammography of a filarial lump in the left breast and found a band-like opacity in the central and upper outer part of the breast.

Ultrasonography Upadhyaya et al. (2006) did ultrasonography using a high-frequency transducer of 11–14 MHz in the patient described above. They found cystic lesions in the central and outer part of the left breast (dilated lymphatics). Within these lesions were seen vigorously moving clusters of small echogenic structures ("filarial dance sign") (Figs. 25.3 and 25.4). Ultrasound-guided fine-

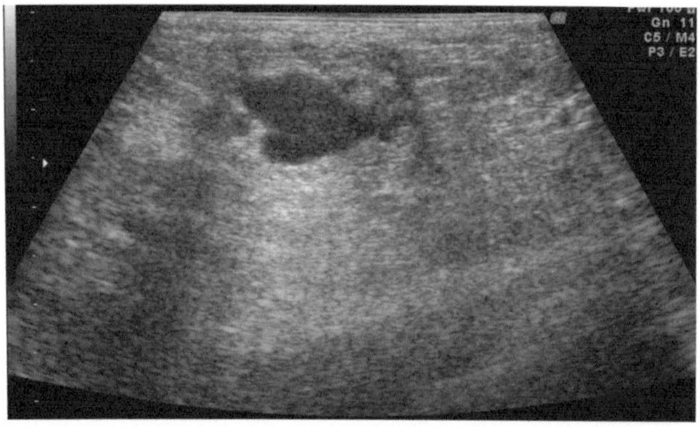

Fig. 25.3 Ultrasonography of breast showing cystic lesions in the breast due to filariasis (Courtesy – Dr. S.S. Sarkar of Sarkar Diagnostics)

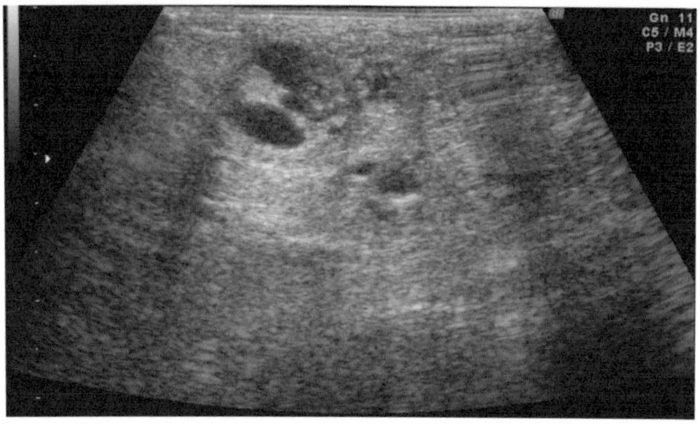

Fig. 25.4 Ultrasonography of the breast showing cystic lesions. Shadows of filarial worms are visible in the lower lesion ("filarial dance sign")

needle aspiration done at the same time showed microfilariae on microscopic examination of the aspirate.

In a late lesion, the dead and fragmented worms may calcify and present as elongated and serpiginous shadows with no evidence of irregularity or pleomorphism. They are not oriented or adjacent to the ducts. Due to their situation in connective tissue unrelated to ducts they can be differentiated from calcification of intraduct carcinoma (Friedman and Kalisher 2002). Hence, in filarial endemic areas, a breast lump may be filarial. Therefore, it must be ultrasonographed for "filarial dance sign."

25.1.3.1 Treatment

The patient is given a course of diethylcarbamazine 100 mg three times daily orally for 3–4 weeks with breast support. The lump may disappear gradually with this treatment. Otherwise, it should be excised.

25.1.4 Filarial Lymph Varix

MacFee described a case of a woman aged 30 years who presented (in May 1925) with a swelling in the lateral half of the right breast that had large tortuous soft fluctuant areas resembling huge varicose veins. She was a migrant to the USA from

British Guyana with a positive history of filariasis. The lesion was aspirated with recovery of straw-colored fluid having live microfilariae seen during microscopic examination. To study the lymph vessels of the breast, an injection of lipiodol was made in June 1928 following which the patient developed fever and chills with elevated local temperature. The swelling gradually reduced and the breast returned to normal (at that time, no specific treatment was available for filariasis).

References

Amaral F, Dreyer G, Figueredo-Silva J, et al. Live adult worms detected by ultrasonography in human Bancroftian filariasis. Am J Trop Med Hyg. 1994;50(6):753–7.

Friedman PD, Kalisher L. Filariasis. Radiology. 2002;222:515–7.

Kinmonth JB. The lymphatics. 2nd ed. London: Edward Arnold; 1982.

Lahiri VL. Microfilariae in nipple secretion. Acta Cytol. 1975;19:154–5.

Lang AP, Luchsinger IS, Rowling EG. Filariasis of breast. Arch Pathol Lab Med. 1987;111:757–9.

MacFee WF. Filarial lymphatic varix of the breast. NY Surg Soc Philadelphia Acad. 1925–1931;135–139.

Mukerjee DR, Gupta A, Sengupta P. Solitary filarial breast lump. J Indian Med Assoc. 1977;69:36–8.

Upadhyaya V, Upadhyaya DN, Sarkar SS. An interesting case of breast filariasis. Indian J Radial Imaging. 2006;16(4):915–7.

Chronic Lymphedema–Elephantiasis of the Vulva

26

Chronic lymphedema–elephantiasis of the vulva is a very uncommon manifestation of lymphatic filariasis. Its incidence is not more than 1–2 % of all the cases of filarial elephantiasis (Khanna and Joshi 1971; Ipyana et al. 2014).

26.1 Etiology

Lymphatic filariasis due to *Wuchereria bancrofti* is the most common cause of chronic lymphedema–elephantiasis of the vulva in tropical and subtropical countries. Chaudhary et al. (2013) reported a case of vulvar elephantiasis of filarial origin. Ipyana et al. (2014) described another case of a 21-year-old female who had massive vulvar elephantiasis of the right labium majus of 2 years' duration. Her blood was positive for microfilariae.

Other causes of vulvar elephantiasis include lymphogranuloma venereum, granuloma inguinale, and metastatic carcinoma of inguinal lymph nodes and its treatment by block dissection, irradiation, or both. Chintamani et al. (2010) have reported two patients with vulvar elephantiasis due to inguinal lymph node tuberculosis. Further, it may be a rare extra-intestinal manifestation of Crohn's disease (Schulman et al. 1987; Fenniche et al. 1997).

26.2 Pathology

The swelling starts in the most dependent and posterior part of the labia and progresses forwards and upwards and may extend into the mons veneris. Posteriorly, it may extend into the perineum but the anal orifice is never involved or distorted.

Grossly, it is a bosselated firm fibrous mass. Microscopically, it shows stratified squamous epithelium with acanthosis and hyperkeratosis. The underlying stroma shows dermal fibrosis and collagenization with mixed inflammatory infiltrate in the

T.C. Goel, A. Goel, *Lymphatic Filariasis*, DOI 10.1007/978-981-10-2257-9_26

form of eosinophils, polymorphs, lymphocytes, macrophages, and plasma cells (Chaudhary et al. 2013). It may show non-caseating granuloma along with foreign body giant cells (Mohan et al. 2012).

26.3 Clinical Features

The patient is usually 30–40 years of age and presents with chronic or recurrently growing swelling and disfigurement of the vulva. The skin is thickened, rough, and dry. The pubic hair become less and less as the disease progresses. The labia majora of one or both sides become firm and nodular (Fig. 26.1). There may be small wart-like swellings, a few of which may be scattered over the pubic region. They have a different consistency at different sites (Ipyana et al. 2014). These swellings are painless. The labia minora are usually not involved (Pani 2013).

Vesicles and fistulae may form on the labia and around the clitoris producing discharge (lymphorrhea), discomfort, pruritus, and dyspareunia. The vaginal orifice may be closed due to swelling of both labia majora (Pani 2013). It may be associated with dragging pain or discomfort, difficulty in walking and psychological distress.

It may also be associated with other manifestations of lymphatic filariasis.

26.4 Investigations

- The blood may show eosinophilia and rarely microfilariae especially if the patient had a recent attack of filariasis. The serological tests for filariasis are usually positive.
- Lymphography, by injection of contrast into the labia, shows dilated lymphatics with obstruction in the inguinal region.

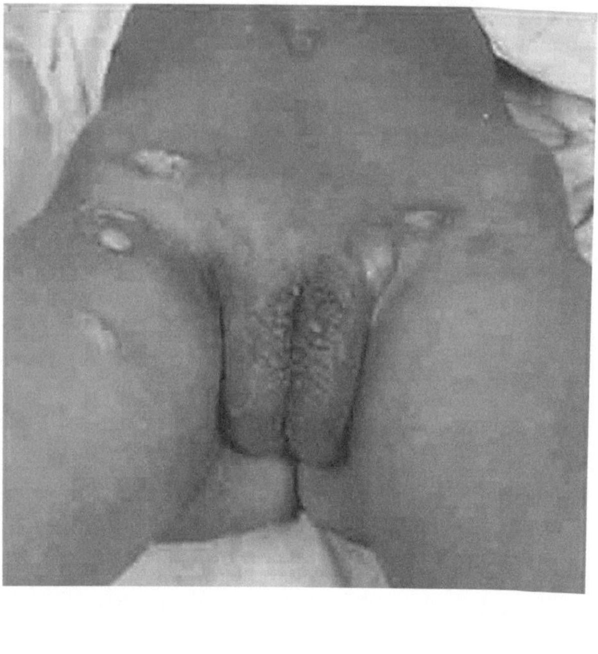

Fig. 26.1 Chronic lymphedema of the vulva (The scars of filarial suppurating lymph nodes are visible on both inguinal regions)

- FNAC or biopsy of the swelling may be done. The needle aspirate may show microfilariae. Biopsy may be done to rule out malignancy. In filarial disease, the histologic findings are nonspecific and nondiagnostic and show chronic inflammation with fibrosis. Hence, the diagnosis is confirmed with the help of serologic tests of filariasis. Mohan et al. (2012) reported a case of vulvar elephantiasis where the filarial antigen test was positive.

26.5 Complications

The most important but rare complication of this manifestation is angiosarcoma (Miller et al. 1998; Kim et al. 2004).

26.6 Treatment

A full course of diethylcarbamazine is given especially if the patient had a recent attack of filariasis. Compression garments may be of help.

Surgical treatment The filarial elephantoid tissue is excised to give near normal shape to the vulva.

In advanced disease, complete or partial excision of the labia majora, reduction of the labia minora, and circumcision of the clitoris may be needed. All this may be combined with reduction of mons veneris (vulvaplasty). The lymphoid condylomata are excised en bloc with the elephantoid tissue and rarely by individual excision and the excised tissue is sent for histopathological examination.

The flow chart given below describes the management of chronic lymphedema–elephantiasis of the vulva:

- Recurrent attacks of fever with rigors and inguinal adenolymphangitis
- Recurrent or progressive swelling of vulva which pits on pressure
- Gradually changes to nonpitting edema and elephantiasis

↓

- Blood may show eosinophilia and microfilariae
- Serological tests for filariasis may be positive
- Lymphography shows inguinal adenolymphatic obstruction
- FNAC or biopsy may be required

↓

Filarial chronic lymphedema-elephantiasis of vulva

↓ (left branch)

- Diethylcarbamazine 100 mg thrice daily orally for 3-4 weeks
- Prevention of further mosquito bite
- Pressure garment
- Symptomatic treatment

↓

- Relief in mild or early disease

↓ (right branch)

Advanced disease

↓

Excision of lymphedematous elephantoid tissue with circumcision of clitoris (vulvaplasty)

Flow Chart 26.1 Management of chronic filarial lymphedema–elephantiasis of the vulva

References

Chaudhary R, Rathi S, Maheshwari A, Nigam S. Vulval elephantiasis of filarial origin: a case report. Indian J Clin Pract. 2013;24(2):160–2.

Chintamani Singh JP, Tandon M, et al. Vulval elephantiasis as a result of tubercular lymphadenitis: two case reports and review of literature. J Med Case Rep. 2010;4:369.

Fenniche S, Mokni M, Haouet S, Ben OA. Vulvar Crohn disease: 3 cases. Ann Dermatol Venereol. 1997;124:629–32.

Ipyana HM, Bonaventura CTM, Januarius H. Vulvar filarial elephantiasis in a Tanzanian woman: rare presentation of lymphatic filariasis: a case report and review of literature. Sudan JMS. 2014;9(4):265–70.

Khanna NN, Joshi GK. Elephantiasis of female genitalia. A case report. Plast Reconstr Surg. 1971;48:379–81.

Kim DL, Huh SH, Hwang JH, Joh JH. Excisional surgery for chronic advanced lymphedema. Surg Today. 2004;34:134–7.

Miller TA, Wyatt LE, Rudkun GH. Staged skin and subcutaneous excision for lymphedema: a favorable report of long-term results. Plast Recontr Surg. 1998;102:1486–98.

Mohan H, Bisht B, Goel P, Garg G. Vulval elephantiasis: a case report. Case Rep Infect Dis. 2012;2012:430745. doi:10.1155/2012/430745.

Pani S. Pani's filariasis. 3rd ed. New Delhi: Jaypee Brothers; 2013.

Schulman D, Beck LS, Roberts IM, Schwartz AM. Crohn's disease of vulva. Am J Gastroenterol. 1987;82:1328–30.

27 Filarial Lymph Varix

It is a localized dilatation and tortuosity of lymphatic vessels and lymph spaces of the lymph nodes (sinuses of the lymph nodes) due to filarial adenolymphatic obstruction. It results in two types of lesions –

1. Lymphangiovarix or lymphangiectasis – It is a localized bunch of dilated and tortuous lymphatics (like a varicocele). It mostly occurs in the spermatic cord.
2. Lymphadenovarix or varicose lymph glands – It is the dilatation of lymph spaces of the lymph node due to obstruction of its efferent lymphatics.

27.1 Lymphangiovarix

It is a localized dilatation and tortuosity of a group of lymphatic vessels which can occur in the spermatic cord, scrotum, lower extremity, upper extremity (Figs. 27.1 and 27.2), breast, and retroperitoneum, but it is most manifest clinically in the spermatic cord.

Pathology The spermatic cord contains a bunch of dilated and tortuous lymphatics containing watery fluid (Fig. 27.3). They may sometimes contain chyle.

Sometimes, there is a multiloculated elongated thin-walled translucent swelling in the cord. It is called "diffuse hydrocele of the cord."

Clinical Features The patient presents with a painless swelling of insidious onset in the spermatic cord (Fig. 27.4). A past history of fever with rigors and inguinal swelling is usually present. There may be some discomfort or heaviness. It may feel like a bag of worms and may have an impulse on coughing like a varicocele. It is translucent (Fig. 27.5). The swelling is maximum in the evening. It reduces gradually on lying down and hence is minimum in the morning upon getting up from the bed.

T.C. Goel, A. Goel, *Lymphatic Filariasis*, DOI 10.1007/978-981-10-2257-9_27

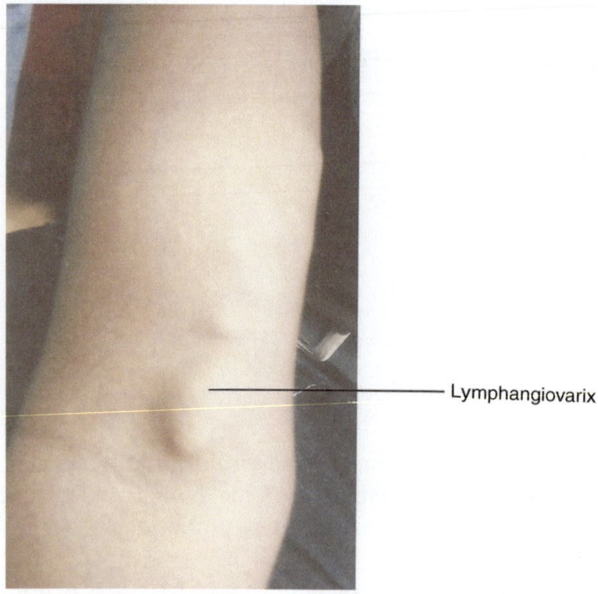

Fig. 27.1 Dilated and tortuous lymphatics (lymphangiovarix) of the right upper arm, which is translucent and shows "filarial dance sign" on ultrasonography (Courtesy – Dr. A.C. Dwivedi)

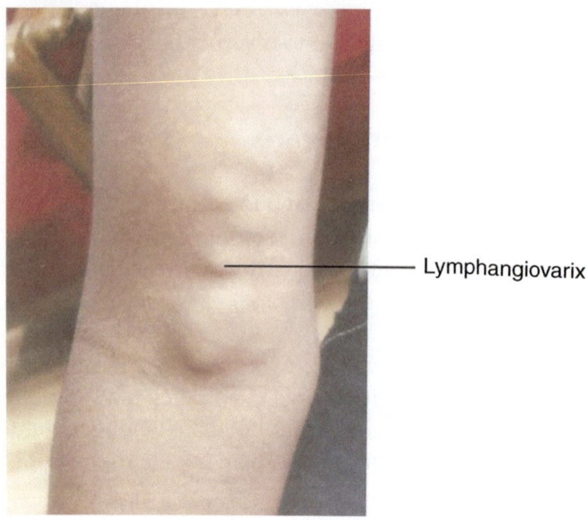

Fig. 27.2 Filarial lymphangiovarix of the right upper arm, which is translucent and shows "filarial dance sign" on ultrasonography (Courtesy – Dr. A.C. Dwivedi)

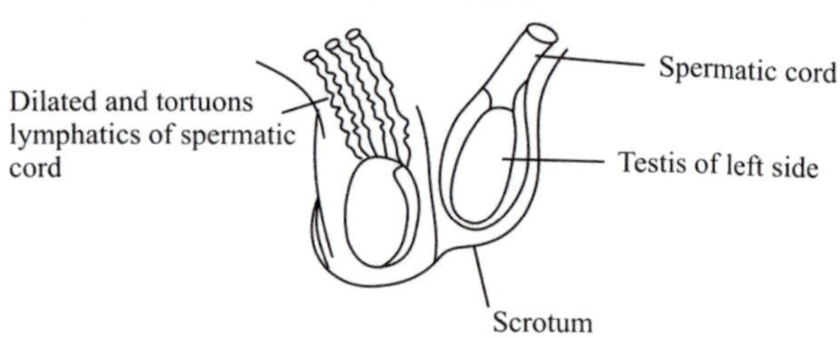

Fig. 27.3 Lymphangiovarix of the right spermatic cord

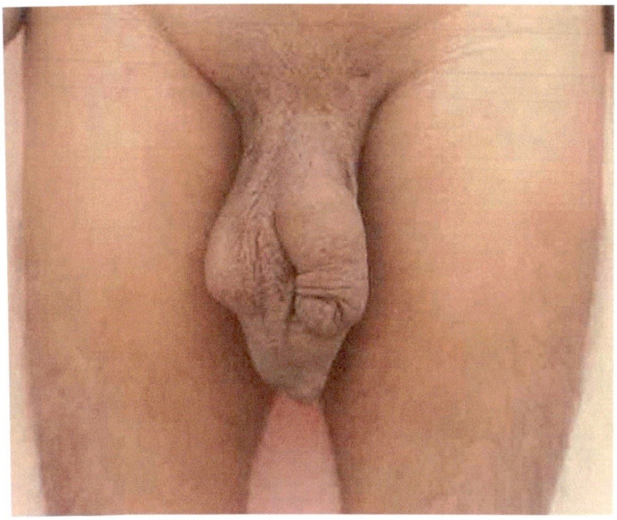

Fig. 27.4 Lymphangiovarix of the left spermatic cord with testis hanging lower down with mild chronic lymphedema of prepuce and distal penis

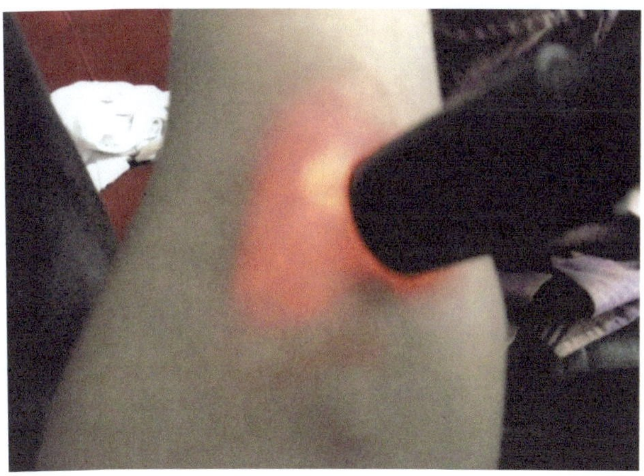

Fig. 27.5 Translucency seen in the lymphangiovarix. This is a picture of the patient shown in Figs. 27.1 and 27.2 (Courtesy – Dr. A.C. Dwivedi)

27.2 Lymphadenovarix

It is the enlargement of a lymph node due to dilatation of its lymphatic spaces caused by obstruction of its efferent lymphatics. It usually affects the inguinal or lymph nodes of the groin on one or both sides. Rarely, axillary lymph nodes are affected.

Fig. 27.6 Lymphadenovarix

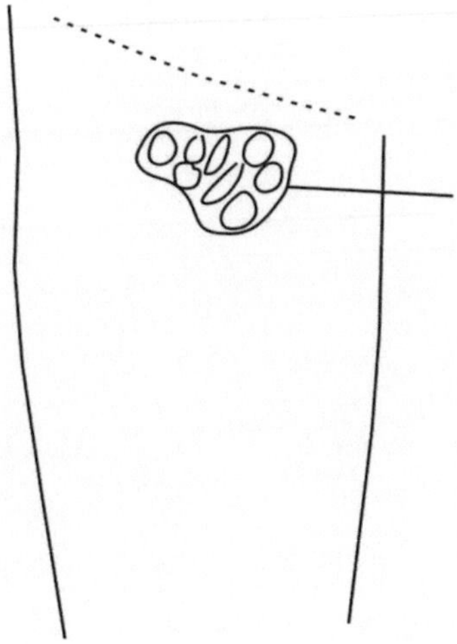

Pathology The affected lymph nodes are enlarged and may be lobulated. The cut surface shows many spaces containing watery fluid (Fig. 27.6). The remnants of a dead filarial worm may be present.

Clinical Features It can occur in both males and females, but more commonly in male adults of about 30–40 years of age. The patient is usually not aware of the existence of this lesion till the enlarged and dilated lymph nodes attain a significant size.

The affected lymph nodes are enlarged, lobulated, soft, cystic, nontender, and translucent. They grow slowly with time and are mobile (not attached to underlying structures or overlying skin). There may be a feeling of coiled rubber tubes interspersed with firm nodules under the skin. They may empty slowly with sustained compression and fill up again slowly after release of pressure. There is no cough impulse.

Kinmonth (1982) mentions about a Negro girl who migrated to Britain from British Guyana 5 years ago and presented with a swelling of the left groin for 3 months. It felt like an enlarged lymph node. Lymphography showed large tortuous inguinal lymphatics. A few months later, the patient came again with a much larger and fluctuant swelling in the left groin below the inguinal ligament. The midnight blood examination revealed swarms of microfilariae bancrofti.

Both these lesions, lymphangiovarix and lymphadenovarix, may be associated with other manifestations of lymphatic filariasis the most common being a hydrocele, lymph scrotum, and chylocele.

27.3 Investigations

The blood may show eosinophilia and microfilariae in the night blood smear. The serological tests for filariasis are likely to be positive.

Ultrasonography of the lesion reveals dilated lymphatics and dilated lymphatic spaces in the lymph nodes. They may show motile adult filarial worms or "filarial dance sign" (Amaral et al. 1994).

Aspiration of the lesion may reveal clear watery or milky fluid (lymph or chyle). It may have microfilariae.

Lymphography It shows extensive abnormalities involving the retroperitoneal lymphatics resembling those found in chyluria. The enormous dilatation and tortuosity of the inguinal and pelvic lymphatics is the most remarkable feature. Irregular diverticuliform projections may be found in the varicose lymphatics. This investigation is quite cumbersome and may further damage the lymphatics. Hence, rarely done now as most of these abnormalities can be visualized by ultrasonography and MRI.

27.4 Treatment

A course of diethylcarbamazine, 100 mg three times daily orally, is given for 3–4 weeks with symptomatic treatment, if any.

A localized large swelling may be excised but the healing may be delayed by lingering lymphatic fistulae (Fig. 27.7).

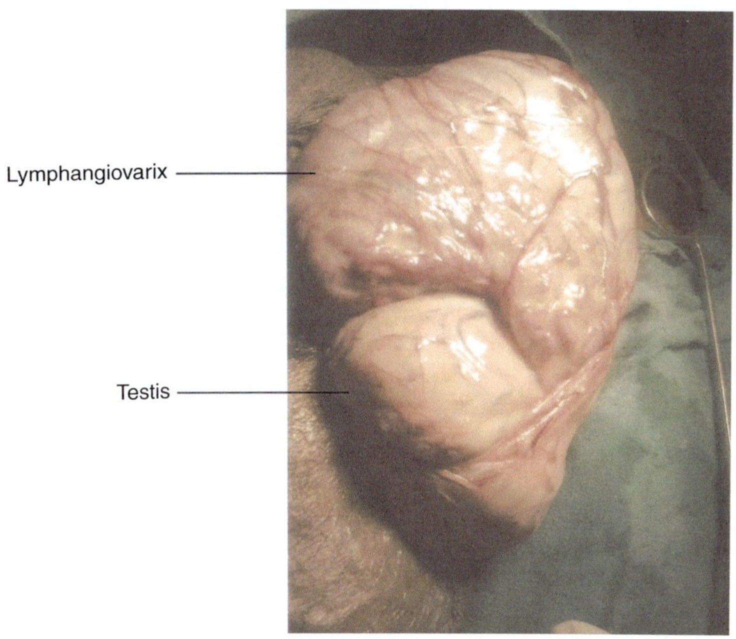

Fig. 27.7 Intraoperative appearance of lymphangiovarix of lower end of right spermatic cord

Recurrent attacks of fever with rigors

- Swelling in the lower part of spermatic cord
- Maximum on standing and reduces slowly on lying down
- Feels like a bag of worms
- Translucent

↓

- Lymphangiovarix

- Single or multiple enlarged lymph node at root of thigh
- Lobulated, soft, nontender and translucent
- Feels like coiled rubber tubes interspersed with firm nodules

↓

Lymphadenovarix

↓

- Blood may show eosinophilia and microfilariae
- Serological tests for filariasis may be positive
- Lesion can be imaged by ultrasonography or MRI

↓

- Diethylcarbamazine 100 mg three thims daily orally for 3-4 weeks
- Prevention of further mosquito bite
- Excision of lesion may result in delayed healing and lymphatic fistulae
- Nodo-venous shunt for lymphadenovarix

Flow Chart 27.1 Management of filarial lymph varix

Nodo-venous shunt (Nielubowicz and Olszewski 1966) may be done to deal with the lymphadenovarix in which the affected lymph node is anastomosed to a vein in the vicinity to drain the obstructed and dilated lymph node. The management of filarial lymph varix is described in the following flow chart 27.1:

References

Amaral F, Dreyer G, Figueredo-Silva J, et al. Live adult worms detected by ultrasonography in human bancroftian filariasis. Am J Trop Med Hyg. 1994;50(6):753.

Kinmonth JB. The lymphatics. 2nd ed. London: Edward Arnold; 1982.

Nielubowicz J, Olszewski W. Special issue for XVth Congress of European Society of Cardiovascular Surgery. J Cardiovasc Surg. 1966;384.

Lymph Scrotum (Superficial Scrotal Lymphangiomatosis) 28

Lymph scrotum is a urogenital manifestation of lymphatic filariasis characterized by the presence of multiple lymphatic vesicles on the surface of scrotum that may rupture easily with leakage of lymph (Aguiar-Santos et al. 2009). Its prevalence in endemic areas is not known, only isolated cases have been reported in the literature (Acton and Rao 1930; Addiss and Brady 2007; Belokar et al. 1983). It is a very crippling complication of lymphatic filariasis (DeVries 2002).

28.1 Etiology

The pathogenesis of lymph scrotum is not well-understood (Dreyer and Piessens 2000; Gyapong et al. 2000). It may occur following surgery for chylocele or hydrocele as it may follow partial excision of sac with "bottleneck" eversion of tunica vaginalis. Out of seven patients with lymph scrotum reported by Aguiar-Santos et al. (2009), two had a past history of hydrocele surgery. Hence, the current recommendation is complete excision of the tunica vaginalis with meticulous attention to cauterization and oversuturing the edge of the excised tunica (WHO 2002). The orientation of skin incision may have a role in the pathogenesis of lymph scrotum. Hence, a longitudinal incision is recommended for treating a filarial hydrocele as it avoids sectioning of superficial lymphatics of the scrotum (DeVries 2002). However, Aguiar-Santos et al. (2009) have reported two cases out of seven cases of lymph scrotum which followed hydrocele surgery with a longitudinal incision.

Acute attacks of dermatolymphangioadenitis (ADLA) due to secondary bacterial infection of lymphatic vessels that are quite superficial is the greatest risk factor for the occurrence of lymph scrotum (DeVries 2002).

T.C. Goel, A. Goel, *Lymphatic Filariasis*, DOI 10.1007/978-981-10-2257-9_28

28.2 Pathology

The superficial lymphatic vessels of skin of the scrotum are dilated and tortuous, and contain lymph (may be chyle). The lymph accumulates in the superficial layers of epidermis resulting in the formation of a large number of vesicles in the scrotal skin. The fluid in these cutaneous lymph cysts is clear like water (lymph) or slightly turbid or may be frank chyle (Figs. 28.1, 28.2, 28.5, and 28.6).

The full evolution of this manifestation takes from 2 to 15 years (Aguiar-Santos et al. 2009).

28.3 Clinical Features

It is one of the uncommon manifestations of filariasis. Ghooi and Khanna (1976) encountered two patients with lymph scrotum out of 90 patients with lymphatic filariasis. In our hospital, two patients with lymph scrotum were admitted out of 1539 patients with lymphatic filariasis admitted during 6 years (1979–1984).

The onset of this manifestation of filariasis is associated with many attacks of fever with rigors (Shenoy et al. 1995). The scrotum is swollen, with its rugosities becoming prominent, giving a silky touch to the scrotum. Later on, multiple cutaneous vesicles varying in size from a pin's head to a marble appear (Figs. 28.3 and 28.4). They are thin-walled, and hence may rupture due to friction leading to raw scrotum and continuous leakage of lymph from the scrotal surface (lymphorrhagia, lymphorrhea).

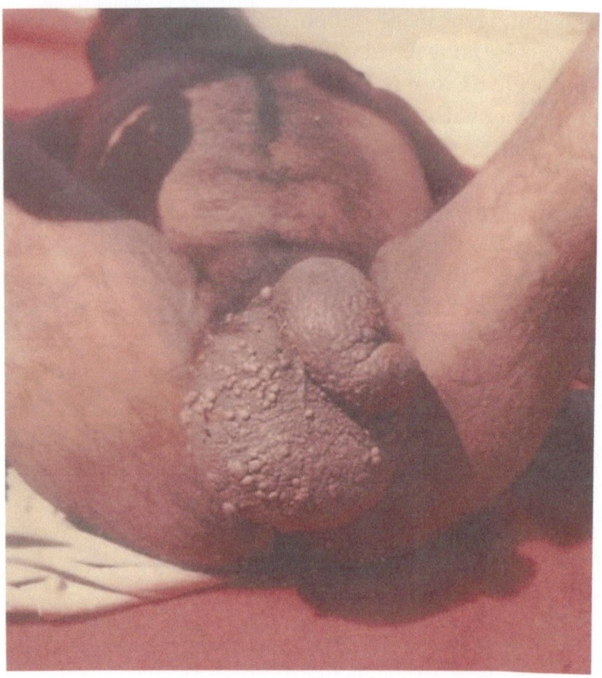

Fig. 28.1 Multiple small vesicles of lymph scrotum caused by filariasis

The drainage is profuse. It is like water and may be straw-colored, milky, or blood-tinged. About 225–280 mL of fluid may be lost in an hour or so leading to exhaustion of the patient (Manson-Bahr and Apted 1982).

The skin of the penis may also be involved including that of the entire shaft but limited by the corona glandis (DeVries 2002).

The lymph scrotum may be associated with other manifestations of filariasis, especially inguinal lymphadenovarix and chyluria.

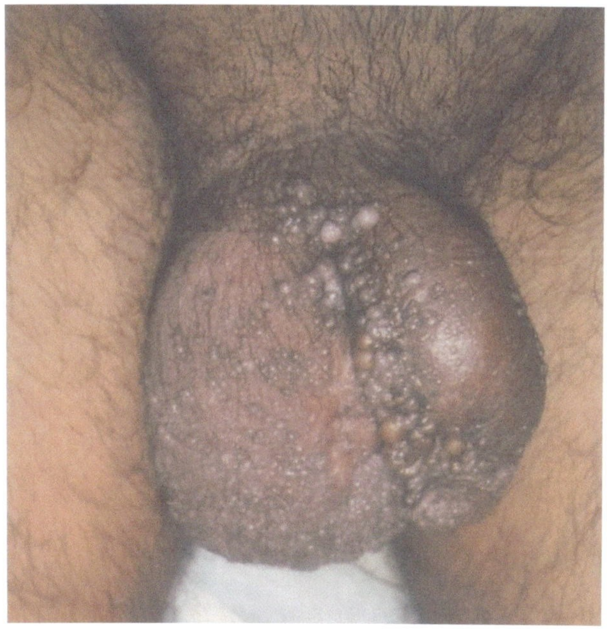

Fig. 28.2 Filarial lymphedema of penis and scrotum with multiple lymph vesicles of scrotum and penis

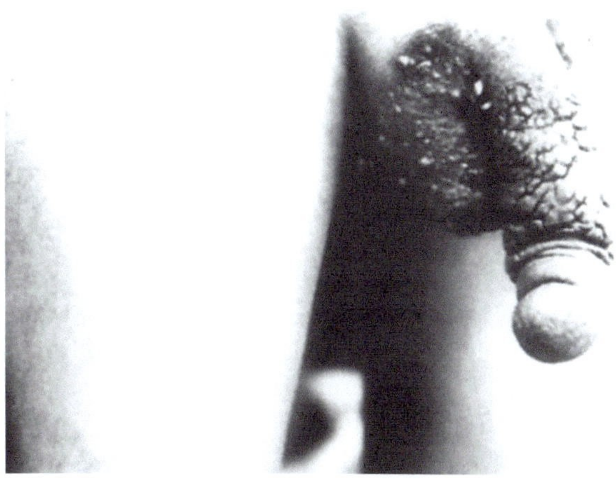

Fig. 28.3 Multiple lymph vesicles of scrotum and penis caused by lymphatic filariasis

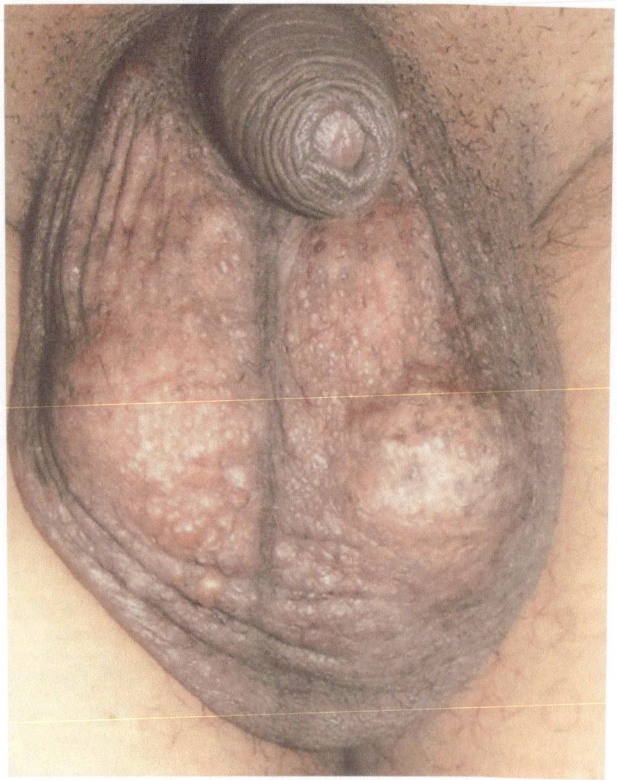

Fig. 28.4 Multiple lymph vesicles of scrotum caused by lymphatic filariasis

28.4 Complications

1. *Infection* – The weeping scrotum invites secondary bacterial/fungal infection which prevents the patient from going to his job and harms social interactions. In order to carry out their routine activities, some patients cover their scrotum with plastic, toilet paper, or cloth (Aguiar-Santos et al. 2009). During attacks of infection, it may not be possible to do sexual intercourse.
2. *Lymphedema–elephantiasis of the scrotum* – Repeated attacks of lymph scrotum with infection gradually results in lymphedema–elephantiasis of the scrotum.

28.5 Investigations

- *Blood* – The blood may show leukocytosis, eosinophilia, and microfilariae (maybe by polycarbonate membrane filtration). It may be sent for culture and sensitivity during acute attacks to find the nature of secondary invading organisms. Serological confirmation of the diagnosis may be required by ELISA and immunochromatographic test (ICT-AD12).

- *Doppler ultrasonography* of the scrotum may show the movements of live adult filarial worms (*Wuchereria bancrofti*) in dilated scrotal lymphatics ("filarial dance sign") (Amaral et al. 1994). Out of seven patients with lymph scrotum as reported by Aguiar-Santos et al. (2009), two patients revealed "filarial dance sign" on scrotal ultrasonography. Other findings include lymphangiectasia in five patients, hydrocele in three patients, nodules in the scrotum of three patients, testicular and epididymal abnormalities in four patients, inguinal adenomegaly in one patient, and scrotal lymphangitis in one patient.
- *Lymphography* – Sen et al. (1969) did lymphography in these patients and found extensive abnormalities in the lymphatics of the inguinal region and retroperitoneum.

28.6 Treatment

A course of diethylcarbamazine (DEC) is given and further mosquito bites are prevented. Doxycycline 200 mg daily orally may be a better drug as it will eliminate the adult worms by killing endosymbiont *Wolbachia* and control secondary bacterial infection as it is a broad-spectrum antibiotic. In regions where coinfection with onchocerciasis is common, a single dose of ivermectin 400 μg/kg and albendazole 400 mg is recommended (Dreyer and Piessens 2000). Other measures include maintenance of local hygiene as done in lymphedema of extremities and antibiotic prophylaxis using benzathine penicillin (Addiss and Brady 2007). The antibiotic therapy may depend on the culture and sensitivity report of the discharge. Locally, a bland antiseptic powder may be used. If the fluid loss is significant, fluid, electrolyte, and nutritional support may be required. If a lymphatic fistula is present, it may be electrocauterized.

Surgical Treatment Most of the patients are relieved by the conservative measures described above. However, surgery may be required in a few cases (DeVries 2002), as this disease is irreversible in nature. The surgical treatment includes excision of diseased skin and subcutaneous tissue. The scrotal raw area is covered by mesh skin grafting and the penile area with full thickness skin grafting. The management of lymph scrotum is summarized in the following Flow Chart 28.1:

28.7 Prophylaxis

- Prevention of filariasis by the measures recommended in the global program for elimination of lymphatic filariasis.
- Adequate surgery of hydrocele in endemic areas – the hydrocele should never be considered simple in patients living in endemic areas (Aguiar-Santos et al. 2009)

- Recurrent attacks of fever with rigors
- Diffuse swelling of scrotum which increases with every attack with prominent rugosities with silk touch
- Large number of vesicles on the scrotum varying from a pin's head to a marble
- They contain lymph, sometimes chyle, and rupture due to friction

↓

Lymphorrhea or chylorrhea

↓

- May result in fluid, electrolyte and nutritional imbalance
- Secondary bacterial and/or fungal infection is common

↓

- Blood may show eosinophilia, microfilariae and leukocytosis
- Serological tests for filariasis are usually positive

↓

- Diethylcarbamazine 100 mg three times daily orally for 3-4 weeks, ivermectin+albendazole in onchocerciasis infested regions
- Prevention of further mosquito bite
- Antibiotics especially doxycycline to control filariasis and secondary bacterial infection
- Maintenance of local hygiene with bland antiseptic powder locally
- Electrocauterization of lymphatic fistula
- Severe problem may require scrotectomy with skin grafting

Flow Chart 28.1 Management of lymph scrotum

and the operative treatment should be done with utmost care with specific stress on the following points:

1. It should be done with a longitudinal incision, though it may occur following this type of incision also.
2. The hydrocele sac should be excised completely with meticulous attention to cauterization of the cut edge and oversuturing (DeVries 2002; WHO 2002).

28.8 Chylous Lymph Scrotum

Sen et al. (1969) described a case of chylous lymph scrotum with oozing milky chyle (chylorrhea) from some ruptured vesicles of the skin of the scrotum. The scrotal skin was velvety and had a number of vesicles containing milky fluid (Figs. 28.5, 28.6, 28.7, and 28.8). A past history of chyluria was present. This manifestation of filariasis can affect the vulva of a woman (Fig. 28.9).

Lymphangiography showed the findings that are seen in patients of chyluria with lymphadenovariceal changes in pelvic lymphatics. The most distinctive finding was the abnormal opacification of lymphatics of anterior abdominal wall and inguino-scrotal lymphatics with retrograde flow extending into scrotal skin.

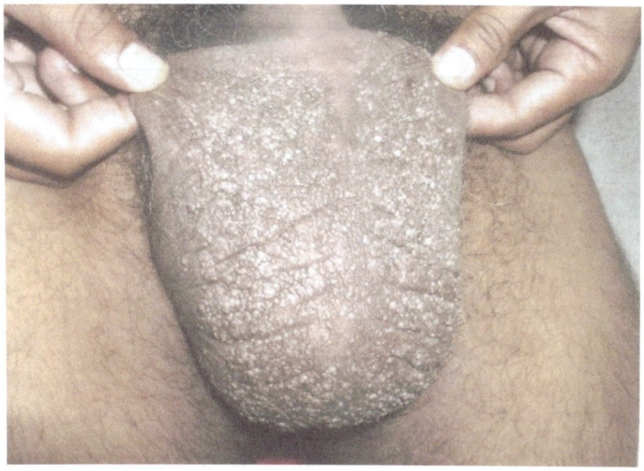

Fig. 28.5 Chylous vesicles of scrotum – a chylous manifestation of filariasis (Courtesy – Professor D. Dalela)

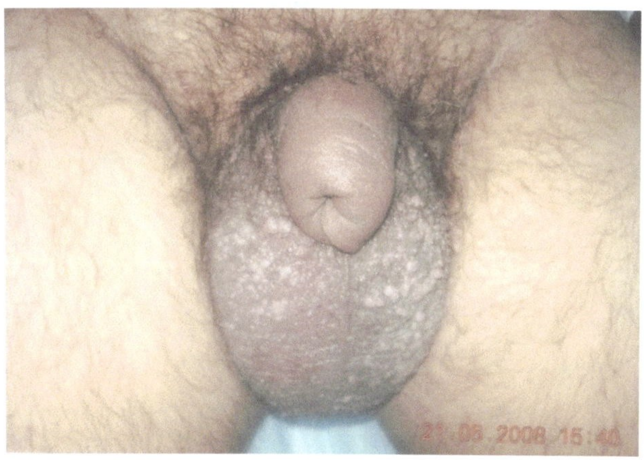

Fig. 28.6 Chylous lymph scrotum with chronic lymphedema of penis (Courtesy – Professor Sandeep Kumar)

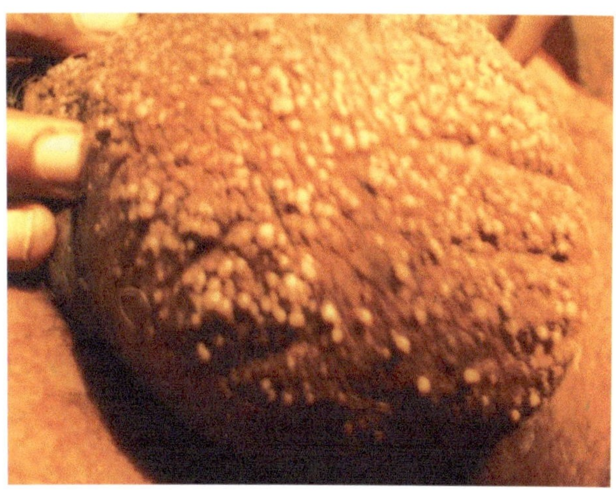

Fig. 28.7 Scrotum studded with chylous vesicles (Courtesy – Professor D. Dalela)

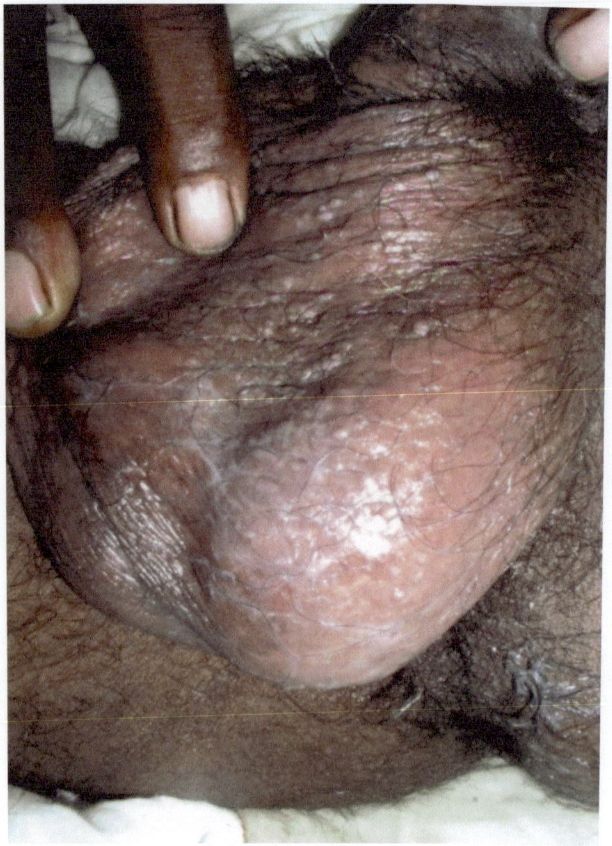

Fig. 28.8 Leaking chyle (chylorrhea) on the skin of scrotum from chylous vesicles of the scrotum (Courtesy – Professor D. Dalela)

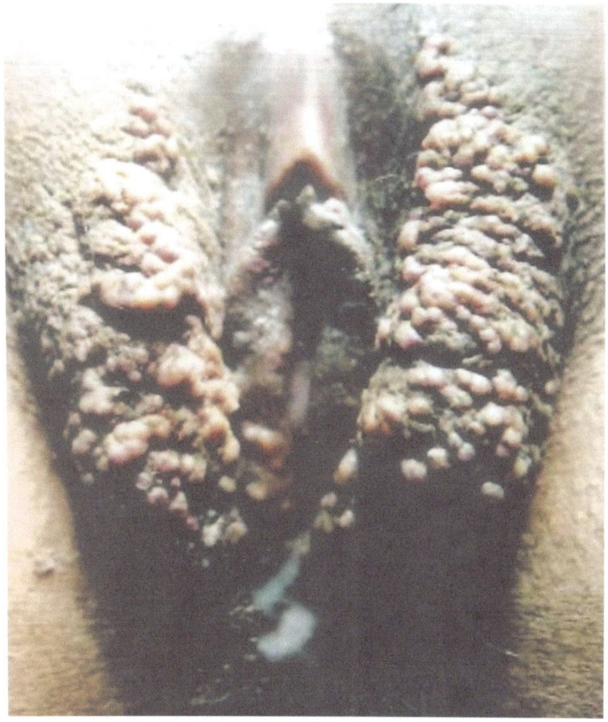

Fig. 28.9 Chylous vesicles of the vulva in a case of lymphatic filariasis

References

Acton HW, Rao SS. The causation of lymph scrotum. Indian Med Gaz. 1930;65:541–6.

Addiss DG, Brady MA. Morbidity management in the Global Programme to Eliminate Lymphatic Filariasis: a review of the scientific literature. Filaria J. 2007;6:2.

Aguiar-Santos AM, Leal-Cruz M, Netto MJ, Carrera A, Lima G, Rocha A. Lymph scrotum: an unusual urological presentation of lymphatic filariasis. A case series study. Rev Inst Med Trop Sao Paulo. 2009;51(4):179–83.

Amaral F, Dreyer G, Figueredo-Silva J, et al. Live adult worms detected by ultrasonography in human bancroftian filariasis. Am J Trop Med Hyg. 1994;50(6):753.

Belokar WK, De Sa O, Amonkar DP, Dharwadkar AM, Priolkar RP. Uncommon manifestations of filariasis. J Postgrad Med. 1983;29:170–4B.

DeVries CR. The role of the urologist in the treatment and elimination of lymphatic filariasis worldwide. BJU Int. 2002;89 Suppl 1:37–43.

Dreyer G, Piessens WF. Worms and micro-organisms can cause lymphatic disease in residents of filariasis-endemic area. In: Nutman TB, editor. Lymphatic filariasis. London: Imperial College Press; 2000. p. 245–64.

Ghooi AM, Khanna T. Surgical manifestations of filariasis. Indian J Surg. 1976;38:150.

Gyapong M, Gyapong JO, Weiss M, Tanner M. The burden of hydrocele in North Ghana. Acta Trop. 2000;77:287–94.

Manson-Bahr PEC, Apted FIC. Filariases. In: Manson's tropical diseases. 18th ed. London: Bailliere Tindal; 1982. p. 148–80.

Sen SB, Chatterjee H, Ramprasad S. Chylous manifestations of filariasis: a clinical and lymphographic study part II. Lymphadenovarix, chylocele and chylous lymph scrotum. Indian J Med Res. 1969;57:1738–44.

Shenoy RK, Sandhya K, Suma TK, Kumaraswami V. A preliminary study of filariasis-related acute adenolymphangitis with special reference to precipitating factors and treatment modalities. SE Asian J Trop Medical Public Health. 1995;26:301–5.

World Health Organization. Surgical approaches to the urogenital manifestations of lymphatic filariasis. Geneva: World Health Organization; 2002. p. 1–29.

Chylous Manifestations (Syndromes) of Lymphatic Filariasis (Filarial Chylous Disease)

29

The filarial infection may affect the chyle-bearing lymphatic pathways and disturb the normal flow of chyle producing some clinical manifestations (syndromes) which are being described in this chapter.

29.1 Chyle-Bearing Pathways

The chyle-bearing pathways start at the lacteal capillary in the mucosal villi of small intestine such as the initial lymphatics of the skin. They drain into the lymphatics of the mesentery, which joins to form intestinal trunks in the root of the mesentery. The intestinal trunks drain into the cisterna chyli situated in front of vertebral L1–L2 bodies. The thoracic duct drains the cisterna chyli into the left jugulo-subclavian venous junction.

There have been mysteries and arguments about the flow of chyle ever since the lacteals were first discovered by Aselli in 1627, who believed that they carried chyle from the intestine to the liver. The true direction of flow to the cisterna chyli and thence through the thoracic duct into the blood stream was not described until 1951 when it was described by Pecquet (Kinmonth 1982).

29.2 Chyle

It is a Greek word which means juice as it is really the "juice" of the food ingested by a person. Chyle is a product of intestinal absorption of digested fats and consists of emulsified fat, albumin, and fibrin (Dowdeswell 1994; Miller 1996) (see Table 29.1 given below). It is an odorless milky white fluid which is bacteriostatic; hence, infection occurs in it infrequently. The intestinal trunks drain it into the cisterna chyli with no interposed lymph glands in between (Last 1963).

T.C. Goel, A. Goel, *Lymphatic Filariasis*, DOI 10.1007/978-981-10-2257-9_29

Table 29.1 Composition of chyle

Component	Content (per 100 mL)
Fats	
Total fat	0.4–5 g
Total cholesterol	65–220 mg
Proteins	
Total protein	2.21–5.9 g
Albumin	1.1–4.1 g
Globulin	1.1–3.1 g
Fibrinogen	16–24 g
Sugars	48–200 g
Electrolytes	Same as in plasma
Cells	
Lymphocytes	400–6800 mm^3
Erythrocytes	50–600 mm^3
Antithrombin globulin	>25 % of plasma concentration
Prothrombin	>25 % of plasma concentration
Fibrinogen	>25 % of plasma concentration

29.3 Dietary Fats

The dietary fats are mainly of two types: long-chain fatty acids and medium-chain fatty acids.

- *Long-chain fatty acids* (>*C12*) – Most dietary fats consist of long-chain fatty acids combined with glycerol as triglycerides. These fatty acids are water-insoluble as they are very hydrophobic. Their absorption entails specialized emulsifying systems predominantly via lymphatics.
  The emulsification of long-chain triglycerides starts in the stomach with the churning action of the antral mill. On entry into the small bowel, their lipolysis occurs by pancreatic lipase with breakdown into fatty acids and monoglycerides. They are then rendered water-soluble by the formation of micelles with bile salts. The entry of lipids into the intestinal mucosal cells is by a passive diffusion process. Within the enterocytes, the triglycerides are re-esterified by an energy-dependent process before they are surrounded by lipoprotein membranes (packaged) to form chylomicrons which are then drained by the lymphatics of bowel (lacteals). About 60–70 % of ingested fat is transported into the blood in this manner through the chyle-bearing pathways.
- *Medium-chain fatty acids* (*C5–11*) – These triglycerides contain 5–11 carbon atoms. They are readily hydrolyzed by pancreatic lipase and their fatty acids are soluble in water and directly absorbed into portal venous circulation (Moncure 1994). They are not resynthesized after uptake by mucosal absorptive cells but enter into the intestinal capillaries and then the portal vessels as free fatty acids. This simple absorptive process has led to their use as an effective albeit expensive

Table 29.2 Differences between long-chain (>C_{12}) and medium-chain (C5-11) including short-chain (<C_5) triglycerides (fatty acids)

Features	Long-chain triglycerides	Medium- and short-chain triglycerides
Aqueous solubility	Low	High
Miscellar solubilization	Required	Not required
Paracellular absorption	Plays a minor role	Likely to play a major role
Biotransformation in enterocytes	CoA ester formation	Does not occur
	Re-esterification	
Form of absorption	Chylomicron triglyceride into the lacteals of the mesentery	Directly into portal venous blood
Fate	Hydrolysis in capillaries by lipoprotein lipase and oxidation in cells to release energy	Hepatic extraction
	Storage after re-esterification	Oxidation to release energy and CO_2

dietary supplement in patients with impaired fat assimilation including chylous manifestations of filariasis.

Short-chain triglycerides (<C5) – They are very much like the medium-chain triglycerides. The differences between various types of triglycerides are given Table 29.2 (Tandon et al. 2012):

After the ingestion of a fatty meal, the volume of intestinal lymph may increase 10 times over its basal flow rate. Starvation and rest diminishes its volume markedly. Thus, the absorption of fat is partitioned between lymph and portal blood (Campbell 1961).

29.4 Chylomicrons

Hewson (1774) observed that the milky fluid seen in the lacteals following a meal leaves a grease spot when dried on a paper. Under the microscope, the milky fluid was seen to contain numerous tiny particles for which Gage (1920) proposed the name chylomicron. Claude Bernard (1856) demonstrated that a fine emulsion of fats occurs in the intestine and he further demonstrated that this depends on the presence of bile and pancreatic lipase. He also observed that lipedemia was present in the systemic circulation following the ingestion of a fat-rich meal.

The chylomicrons are stable oil droplets which are readily seen during fat absorption using light microscopy. They are formed in the enterocytes and are exocytosed across the basolateral membrane of the enterocytes and enter the central lacteal of the villi. From there, they pass into larger lymphatics of the mesentery and thence to the thoracic duct and ultimately into the left jugulo-subclavian vein junction.

The chylomicrons have a diameter of 0.05–1 μm, have an oily interior consisting of triglycerides, cholesterol esters, and trace lipids (vitamins, xenobiotics) and a

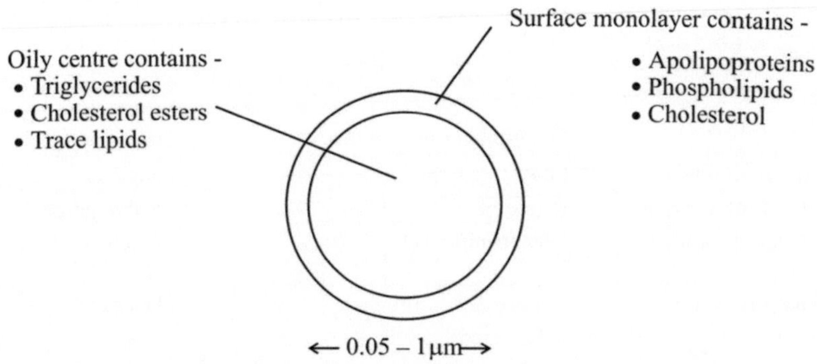

Fig. 29.1 Structure and composition of a chylomicron

stabilizing surface monolayer with apolipoproteins, phospholipids, and cholesterol (Fig. 29.1). The exact composition of chylomicrons is described below (Pratibha 2012) –

Triglycerides – 90 %
Cholesterol esters – 1–3 %
Cholesterol – 1 %
Protein – 1.5 %
Phospholipids – 6.5 %

During fat absorption, the central lacteals show rhythmic contractions which pump the contained chyle through the lymphatics of the mesentery into the thoracic duct.

The blood, 3–6 h after a fat-rich meal such as thick cream, shows milky plasma which on microscopy shows very small fat particles, i.e., chylomicrons (Campbell 1961).

29.5 Chylous Reflux

It is the flow of chyle in the chyle-bearing lymphatics opposite the normal direction of flow (backflow). It usually occurs through the dilated (almost varicose) valveless megalymphatics.

29.6 Chylous Manifestations of Lymphatic Filariasis

Following obstruction in the chyle-bearing pathways, there occurs regurgitation of chyle (chylous reflux) into the connecting lymphatics of nearby organs and cavities, which become dilated and tortuous. The dilated lymphatics may rupture due either

Table 29.3 Etiopathogenesis of various chylous manifestations

Site of obstruction	Mechanism	Manifestation
Cisterna chyli or above	Pyelo-lymphatic backflow	Chyluria
	Ilio-inguinal backflow	
	Inguino-scrotal backflow	Chylocele
		Chylous scrotum
		Chylous fistulae and chylorrhea (scrotum)
		Chylous lymphangiovarix
		Chylous cyst of spermatic cord
	Backflow into lower extremity	Chylous lymphadenovarix
		Chylous vesicles and fistulae of lower extremity
		Chylorrhea
		Chylous arthritis of knee
Upper part of thoracic duct	Thoracic backflow	Chylothorax due to ooze from pleural surface of lung
		Chylopericardium (rare) due to ooze from inner surface of pericardium
Base of mesentery	Intestinal backflow	Chylous ascites from transudation of chyle from peritoneal surface
		Chylous diarrhea from rupture of dilated lacteals into the lumen of bowel

to their thin walls or chylous hypertension resulting in leakage of chyle into the affected organ or cavity producing some clinical manifestations as described below in Table 29.3 (Servelle 1963).

As shown in Table 29.3, the type of chylous manifestation depends on the site of obstruction and the direction of reflux which in turn depends on the path of least resistance (Fig. 29.2).

Whereas chyluria, chylous lymph varix, chylocele, and chylorrhea are well-recognized complications of filariasis, it is not generally recognized that chylous arthritis of knee joint occurs in this parasitic infection (Sen and Ellapan 1968).

29.7 Incidence

The chylous manifestations of filariasis are not common. Ghooi and Khanna (1976) did not find even a single case of chylous manifestation amongst 90 cases of lymphatic filariasis. At our hospital, only two chylous manifestations, i.e., chyluria and chylocele were seen, and during a period of 5 years (1979–1983), 39 cases of chyluria were recorded out of a total of 1236 patients of filariasis. Approximately 1 % of all hydroceles operated were chyloceles. The senior author (TCG) has seen a case of chylous ascites also.

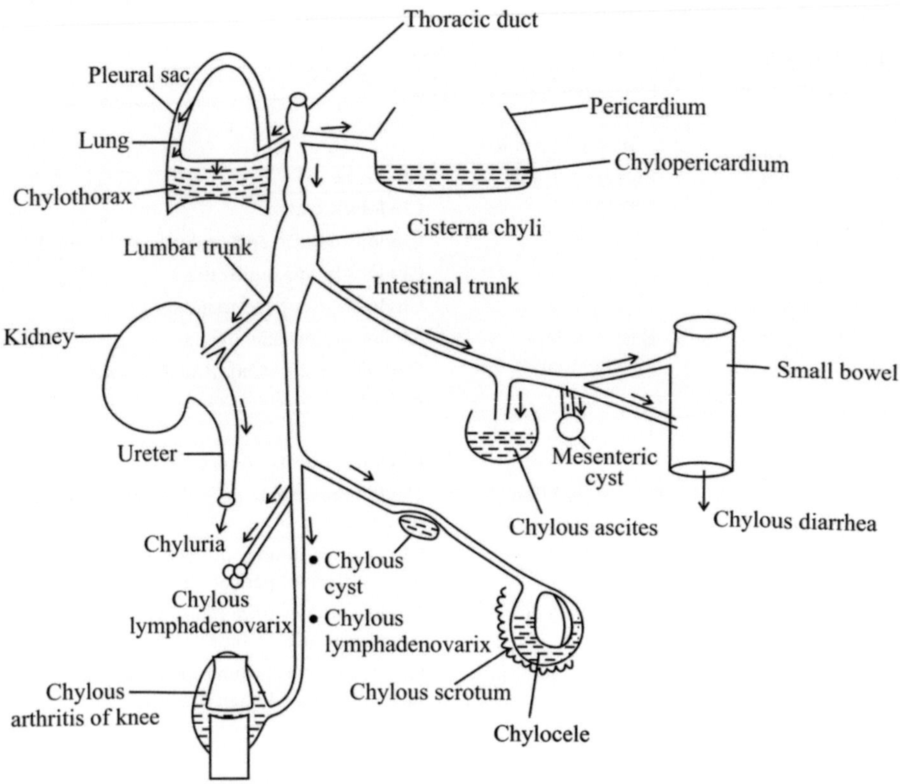

Fig. 29.2 Chylous reflux and chylous manifestations of lymphatic filariasis

29.8 Pathology

Servelle (1963) found definite evidence of structural abnormality of thoracic duct in patients of chylous manifestations. Most of the patients showed a successive progression of chylous reflux starting in more proximal vessels such as gonadal, renal, and abdominal; then progressing to groin, lower abdominal, and scrotal lymphatics; and finally terminating in the chylous manifestations. However, Sen et al. (1969) failed to confirm the existence of a localized organic obstruction in the thoracic duct.

References

Aselli G. De lactibus. Milan. 1627.

Campbell J. Fat metabolism. In: Best CH, Taylor NB, editors. The physiological basis of medical practice. 7th ed. Baltimore: Williams & Wilkins; 1961. p. 845–6.

Bernard C 1856. Quoted by Campbell J. Fat metabolism. In: Best CH Taylor NB, editors. The physiological basis of medical practice. 7th ed. Baltimore: Williams & Wilkins; 1961. p. 845–6.

Dowdeswell IRG. Pleural diseases. In: Stein JH, Sande MA, editors. Internal medicine. 4th ed. St. Louis: Mosby; 1994. p. 1760.
Gage 1920. Quoted by Campbell J. Fat metabolism. In: Best CH, Taylor NB, editors. The physiological basis of medical practice. 7th ed. Baltimore: Williams & Wilkins; 1961. p. 845–6.
Ghooi AM, Khanna T. Surgical manifestations of filariasis. Indian J Surg. 1976;38:150.
Hewson 1774. Quoted by Campbell J. Fat metabolism. In: Best CH, Taylor NB, editors. The physiological basis of medical practice. 7th ed. Baltimore: Williams & Wilkins; 1961. p. 845–6.
Kinmonth JB. The lymphatics. 2nd ed. London: Edward Arnold; 1982.
Last RJ. Lymphoid tissue. In: Anatomy, regional and applied. 3rd ed. London: J & A Churchill Ltd; 1963. p. 25–7.
Miller Jr JI. Diagnosis and management of chylothorax. Chest Surg Clin N Am. 1996;6:139–48.
Moncure AC. Chylothorax. In: Morris PJ, Malt RA, editors. Oxford Textbook of Surgery Vol I. New York: Oxford University Press; 1994. p. 1933–5.
Pratibha KM. Digestion and absorption. In: Tandon OP, Tripathi Y, Kumar A, Ravi K, Mandal MB, Venkatesh D, editors. Best and Taylor's physiological basis of medical practice. 13th ed. New Delhi: Wolters Kluwer; 2012. p. 777–8.
Servelle M. Pathology of thoracic duct. J Cardiovasc Surg. 1963;4:702–27.
Sen SB, Ellapan S. Chylous manifestations of filariasis: A clinical and lymphographic study. Part 1. Filarial chyluria. Indian J Med Res. 1968;56:1535–45.
Sen SB, Chatterjee H, Ramaprasad S. Chylous manifestations of filariasis: A clinical and lymphographic study. II. Lymphadenovarix chylocoele and chylous lymph scrotum. Indian J Med Res. 1969;57(9):1738–44.
Tandon OP, Tripathi Y et al. Digestion and absorption of fact. In: Physiological Basis of Medical Practice. 13th edition. New Delhi: Wolters Kluwer; 2012. p. 776–779.

30 Chyluria

Chyluria is defined as the passage of intestinal lymph (chyle) in urine due to chylous reflux into the urinary tract caused by filarial obstruction of chyle-carrying pathways. It is a late sequel of lymphatic filariasis.

Chyluria is not an uncommon presentation of filariasis in endemic areas. It mostly affects the economically weaker sections of society, and occurs in 1–2 % cases of filariasis 10–20 years after the initial infection, when active filariasis is no longer demonstrable (Pandey 1994). Yamauchi (1945) described this interval to be 1 month to 54 years. Its incidence in Pondicherry (India) is over 4 % of all filarial disease (Sen and Ellapan 1968).

Chyluria has been recognized since ancient times. Charak (300 BC), an ancient Indian physician, described it as "shuklameha" (शुक्लमेह). Hippocrates (400 BC) and Galen regarded it as a serious problem as it was associated with fever and convulsions and often culminated in death. Although Pecquet (1651) discovered and described the lymphatic system, it was not until 100 years later that Morgagni showed chyluria to be due to a disturbance in the lymphatic circulation.

30.1 Etiology

Etiologically, chyluria is of two types—parasitic and nonparasitic—the causes of which are described below (Dalela 2005; Sharma and Hemal 2009).

- *Parasitic chyluria* (primary or tropical) due to parasitic infections
  1. *Wuchereria bancrofti*
  2. Other parasites—*Taenia echinococcus*, *Taenia nana*, *Ankylostoma duodenale*, *Trichinella spiralis*, malarial parasites
- *Nonparasitic chyluria* (secondary or nontropical)
  1. Congenital
  2. Lymphangioma of urinary tract
  3. Megalymphatics with urethral or vesical fistulae

T.C. Goel, A. Goel, *Lymphatic Filariasis*, DOI 10.1007/978-981-10-2257-9_30

4. Stenosis of thoracic duct
5. Retroperitoneal lymphangiectasia
6. Traumatic lymphangio-urinary fistulae
7. Obstruction of thoracic duct and/or thoracic and retroperitoneal lymphatics due to tumors, granulomas, and aortic aneurysm
8. Other causes—pregnancy, diabetes, pernicious anemia, nephrotic syndrome

Out of the above list, the most common cause is lymphatic filariasis (90 %), hence the chyluria is considered filarial unless proved otherwise. For the same reason, the chyluria is an uncommon symptom in western countries.

The endemic occurrence of chyluria in filarial infested regions and demonstration of this parasitic in the blood, lymph, or urine in chyluric individuals by various workers supports this view.

30.2 Pathophysiology

The lymphatics of the kidney follow the renal vein and end in the lateral aortic (para-aortic) glands. The efferents from these glands form the lumbar trunks on either side.

The intestinal trunks comprise large vessels which receive lymph from the gastrointestinal tract.

The lumbar trunks and intestinal trunks drain into the cisterna chyli.

The dilatation and tortuosity of retroperitoneal lymphatics including intestinal and renal lymphatics has long been recognized in patients with chyluria. The pathogenesis of chyluria is not exactly understood. It is explained by two theories:

1. *Obstructive theory* (Aye and Aung 1975) the filarial infection produces obliterative lymphangitis and lymphatic hypertension, which subsequently generate varicosity and collateral formation. Once the lymphatics are dilated, their valves fail adding to reflux and further dilatation and leakage of chyle into the urinary system (lymphatico-renal shunt).
2. *Regurgitative theory* (Ngan and Leong 1977) the toxins released from dying adult worms in the lymphatics lead to some kind of weakness in the lymphatic wall (ectasia), which in turn leads to impairment of valvular mechanism. Direct inflammatory damage to valves may cause additional effects. Hence, regurgitation of chyle from chyle-bearing lymphatics results in varicosity and rupture of dilated lymphatics into the renal calyces or pelvis. Definite inadequacy of the lymphatic valves exists since retrograde flow is frequently seen extending down the prevertebral and paravertebral regions as seen by retrograde pyelography.

30.3 Unilateral Disease

The chyluria is usually unilateral being more common on the left side. The classical cisterna chyli is present in about 47 % of people in which the lumbar lymphatic trunks and intestinal trunks drain.

When the cisterna chyli is absent, the intestinal trunks drain into the lumbar trunk of onc side (more commonly on the left) or directly into the thoracic duct either as a single trunk or as multiple smaller channels. This explains unilateral chyluria, which is more common on the left side.

30.4 Pathology

The kidney appears normal or slightly enlarged with many dilated or varicose lymphatics in the hilum and/or around it. The abnormal communications with the lymphatics are present in the renal pelvis or calyces.

The route from the intestinal lymphatics (lacteals) to the renal lymphatics has been the subject of much speculation. It is agreed that the chyle first travels from lacteals to the cisterna chyli or thoracic duct and then, because of obstruction and/or valvular insufficiency, there occurs retrograde flow to the upper lumbar glands which drain the renal lymph. Further retrograde flow is frequently seen extending down the prevertebral and paravertebral regions (Dalela 2005).

It is also believed that retroperitoneal lymphatics receiving intestinal lymph are obstructed by inflammatory fibrosis produced by this parasite short-circuiting chyle from the intestinal lacteals to renal lymphatics which rupture subsequently.

The leak may occur in any part of the urinary tract but the kidneys are the most common site. Rarely the fistulous communication may be present in the trigone of the urinary bladder (Edwards 1982) and in the posterior urethra (Pope 1909). The fistulous communications may be bilateral or at multiple sites.

Sometimes there is a network of tensely distended lymphangiovenous mass embedding the ureter from the pelvi-ureteral junction to its entry into the bladder (Prasad et al. 1977).

The chyluria is not a disease of the urinary system and does not have any deleterious effect on the urinary organs. However, recent histopathological studies of biopsy specimens of kidney have shown membranous nephropathy, mesangioproliferative nephropathy, endothelial cell proliferation, and mild mononuclear cell interstitial infiltration. Ultrastructural studies have shown immune complex type glomerulonephritis (filarial nephropathy).

How far these changes affect the course of chyluria is not known as they are the effects of filariasis and not of chyluria per se.

30.5 Clinical Features

Age and sex Chyluria commonly occurs in the second and third decades of life and the majority of patients are male (86 %).

The onset is usually sudden but it may occur intermittently for many years in mild form. It may sometimes start gradually. It frequently appears without warning, may be with pain in the back, and aching sensations about the pelvis and groins, probably due to distension of preexisting varix (Manson-Bahr and Apted 1982).

Aggravating and relieving factors The exercise and trauma may initiate or accentuate it, whereas bed rest may improve or even arrest it temporarily.

The symptoms and signs of chyluria can be divided into three groups (Bhuta et al. 1978)—those due to the presence of chyle in urine, those due to the loss of chyle (and blood) in urine, and those due to its causative disease, i.e., filariasis and its other manifestations.

30.5.1 Those Due to Presence of Chyle in Urine

1. Passage of milky urine; sometimes blood is mixed with chyle when the patient passes pink milky urine (hematochyluria). It is usually intermittent and most prominent in the morning (Nutman and Weller 2012). Klousia et al. (1977) have described a 25-year-old male who presented with intermittent gross hematochyluria.
2. Frequency of micturition, dysuria, and urgency.
3. Clot colic which is usually due to chylous clots (solid masses of cheese-like consistency) passing down the ureter. In hematochyluria, the clot consists of chyle and blood.
4. Retention of urine due to the formation of a large chylous clot in the bladder and when the clots are passing through the urethra and get stuck up there.

30.5.2 Those Due to Loss of Chyle (and Blood) in Urine

If the chyluria is mild and intermittent, the general health of the patient is not impaired. However, if it is severe and continuous, a considerable amount of fat is lost, which may amount to 15 % of lymphatic drainage of the gut when the patient suffers from nutritional deficiency and anemia as seen in patients with malnutrition and weight loss. It also produces a state of immunosuppression as the chyle is rich in lymphocytes (Dusmet 2005).

30.5.3 Those Due to Filariasis

About 70 % patients with chyluria have genital manifestations such as epididymo-orchitis (Kanetkar et al. 1966), funiculitis, and hydrocele; 25 % have chronic lymphedema of extremities; and 5 % have other manifestations like cellulitis and abscesses. A past history of filariasis or its complications have been documented in 10 % of patients.

30.6 Differential Diagnosis

The differential diagnosis of chyluria includes gross pyuria, phosphaturia, passage of amorphous urates and caseous material, and pseudochyluria.

30.7 Investigations

30.7.1 Urine

A diet rich in fat a day or night before the examination of urine enhances chyluria and helps in its detection. A fresh sample of urine looks white like milk and, if kept for some time, may convert into a semisolid gel that contains blood and fibrin clots. If the urine is passed into a glass and allowed to stand for some time, it separates into three layers. At the top, there is a cream-like pellicle; at the bottom, there is a scanty reddish sediment consisting of cells and debris; and in the middle, there is a reddish white layer with fibrin (Manson-Bahr and Apted 1982).

Microscopic examination shows a variable number of red blood cells and small lymphocytes. Fat droplets of varying sizes can be seen. Chylomicrons are seen directly under the microscope with dark ground illumination or stained with Sudan red III. Casts and cylindroids are usually absent.

Ether test An equal amount of ether is added to urine and the mixture is shaken vigorously for a few minutes. It results in the clearance of opacity of urine. Goel et al. (2004) found lymphocyturia a more sensitive test to diagnose chyluria than the ether test.

Sudan red III test Oral ingestion of fat labelled with Sudan red III (10 g of butter with 100 mg of Sudan red III) causes orange–pink coloration of chyluric urine within 2–6 h. One limitation of this test is that Sudan red III is costly and not available freely. It does not make the normal urine red (Pandey 1994).

Methylene blue test Staining of fresh urinary deposit with one or two drops of 1:1300 methylene blue reveals small lymphocytes (single or clumps).

Biochemical examination Now the focus is being shifted to biochemical and electrophoretic analysis of urine to detect the lipid constituents (triglycerides) and albumin. Triglycerides are invariably present in urine even if the urine is grossly clear, and even if the chyluria is continuous or intermittent and mild or severe. The estimation of urinary triglycerides is 100% sensitive and specific for chyluria. The levels of chylomicrons, triglycerides, and cholesterol in urine may point to the degree or extent of abnormal communication. Postprandial urinary lipids, especially triglycerides ranging from 10 to 1955 mg/dL, might be used as a marker in clinical evaluation of chyluria.

The urinary albumin is abnormally high in most of the cases. The urine is acidic in reaction becoming alkaline on exposure to air.

Immunoelectrophoresis of urine shows globulins of various types including apolipoprotein A-48 of intestinal origin.

The urine may sometimes contain gross blood with chyle (hematochyluria). It may contain microfilariae. They were present in 4 out of 18 cases in the series reported by Kanetkar et al. (1966) and in 17 out of 40 cases in the series by Bhuta et al. (1978).

30.7.2 Blood

It usually reveals eosinophilia and anemia. It may be positive for microfilariae, especially during an acute attack. The plasma proteins and triglycerides are reduced in most of the cases. The albumin–globulin ratio is reversed (Tanagho and Kane 2013).

30.7.3 Urethrocystoscopy

It often shows the chylous efflux from one or sometimes both ureteral orifices (Figs. 30.1 and 30.2). A fatty meal on the previous day/night enhances the results. Rarely the chylous efflux is seen from the urinary bladder or even posterior urethra. It is best seen when the irrigant flow is stopped and the bladder is semifilled.

In mild chyluria, ureteral catheterization and split urinalysis for chyle may be performed.

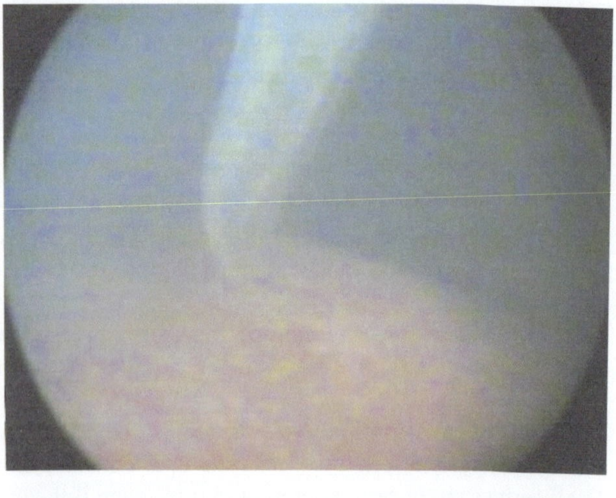

Fig. 30.1 Chylous efflux from the right ureter as seen during cystoscopy. (Courtesy of Professor D. Dalela)

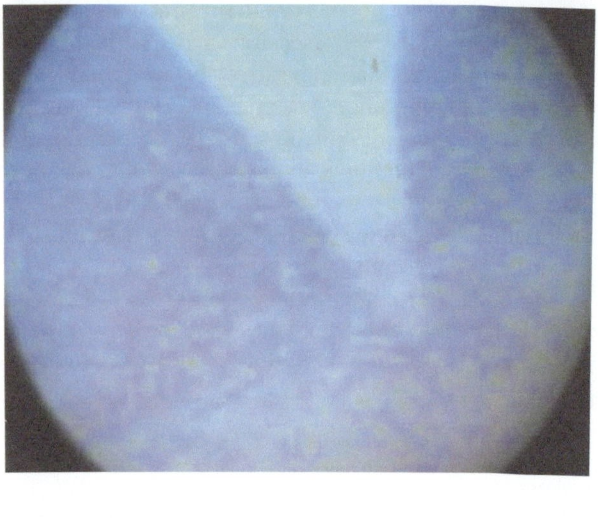

Fig. 30.2 Chylous efflux as seen during cystoscopy. (Courtesy of Professor D. Dalela)

30.7.4 Retrograde Pyelography (RGP)

Retrograde pyelography under fluoroscopic control and spot films often demonstrates pyelo-lymphatic backflow.

Once the side of chylous efflux is found during cystoscopy, a 5–6 F ureteral catheter is passed under fluoroscopic guidance into the renal pelvis and a radiograph is taken with the patient in 20° Trendelenburg position. The contrast is put into the renal pelvis allowing gravity-propagated filling of renal pelvis and not filling with pressure. Then, the films are taken to see the pyelo-lymphatic fistulae (Figs 30.3, 30.4, and 30.5).

The filling of renal pelvis with pressure must be avoided as it is painful to the patient and may open up the pyelo-venous or pyelo-sinus channels, which may cause adverse reactions. In a modification described by Goel et al., 2.5 mL gadolinium (instead of radiographic contrast material) mixed with 5 mL normal saline is instilled and then coronal fat suppressed T2 and T1 MR sequences are taken. The advantages of this technique include no radiation exposure and no risk of contrast-related complications. Another advantage is simultaneous detailed intra-abdominal evaluation to diagnose the cause of chlyuria especially in non-endemic countries (Goel et al. 2014).

30.7.5 Lymphangiography

It is a radiographic visualization of retroperitoneal lymphatics by the injection of contrast (ultrafluid lipiodol) into a lymphatic of the dorsum of foot. It may be a

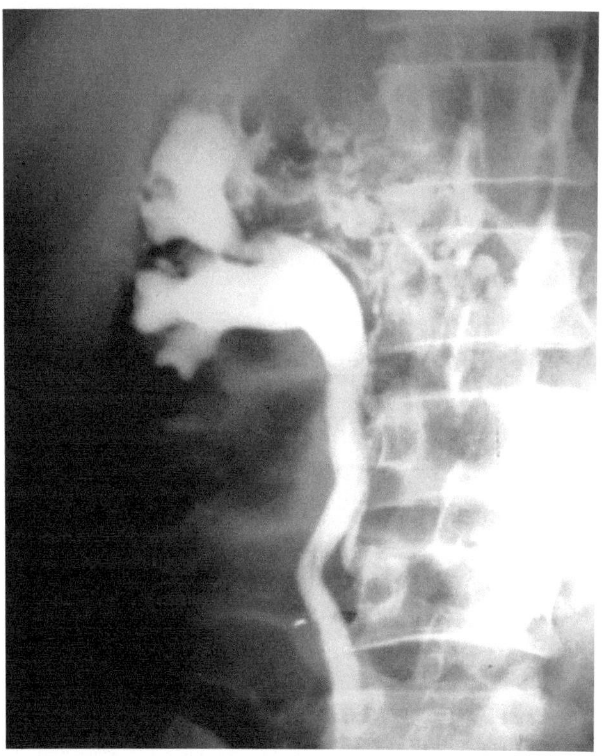

Fig. 30.3 Retrograde pyelogram (RGP) showing pyelo-lymphatic backflow on the right side. (Courtesy of Professor D. Dalela)

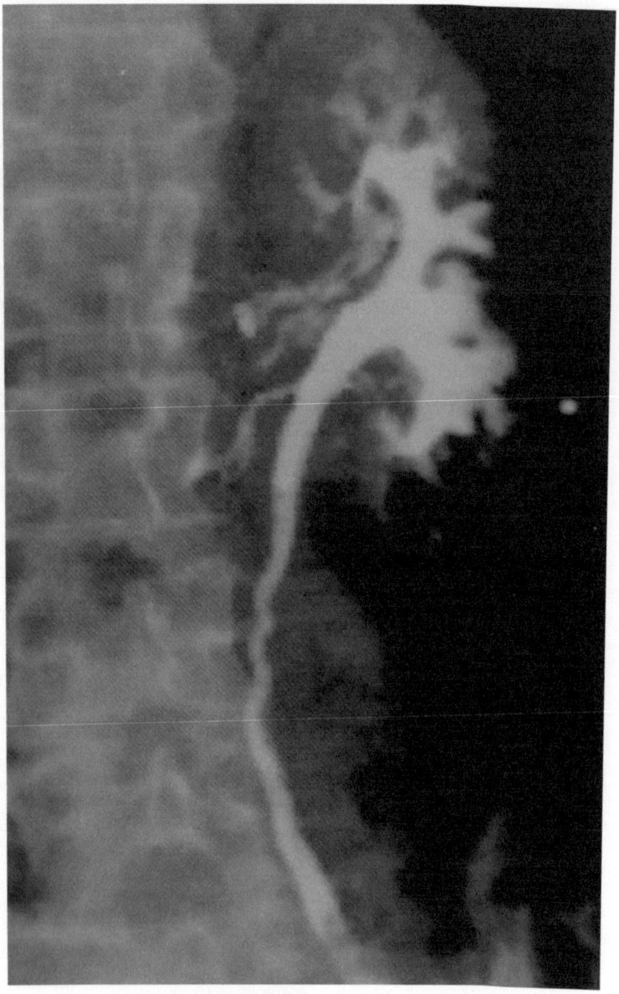

Fig. 30.4 Retrograde pyelography showing pyelo-lymphatic fistulae on the left side

unilateral or bilateral procedure, but mostly unilateral lymphangiography is done, the advantages of which are

1. It is easy to identify crossover channels
2. The discomfort and pain are less
3. It saves time
4. The lymphatics of other limb are not injured

It shows numerous dilated and tortuous lymphatics around the renal hilum communicating with paravertebral lymphatics and the contrast outlining a major or minor calyx. The contrast may enter the pelvi-calyceal system in 40 % of patients and may be followed into the urinary bladder. Other findings which may be present include tortuous and beaded thoracic duct (it is normal in most of the patients), round granular

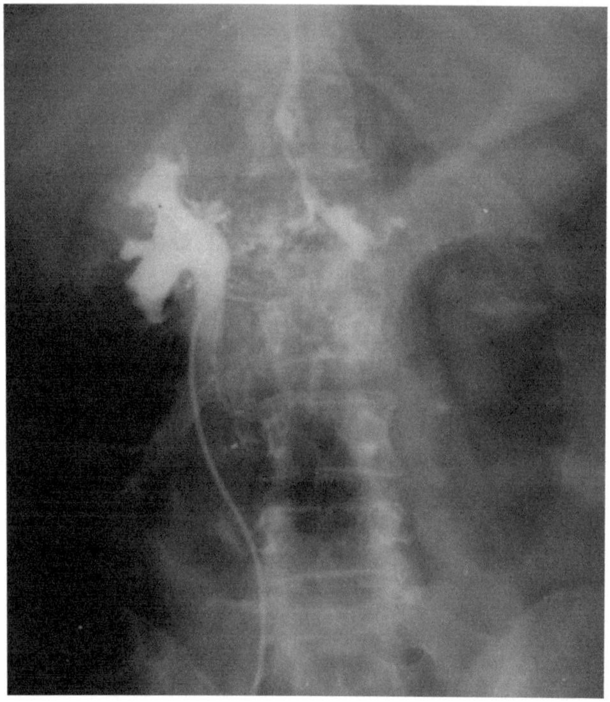

Fig. 30.5 Right-sided retrograde pyelography showing pyelo-lymphatic backflow and fistulae

enlarged para-aortic nodes, skipping of lymphatic chain (in advanced disease), dilated cisterna chyli, abnormal lymphatics along the line of the ureter, and accelerated transit of contrast from foot to thoracic duct. The infra-inguinal lymphatics are normal.

As this investigation is time-consuming, technically demanding, and invasive and may further damage lymphatics, it is not done routinely.

Sen and Ellapan (1968) could visualize the thoracic duct in 10 out of 12 patients with chyluria. The thoracic duct was always abnormal, and four grades of ductal abnormalities were recognized:

Grade I—terminal 5–8 cm tortuous and dilated duct narrowing abruptly at its termination seen in two cases

Grade II—a segmental opacification 2–3 cm long was seen in two patients

Grade III—entire duct opacified, dilated, and wavy in three patients

Grade IV—opacification of grossly dilated commencement of the duct (or it was opacified when the contrast was forced through the pyelo-lymphatic fistulae during retrograde pyelography)

Akisada and Tani (1970) did a lymphographic study in 34 cases of filarial chyluria and 3 cases of prechyluria and described six types of lymphatico-pelvic fistulae

1. Cystic type
2. Circular and semicircular type
3. Vermiform plexus type

4. Arborization type
5. Indeterminate type
6. Type without fistulae

30.7.6 Lymphoscintigraphy (Lymphangioscintigraphy)

It is the radioisotopic visualization of the lymphatic system. It gives useful information about the function of lymphatics (and the site of fistulae) rather than full anatomical details. It is a useful, noninvasive, safe, quick, and simple technique using Tc-99 m human serum albumin sulfur colloid, Tc-99 m diethylenetriamine pentaacetic acid and Tc-99 m antimony sulfide colloid or dextran. It is the investigation of choice to localize the site of fistulae and assess the extent of reflux, and later on to detect recurrence on follow-up. It allows functional assessment of lymphatic transport and depiction of regional lymph nodes. It has no known side effects, but it is not freely available. The differences between the lymphangiography and lymphoscintigraphy are given in the following Table 30.1:

30.7.7 Immunological Studies

ELISA It is useful in confirming the etiological diagnosis where it is suspected to be filarial. It is based on the humoral immune response of host to filarial antigen. IgG antibodies against microfilarial excretory–secretory (mf ES) antigens have been detected in 89 % of patients with genital manifestations, 87 % with lymphedema, 67 % with lymphadenitis, and 60 % with other clinical manifestations. It has 85 % specificity and 95 % sensitivity. It is interesting to note that it is positive in 3 % endemic normals (Mehta et al. 1999).

A study by Date et al. (1981) in 11 patients with chyluria showed lymphocytopenia, decrease in T-cells, low serum IgA concentration, and suppression of delayed hypersensitivity responses to intradermally injected antigens. The similarity of

Table 30.1 Differences between lymphangiography and lymphography

Features	Lymphangiography	Lymphoscintigraphy
Definition	Radiographic visualization of lymphatics	Radioisotopic visualization of lymphatics
Contrast used	Ultrafluid lipiodol	Tc-99 m serum albumin sulfur colloid
Requirements	More demanding in terms of labor and time	Less demanding in terms of labor and time
Image resolution	Good	Poor
	Gives full anatomical details of lymphatic system	Gives full information about the function of lymphatic system
Complications	Painful invasive procedure	Noninvasive, not painful procedure
	Causes further damage to lymphatics	Not damaging to lymphatics

findings in chyluria with intestinal lymphangiectasia and thoracic duct fistula suggests that the immune deficiency may be due to loss of lymph in urine.

The immune function in filarial chyluria is impaired as regards T-lymphocyte subsets. The percentage of CD3+/CD4+ cell is significantly decreased. The ratio of CD4+/CD8+ is under 1.0 (Gu et al. 2000). Both cell-mediated and humoral immunity are low. The OKT3 and OKT4 levels are commonly low, and OKT8 is higher than normal with OKT4/OKT8 ratio reversed (Xing et al. 1994).

Golestaneh et al. (2009) have described a young man who had prolonged and severe chyluria and presented with acute myocardial infarction. He had hypoalbuminemia, increased production of factor VIII, increased clotting tendency, and secondary polycythemia.

30.7.8 Intravenous Urography (IVU)

It may be done to visualize the urinary tract, but it is usually not required in most of the patients. Rarely it may show increased renal size in severe disease due to chylous clot obstruction. It may also show dilated paracalyceal lymphatics (with ureteral pressure).

IVU or some sort of functioning study must be done before (and after) operation (Yu et al. 1978) as there are reports of loss of renal function following pyelolymphatic disconnection.

30.7.9 Ultrasonography

It is usually normal. In hematochyluria, it may show echolucent areas with hematochylous clot (heterogenous shadow) in the urinary bladder, which has to be differentiated from carcinoma of the bladder (Fig. 30.6).

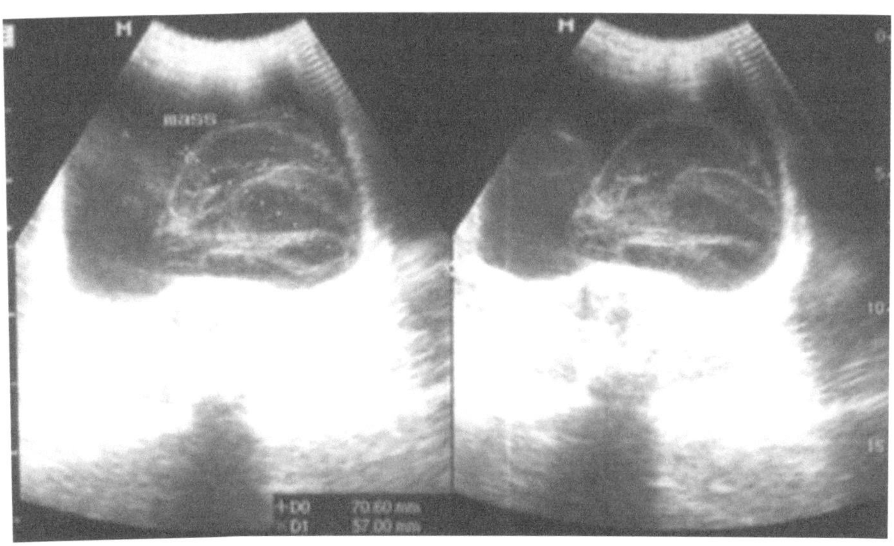

Fig. 30.6 Ultrasonography showing hematochylous clot in urinary bladder

30.7.10 CT Scan

On CT scan of the abdomen, the dilated lymphatic channels may mimic a mass of confluent low-density lymph nodes. The chyle in the urinary bladder may also be seen.

30.7.11 MRI

It shows the lymphatic channels as a meshwork of multiple tortuous tubular fluid-filled structures in the retroperitoneum of the abdomen and pelvis. On T1W axial imaging, these channels are seen as numerous interconnected small nodular and streaky intensities and, on T2W axial imaging, as a cloak of diffuse homogenous hyperintensity (Govil et al. 2007).

30.7.12 Renal Biopsy

It has hardly any practical clinical value. It is mainly done for academic and research purposes and usually shows immune complex type of glomerulonephritis (Date et al. 1981).

30.7.13 Other Investigations

In lymphatic filariasis, serum type I collagen and type III procollagen are decreased. On the other hand, serum hyaluronon (linked to perilymphatic granulomatous inflammation) and serum eosinophil cationic protein are significantly increased in filarial chyluria (Esterre et al. 2006).

30.8 Diagnosis

The steps to make a complete diagnosis are described in the following Table 30.2 and Flow chart 30.1 (Dalela 2005):

30.9 Grades of Chyluria

Hemal and Gupta (2002) described the grades of chyluria based on the findings of retrograde pyelography as described below (with its clinical features):

- *Mild chyluria* is characterized by involvement of a single calyx on retrograde pyelography.
  It is seen in 34–50 % of cases of chyluria and is characterized by (1) intermittent milky urine and (2) no colic, no chylous coagulum, no urinary retention, and no weight loss.

Table 30.2 Steps to make a complete diagnosis of chyluria

Step I	Confirmation of chyluria by detailed examination of urine	Gross inspection—milky white color
		Ether test
		Dark ground illumination—lymphocyturia
		Sudan III staining—orange–red color
		Urinary triglyceride estimation, present even if urine is clinically clear
Step II	Localization of site of chyle leakage in urinary tract	Cystoscopy following fatty diet to see the chylous efflux from ureteral orifice
		Retrograde pyelography to see pyelo-lymphatic backflow (fistulae)
		Lymphangiography to see numerous dilated tortuous lymphatics around hilar region (not done routinely)
		Lymphoscintigraphy, if facilities are available
Step III	Confirmation of etiological diagnosis (mostly it is filarial)	Urine may show microfilariae
		Blood shows eosinophilia and may be positive for microfilariae
		Immunological tests for filariasis including ELISA
		Investigations for other causes if filariasis is not confirmed
Step IV	To find the effect on nutrition and immune function	Serum proteins including albumin ↓
		Hemoglobin ↓
		Serum lipids ↓
		$CD3^+$ $CD4^+$ decreased
		Ratio of $CD4^+/CD8^+$ under 1.0
		Cell-mediated and humoral immunity ↓
		OKT4/OKT8 ratio reversed

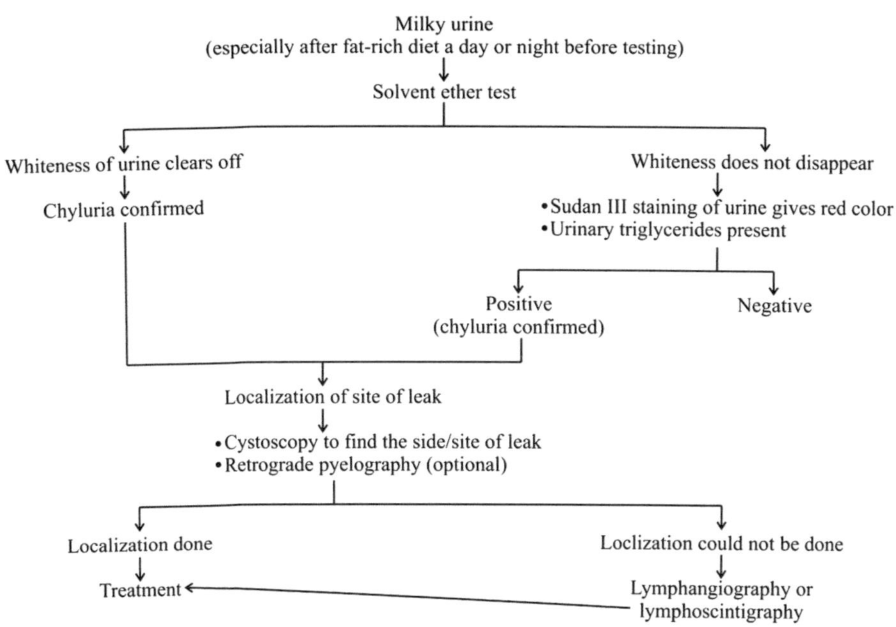

Flow chart 30.1 Diagnostic algorithm for chyluria

- *Moderate chyluria* is characterized by the involvement of two or more calyces on retrograde pyelography.
  It is seen in 33–40 % of patients with chyluria and is characterized by (1) intermittent or continuous milky urine, (2) occasional clot colic, chylous coagulum, and (3) no urinary retention and no weight loss.
- *Severe chyluria* is characterized by the involvement of most calyces with or without involvement of ureter on retrograde pyelography.
  It is seen in 15–26 % of cases and is characterized by (1) continuous passage of milky urine with clot colic, (2) chylous coagulum/urinary retention, and (3) weight loss.

30.10 Treatment

No treatment is necessary for chyluria if there is no disturbance in general health (Maged 1967) and in mild intermittent chyluria as it may recover spontaneously with passage of time in many patients. Ohyama et al. (1979) noted spontaneous remission in 36 out of 72 patients with chyluria.

Chyluria often occurs in conjunction with some other condition which increases the burden on the lymphatic system or causes impediment to the lymphatic drainage. Hence, it can be effectively managed by the treatment of this coexistent problem, which should be managed first in such patients. Koga et al. (1990) found 132 patients in a series of 323 patients with chyluria in whom the chyluria was apparently precipitated by some other condition. It disappeared following treatment of coexistent problem such as congestive heart failure, cirrhosis of liver, pregnancy.

- A course of diethylcarbamazine 6 mg/kg in three divided doses after food is given over a period of 10–14 days which reduces the microfilaremia levels by approximately 80–90 % in several days. Initially, a lower dose (1–3 mg/kg) once a day is given to decrease the side effects of this drug in case of a heavy parasitic load. The side effects of this drug may be systemic and local.

The systemic reactions include fever, headache, myalgia, vomiting weakness, and asthma. They usually result from rapid destruction of microfilariae and perhaps adult worms. The local reactions include lymphadenitis, abscess formation, and transient lymphedema. These symptoms occur within 2 days, often within 24 h after the start of treatment, and persist for 3–4 days. Another course can be given 1 month following completion of the first course.

Dietary modification Dietary modifications play a major role in the treatment of chyluria with the aim to prevent undernutrition and to minimize chyle production and its leakage in the urine. This is done by a diet excluding normal fat and supplemented by medium-chain triglycerides (<12 carbon atoms) and high protein content. Commercial medium-chain triglycerides (MCTs) are unpalatable, and hence require nasogastric tube feeding (Henry and Thompson 2005). Coconut oil is a good natural source of MCTs where there is not much problem of taste; hence, it may be used in cooking. MCTs are absorbed directly into the portal venous system of the liver bypassing the intestinal lymphatics (Geliebter et al. 1983). Obligatory oxidation of these fats in the liver leaves almost no MCT derivative for incorporation in the body fat or general circulation through other organs.

Fat restriction with total fat consumption to 50 g a day reduces the urinary losses of triglycerides, phospholipids, cholesterol, and free fatty acids significantly.

In heavy chyluria, parenteral administration of specialized products with MCT formulas along with albumin has been done with relief. In cases of intractable chyluria, total parenteral nutrition with enteric rest is usually prescribed (Buttiker et al. 1999).

Ansari (2005) has described general guidelines for dietary modification in Indian patients with chyluria as given below.

1. The amount of fat (oil and ghee) in the diet should be as low as possible, i.e., around 50 g a day.
2. Coconut oil, which contains medium-chain fatty acids, should be used as a cooking medium.
3. Avoid putting "ghee" in "daal" and applying butter or "ghee" on bread or "roti."
4. Use skimmed milk—cow's milk is better than that of a buffalo. If only buffalo milk is available, it should be boiled, cooled, and refrigerated for 12–24 h, and then the top creamy layer is removed. The bottom layer of this milk can be consumed by a patient with chyluria.
5. Deep-fried foods like "paratha," "poori," "kachauri," "bhatura," "daal-moth," and "chaat" are avoided.
6. Cake, pastry, and cream biscuits are avoided.
7. Fat-rich sweets like "jalebi," "imarti," "gulabjamun," and "khoya sweets" are avoided.
8. Fatty dry fruits are avoided.
9. A nonvegetarian should not take whole eggs more than once or twice during a week. Avoid the yellow part. Boiled egg is better than omelette. Mutton should be avoided; fish and chicken are better.
10. No restriction on salt, sugar, and spices. Hence, the diet should include "roti," "daal," "dalia," "rice," cornflakes, vegetables, and fruits.

In addition to the above measures, the patient is given plenty of water to prevent chylous clot colic.

Many patients with chyluria are relieved with these measures when no further treatment is required. It must be noted that spontaneous remissions are also known to occur (Ohyama et al. 1979). Tanagho EA and Kane CJ (2013) have described them to occur in 50 % of patients.

An abdominal binder may be tied around the abdomen in an acute attack to reduce the loss of chyle (Sharma and Hemal 2009). It raises the intra-abdominal pressure sufficiently to stop the leak of low-pressure lymphatic fluid.

Cystoscopic bladder wash may be indicated in patients with retention of urine due to chylous or hematochylous clots. Hematinics, multivitamins, and green leafy vegetables are recommended to correct the deficiency caused by hematochyluria. Goyal et al. (2014) have tried to find out the factors that predict response to medical management. They reported that patients with higher grade disease and higher urinary cholesterol loss were predictors of poor response.

30.10.1 Renal Pelvic Instillation Sclerotherapy (RPIS)

Chyluria is a debilitating problem that causes morbidity, but is not life-threatening. Hence, the treatment of chyluria should be safe, effective, and minimally invasive. RPIS is one such treatment.

It is the cornerstone of treatment of chyluria in which a sclerosant is injected under fluoroscopic guidance in the renal pelvis which blocks the lymphatic fistulae by an inflammatory reaction followed by fibrosis. The sclerosants used are described below

1. Silver nitrate: 0.1–3.0 %
2. Povidone iodine: 0.2 %
3. Sodium iodide: 15–25 %
4. Potassium iodide: 10–25 %
5. Dextrose: 50 %
6. Meglumine diatrizoate (urografin): 76 %
7. Hypertonic saline: 3 %
8. Combination therapy

Renal pelvic instillation therapy is indicated when the conservative measures described above fail to give relief in chyluria.

Technique A 0.1–1.0 % solution of silver nitrate is made in distilled water and kept in a clean bottle wrapped in thick black paper and stored in a dark room. It is used after autoclaving.

Under local anesthesia and sedation, cystoscopy is done and the side of the chylous efflux is found. A fatty meal taken on the previous night facilitates the identification of leaking side. A bulb ureteral catheter is passed into the ureter of the affected side under C-arm fluoroscopy to put its tip in the renal pelvis and retrograde pyelography is done to see the pyelo-lymphatic fistulae. The capacity of the renal pelvis is measured, and the sclerosant solution is instilled slowly with an amount equal to the capacity of renal pelvis, i.e., 7–10 mL (Fig. 30.7). During instillation, the head of the patient is held down by 20° and instillation is done without pressure avoiding overdistension of the pelvis. The whole procedure is done under strict aseptic precautions and the patient is given intravenous lasix to wash out $AgNO_3$ as well as antibiotics and analgesics for 5 days. The pelvis may be irrigated with distilled water after the procedure.

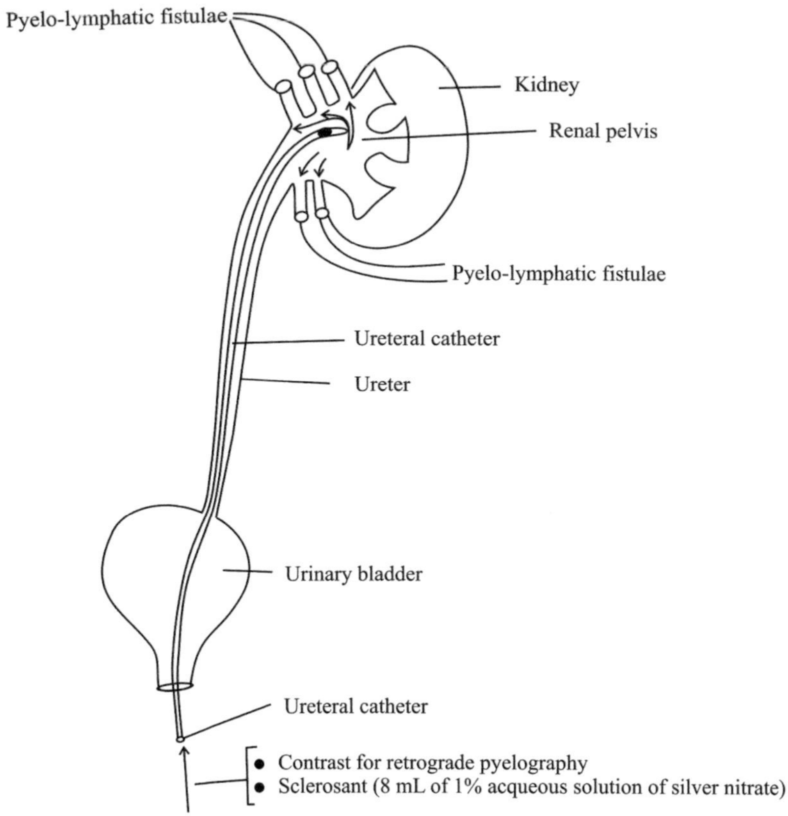

Fig. 30.7 Technique of retrograde pyelography (RGP) and sclerotherapy in renal chyluria

Mechanism of action The sclerosant enters the lymphatics through the pyelo-lymphatic fistulae resulting in chemical inflammation and edema of fistulae. Finally, the fistulae are occluded permanently by fibrosis.

Precautions The precautions to be taken during silver nitrate instillation therapy are given below:

1. A freshly prepared solution should be used in each patient.
2. The renal pelvis and the ureteral catheter must not be washed with plain water or normal saline as it results in precipitation of silver chloride, which may cause ureteral obstruction. They should be washed with distilled water.
3. No pressure should be used when the silver nitrate is being instilled as it may open pyelo-venous backflow leading to systemic reactions.

Dosage schedule Many protocols have been described but a protocol consisting of eight hourly instillations for 3 days (a total of nine doses) is most popular. Other dosage schedules are 12 hourly instillations for 2 days or weekly for 6–8 weeks. In bilateral efflux, a gap of 6–8 weeks is recommended between the treatments of two sides.

Results Sclerotherapy at a total of nine doses is effective in 60–80 % of cases. The patients with early recurrence do not fare better with a second course of RPIS in comparison with patients with delayed recurrence (Singh and Srivastava 2005). Overall, the sclerotherapy is effective in curing about 85 % cases of chyluria (see Table 30.3 and Flow chart 30.2 given below)

Disadvantages The disadvantages of use of silver nitrate are as follows:

1. The solution has to be stored in the dark to prevent its degradation.
2. It has to be autoclaved before use.
3. It is difficult to maintain the exact concentration of solution because of autoclaving.

Table 30.3 Results of silver nitrate sclerotherapy in chyluria

Authors (year)	Response rate		Follow-up (months)	Recurrence rate
Yu et al. (1978)	119/161	74 %	–	26 %
Ohyama et al. (1979)		62.5 %	2–115	37.5 %
Okamoto and Ohi (1983)	129/217	59.4 %	24	40.6 %
Tan et al. (1990)	46/55	83.6 %	24	16.4 %
Sabnis et al. (1992)	51/62	82 %	24–84	18.0 %
Dalela et al. (1992)		70 %	–	30.0 %
Goel et al. (2004)	40/44	81 %	24	19 %
Suri and Kumar (2005)	40/44	91 %	28.4	21 %

Chyluria

↓

Cystoscopy after fatty meal to find the side of chylous efflux

↓

Ureteral catheterization of the leaking side under C-arm fluoroscopy
(may be with retrograde pyelography to see the fistulae)

↓

Instillation of 8-10 mL of 0.1-1.0 % of silver nitrate solution in distilled water without pressure 8 hourly for 3 days (9 doses)

↓

Entry of sclerosant into lymphatic fistulae

↓

Immediate blockage of lymphatic fistulae by acute chemical inflammation i.e., inflammatory edema

↓

Immediate relief

↓

Delayed closure of lymphatic fistulae by postinflammatory fibrosis

↓

Permanent (delayed) relief

Flow chart 30.2 Silver nitrate instillation sclerotherapy in chyluria

4. The solution has to be prepared fresh for each patient. It may result in 8–24 h delay in starting therapy.

Complications The complications of 0.1–1.0 % silver nitrate instillation therapy include flank pain, fever, nausea, vomiting, and occasional hematuria. Spillage of the sclerosant at the pelvi-ureteral junction or at the ureter level may cause stricture formation. There are reports of renal papillary necrosis, arterial hemorrhage, and acute renal failure after pelvi-calyceal system cast formation (Sabnis et al. 1992; Mandhani et al. 1998).

Recurrence Recurrence of chyluria occurs in 15–20 % of patients. Early recurrence could be due to inadequate sclerotherapy, release of chyle from the opposite kidney, and the presence of chylo-lymphatic fistulae in lower ureter or urinary bladder. Late recurrence is due to recanalization of obstructed or sclerosed lymphatics in treated kidney (see the Table 30.4 below):

The recurrences are managed with an alternative sclerosant instillation, e.g., povidone iodine, removal of cause, if any, or surgical treatment.

Silver nitrate at 1 % Sabnis et al. (1992) treated 62 patients with chyluria over 8 years with instillation of 10–15 mL of 1.0 % silver nitrate every half an hour for four times (one course), repeated if required after 6 weeks. In bilateral disease, the opposite side was treated after 6 weeks. It gave 80–85 % permanent remissions. The complications were minor such as flank pain, hematuria, nausea, and vomiting 24–48 h after treatment. There were no major problems.

Silver nitrate at 3 % The experience with silver nitrate at 3 % is not good. Many authors have reported severe to fatal complications with the use of 3 % silver nitrate. Mandhani et al. (1998) have reported a case where bilateral simultaneous 3 % silver nitrate instillation was done elsewhere who presented with anuria and acute renal tubular necrosis. This patient was treated with percutaneous nephrostomy with right Davis intubated ureterotomy with DJ stent and left ileal replacement. During exploration, both ureters were cord-like with black deposits. The patient died of septicemia 15 days after operation. Srivasta et al. (1998) reported a case of massive arterial hematuria following 3 % $AgNO_3$ instillation. It required coil embolization of ruptured intra-renal aneurysm.

Silver nitrate at 5 % Kumar and Bhat (1975) treated 45 patients with chyluria by instillation of 5 % silver nitrate in the renal pelvis with the disappearance of chyluria in

Table 30.4 Causes of recurrence

Early recurrence	Late recurrence
Inadequate sclerotherapy	Recanalization of sclerosed or obstructed lymphatics
Release of chyle from the opposite kidney	
Presence of chylo-lymphatic fistulae in lower ureter, urinary bladder, or posterior urethra	

41 patients. Pandey (1985) reported his experience of treating over 200 patients with chyluria with unilateral instillation of 10–15 mL of 5 % $AgNO_3$ using ureteral balloon catheter to block the pelvi-ureteral junction. It was followed by aspiration of $AgNO_3$ and distilled water washout. The complications reported include anaphylactic reaction, renal cortical and perinephric abscess, ureteral stricture, and chemical cystitis.

Povidone iodine instillation therapy Povidone iodine is a water-soluble nonionic surfactant polymer (polyvinyl pyrrolidone) which releases iodine slowly. It has antibacterial and antifungal activity and is safe and effective. A freshly prepared 0.2 % solution in distilled water should be used every time. The results of some series are given in the following Table 30.5:

The advantages of povidone iodine sclerotherapy include: (1) it is cheap and readily available, (2) it has antibacterial and antifungal properties, hence there is no need to autoclave it, and (3) it hardly has any side effects that are seen with $AgNO_3$ sclerotherapy. However, its long-term results are awaited before declaring it as the sclerosant of first choice for chyluria.

Combination sclerotherapy The combination therapy consists of the use of a mixture of two sclerosants in the hope of getting a better and stronger fibrotic response. One method is to combine 5 mL of 0.2 % povidone iodine with 5 mL of 50 % dextrose for instillation in renal pelvis. This therapy is considered safe, and it provides a better and stronger fibrotic response. Nandy et al. (2004) treated 46 patients with chyluria with this method with a response rate of 87 % with 13 % recurrences on a follow-up of 24 months.

Sharma et al. (2008) treated 40 patients with chyluria with renal pelvic instillation using a solution containing povidone iodine with a contrast agent diluted with sterile water at a ratio of 1:1:3—unilateral in 26 cases (10 on the right side and 16 on the left side) and bilateral in 14 patients who had bilateral efflux. Immediate clearance was observed in 39 and recurrence occurred in 5 cases. They were treated again with the same technique with satisfactory results.

Suri and Kumar (2005) treated 21 patients with 50 % dextrose instillation with high immediate failure (57 %) and 38 % recurrence rate. Hence, they stopped using this method further. Subsequently, they treated 44 patients with 1 % silver nitrate and 41 with 0.2 % povidone iodine. Forty patients in the $AgNO_3$ group (91 %) and 40 patients in the povidone iodine group (98 %) showed immediate clearance but it recurred in a few patients in each group. The cumulative success rate after two courses of RPIS was 82 % (36/44) in the $AgNO_3$ group and 83 % (34/41) in the povidone iodine group. Five patients (11 %) in the first group had

Table 30.5 Results of povidone iodine instillation therapy

Authors (year)	Response rate		Follow up (months)	Recurrence rate
Shanmugam et al. (1988)	5/5	100 %	6	–
Goel et al. (2004)	36/41	88 %	24	12
Nandy et al. (2004)	40/46	87 %	24	13

significant flank pain with each instillation requiring injectable analgesia while one patient (2 %) in the second group had flank pain requiring an injectable analgesic.

Concluding, sclerotherapy is a safe, effective, and minimally invasive treatment for chyluria. Recurrence after the first course of sclerotherapy should be treated with a second course of sclerotherapy. The time of recurrence after the first course is important as the patients who have a shorter chyluria-free duration fare poorly with a second course of sclerotherapy. Both sides should not be instilled in one sitting.

30.10.2 Surgical Treatment

Most patients with chyluria are relieved by the therapeutic measures described above. It is only 20 % of the chylurics who are not relieved by the treatment already described that require surgical help (Karanjavala 1979). The indications for surgery are

1. Failure of nonoperative treatment that includes a course of diethylcarbamazine, dietary modification, and two or more courses of instillation sclerotherapy
2. Weight loss, significant hypoproteinemia, anasarca, recurrent clot retention, persistent clot colic, hematochyluria, and recurrent urinary tract infection due to chyluria

The operative procedures that are available are pyelo-lymphatic disconnection, uretero-lympholysis (Patna operation), Cockett and Goodwin (1962) procedure, microsurgical techniques, renal autotransplantation, and nephrectomy.

Pyelo-lymphatic disconnection It is the most commonly performed procedure first described by Katamine (1952) and later modified by many workers (Yu et al. 1978; Okamoto and Ohi 1983). Katamine named this operation as interruption of renal pedicle lymphatics. The patient is given a fat-rich diet 24–36 h before operation to facilitate intraoperative recognition of lymphatic communications.

Under general anesthesia, the kidney is exposed by an extra-peritoneal standard flank incision. Turner Warwick 11th rib approach may be used. The kidney is freed all round and the varicose lymphatics of the renal hilum coursing along the renal vessels are dissected, ligated, and excised. The whole renal pedicle is bared along its entire circumference at least one centimeter in length. If a lymphatic is torn or injured during dissection, it should be ligated by fine absorbable suture rather than blocking it by electrocoagulation as the latter is ineffective because of the very thin cellular walls of these lymphatics. Mannitol 100 mL of 12.5 % is given by intravenous drip before dissecting around the renal hilum to prevent arterial spasm and transient renal ischemia.

The hilar stripping is continued up to 3–4 cm of the proximal ureter, which is the site of a majority of lymphatic shunts. The results of various workers of pyelo-lymphatic disconnection by open operation are given in the following Table 30.6:

Recurrence can occur after pyelo-lymphatic disconnection as was seen in 41 out of 160 patients (25.6 %) operated on by Okamoto and Ohi (1983). It occurred from contralateral and undetermined sites. Postoperative contralateral chyluria is believed to result from the pressure of chylous lymphostasis near the opposite renal pedicle lymphatics, causing a reflux of lymph into the unoperated kidney (Yu et al. 1978).

The pyelo-lymphatic disconnection operation destroys the pyelo-lymphatic backflow mechanism of the kidney. Kaufman and Goodwin (1958) showed that an effective pyelo-lymphatic backflow protects the kidney from the lethal effects of back pressure (obstructed uropathy) as this mechanism permits the escape of fluid from an obstructed kidney.

However, it is a relatively minor consideration when the life of the patient is threatened by the metabolic problems of severe chyluria.

The pyelo-lymphatic disconnection is a palliative measure as it does not correct the lymphatic hypertension. However, it gives dramatic relief in chyluria similar to that given by Crile–Boerema procedure in bleeding esophageal varices (Kanetkar et al. 1966).

Minimally invasive approach With the advent of laparoscopy, the problem of chyluria is now being managed with both transperitoneal and extraperitoneal endoscopic (retroperitoneoscopic) methods. The results of some of the authors are given in the following Table 30.7

Table 30.6 Results of pyelo-lymphatic disconnection

Authors (year)	Number of cases	Complete relief	Improved	No change
Okamoto and Ohi (1983)	383	375 (97.9 %)	5 (1.3 %)	3 (0.8 %)
Karanjavala (1979)	38	28 (73.7 %)	10 (16.3 %)	Nil
Punekar et al. (1997)	78	69 (88 %)	–	9 (12 %)
Chang et al. (1973)	13	12 (92.3 %)	–	1 (7.7 %)

Table 30.7 Results of minimally invasive methods in chyluria

Author (year)	Number of cases	Results	Follow-up
Gomella et al. (1998)	1	Complete relief	2 years
Jiang et al. (2003)	6	100 %	1–1.6 years
Gupta (2005)	12	100 % Recurrence in two patients from opposite sides which were treated by operation on that side later on	4–54 months (average 31 months)

Gupta's (2005) operative technique consisted of nephro-lympholysis, uretero-lympholysis (mobilization of ureter up to common iliac vessels), hilar lymphatic vessel stripping, fasciectomy (removal of perinephric fat), and nephropexy (fixation of renal capsule to psoas fascia at the upper, middle, and lower poles).

Tang et al. (2014) did renal pedicle lymphatic disconnection in 15 patients by retroperitoneoscopic method without fasciectomy and nephropexy. Avoidance of fasciectomy keeps the kidney adherent to posterior parietes, preventing the complication of nephroptosis, renal torsion, injury to accessory renal artery, and excessive capillary bleeding.

Patna operation Prasad et al. (1977) introduced the "ureter in a lymphatic tunnel concept" which is formed by a pampiniform plexus of tensely distended lymphatics and blood vessels and connective tissue around the ureter in close proximity to the abdominal aorta up to the uretero-vesical junction. It is markedly fragile and has many lymphatic lakes. It is considered responsible for chyluria. Hence, they did lymphatic disconnection of abdominal ureter only (Patna operation) without renal hilar disconnection. They treated 15 patients in this manner. Eight had surgery on the right side, and seven had bilateral operation—one had synchronous procedure and the rest had contralateral operation after 2 months. The overall success of this procedure was 93 % with one recurrence.

The routine stripping of the whole ureter up to the urinary bladder is not recommended as most of the leaks occur around the renal hilum. If there is an obvious leak at the bladder level on lymphoscintigraphy or pedal lymphangiography, dissection up to bladder level is mandatory.

Omental wrapping after pyelo-lymphatic disconnection Dalela et al. (2004) used greater omentum to wrap around the renal vessels after disconnection in chyluria to minimize morbidity and recurrence. It reduces lymphorrhea from the wound and incidence of lymphocele formation, recurrence, and fibrosis.

Microsurgical procedures In these operations, the obstructed lymphatic system is anastomosed to the venous system by microsurgical technique to decrease the renal lymphatic hypertension and lymphangiectasis to facilitate healing of lymphatic fistulae at renal papillae. There are many procedures in this group.

1. Cockett and Goodwin (1962): It includes the anastomosis of a single dilated hilar lymphatic to a spermatic or gonadal vein in the vicinity in end-to-side fashion. The disadvantages of this procedure include increased operating time and need for special facilities, and it is technically demanding.
2. *Lymphangio-venous anastomosis*: It is the anastomosis of a small vein in the inguinal region, dorsum of foot, leg, or thigh to a nearby lymphatic. It is a technically challenging procedure, more so in females as the vessels are thin. Zhao et al. (1988), in their series of cases, observed that 90 % of lymphatics had a diameter of less than 1 mm and the vessel wall consisted of one layer of endo-

thelial cell, making magnification mandatory for successful performance of this operation. Another difficulty includes finding a vein of adequate diameter locally.

In men, the anastomosis is done in the inguinal region, and in women, either in the dorsum of the foot or in the leg or thigh using end-to-end anastomosis. Usually, three to four anastomoses are done using four to six interrupted 9–10/0 nylon sutures.

If the lymphatics are less than 0.1 mm, a bundle of lymphatics is cut and inserted into a vein of appropriate size with a few anchoring sutures but it is usually difficult to find a vein of adequate diameter.

3. *Lymphadeno-venous anastomosis*: Ji et al. (1993) performed lymph node–saphenous vein anastomosis wherein they made a 2–3 mm diameter hole into the medulla of the lymph node and after confirmation of efflux of lymph it is anastomosed to the obliquely cut end of a tributary of saphenous vein with ligation of distal end. Generally, a single anastomosis using six to seven interrupted sutures is sufficient (Xu et al. 1991). The success rate of microsurgical procedures varies from 60 to 83 %. Xu et al. (1991)) have reported their experience of both these microsurgical procedures as given below (Table 30.8):

   The last two procedures are recommended in old and debilitated patients. Other advantages include no need to do lymphangiography and cystoscopy.

Renal autotransplantation Brunkwall et al. (1990) did renal autotransplantation in a patient with Klippel–Trenaunay–Weber syndrome who had failed pyelo-lymphatic disconnection done 3 months earlier. Following autotransplantation, he was asymptomatic for more than 12 months.

30.11 Other Treatments

Medical treatment Somatostatin has been used with benefit in posttraumatic chyluria due to lympho-renal fistula (Campieri et al. 1996; Giordano et al. 1996). Chyluria after radical nephrectomy has been treated successfully with *N*-butyl-2-cyanoacrylate (Tuck et al. 2000).

Surgical treatment Excision of perinephric fascia and fat (Gerota's fasciectomy) on both sides in two stages has been reported to result in complete resolution of chyluria (Pool et al. 1991).

Table 30.8 Results of microsurgical procedures

Procedure	Number of cases	Results		
		Complete cure	Improved	No relief
Lymphangio-venous anastomosis	50	30 (60 %)	6 (12 %)	14 (28 %)
Lymphadeno-venous anastomosis	12	6 (50 %)	2 (16.7 %)	4 (33.3 %)

Endoscopic therapy Chyluria was treated in five patients successfully with endoscopic coagulation using guide tube methods (Yagi et al. 1998). It can be easily done if the fistulous openings are present in the lower urinary tract.

30.12 Lymphuria

Lymphuria is a symptom characterized by the passage of lymph in urine. Similar to chyluria, it occurs due to the rupture of a lymph varix into the urinary tract anywhere from a calyx down to the urinary bladder including the ureter with escape of lymph into the urinary tract.

Clinical features It frequently appears without warning, but usually appears following pain in the back and aching sensation about the pelvis and groins probably caused by distension of the preexisting varix (Manson-Bahr and Apted 1982). The patient may have dysuria, frequency, and there may be retention of urine due to the presence of lymphous coagula. As the patient passes milky urine, this syndrome is labelled as chyluria till the examination of urine confirms it otherwise.

Urine examination The urine is thick, turbid, and may form a coagulum on prolonged standing. As the urine does not contain any fat, the turbidity does not disappear by the addition of xylol, ether, or chloroform. The Sudan III stain is negative. It contains protein which may be significant like that of nephrotic syndrome. The microscopic examination shows the absence of chylomicrons and the presence of plenty of lymphocytes and red blood cells.

The plain radiography of abdomen and intravenous pyelography are normal.

Ravichandran et al. (1982) reported the lymphographic findings in lymphuria—there is lymphangiectasis of pelvic and abdominal lymphatics and abnormal lymphatico-renal communications. The cisterna chyli and thoracic duct are normal.

It is investigated further like chyluria and treated on similar lines.

References

Akisada M, Tani S. Lymphagio-adenopathy in filariasis. Trans R Soc Trop Med Hyg. 1970;64: 884–94.

Ansari MS. Medical treatment of filariasis and chyluria. Indian J Urol. 2005;21:24–6.

Aye UT, Aung STT. Chyluria. Clin Radiol. 1975;26:237–42.

Bhuta KM, Rajdeo HP, Delima RJ, Vaze ML. Chyluria. Ind J Surg. 1978;40:608.

Brunkwall J, Simonsen O, Bergqvist D, Jonsson K, Bergentz SE. Chyluria treated with renal autotransplantation: a case report. J Urol. 1990;143(4):793–6.

Buttiker V, Fanconi S, Burger R. Chylothorax in children: guidelines for diagnosis and management. Chest. 1999;116:682–7.

Campieri C, Raimondi C, Dalmastri V, Sestigiani E, Neri L, Giudicissi A, et al. Post-traumatic chyluria due to lymphorenal fistula regressed after somatostatin therapy. Nephron. 1996;72: 705–7.

Chang CY, Yu HN, Lapides CH. Surgical treatment of chyluria. J Urol. 1973;109:299–302.

Charak Samhita (300 BC): Commented by Sastri KN and Chaturvedi CN. 2nd ed. Varanasi: Chowkhamba Vidya Bhawan; 1969. p. 635.
Cockett AT, Goodwin WE. Chyluria: attempted surgical treatment by lymphatic venous anastomosis. J Urol. 1962;88:566–8.
Dalela D, Kumar A, Ahlawat R, Goel TC, Misra VK, Chandra H. Routine radioimaging in filarial chyluria – is it necessary in developing countries? Brit J Urol. 1992;69:291–3.
Dalela D, Gupta VP, Goel A, Singh KM. Omental wrap around the renal pedicle: an adjunctive step to minimize morbidity and recurrence after lymphorenal disconnection for chyluria. BJU Int. 2004;94:673–4.
Dalela D. Issues in etiology and diagnosis making of chyluria. Indian J Urol. 2005;21:18–23.
Date A, John IJ, Chandy KG, et al. Abnormalities of the immune system in patients with chyluria. Brit J Urol. 1981;53:384–6.
Edwards JM. Surgery of the lymphatics. In: Bevan PG, editor. Reconstructive procedures in surgery. Oxford: Blackwell Scientific Publications; 1982. p. 380–2.
Esterre P, Plichart C, Huin-Blondey MO, et al. Circulating fibrosis markers, eosinophil cationic protein and eosinophil protein X in patients with Wuchereria bancrofti infection: association with clinical status. Parasite. 2006;13(2):165–70.
Geliebter A, Torby N, Braco EF. Over feeding with medium chain triglycerides diet results in diminished deposition of fat. Am J Clin Nut. 1983;37:1–4.
Giordano M, Crillo D, Baron I, Sorrentino F, Tomasino G, Cicchella T, et al. Treatment of post-traumatic chyluria with subcutaneous octreotide administration. Nephrol Dial Transplant. 1996;11:365–7.
Goel A, Goyal NK, Parihar A, Singh R. Magnetic resonance-retrograde pyelography: a novel technique for evaluation of chyluria. Indian J Urol. 2014;30:115–6.
Goel S, Mandhani A, Srivastava A, Kapoor R, Gogoi S, Kumar A, et al. Is povidone iodine an alternative to silver nitrate for renal pelvic instillation sclerotherapy in chyluria? Br J Urol. 2004;94:1082–5.
Golestaneh L, Karam S, et al. Hypercoagulability in a patient with chronic chyluria, proteinuria and hypoalbuminemia. Nephrol Dial Transplant. 2009;24:3240–3.
Gomella LG, Shenot P, Abdel-Meguid TA. Extraperitoneal laparoscopic nephrolysis for treatment of chyluria. Br J Urol. 1998;81:320–1.
Govil S, Justus A, Lakshminarayanan R, Nayak S, Devasia A, Gopalkirshnan G. Retro-peritoneal lymphatics on CT and MRI. Abdom Imaging. 2007;32:53–5.
Goyal NK, Goel A, Sankhwar SN, Singh V, Ali W, Natu SM, et al. Factors affecting response to medical management in patients of filarial chyluria: a prospective study. Indian J Urol. 2014;30:23–7.
Gu XT, Gao ZG, Shen BR, et al. Changes in T-lymphocyte subsets of peripheral blood in patients with filarial chyluria. Zhongguo Ji Sheng Chong Xue Yu Ji Sheng Chong Bing Za Zhi. 2000; 18(2):103–5.
Gupta NP. Retroperitoneoscopic management of intractable chyluria. Indian J Urol. 2005;21:63–5.
Hemal AK, Gupta NP. Retroperitoneoscipic lymphatic management of intractable chyluria. J Urol. 2002;167:2473–6.
Henry MM, Thompson JN. Chylothorax. In: Henry MM, Thompson JN, editors. Clinical Surgery. Second edition. Edinburgh: Elsevier Saunders; 2005. p 264.
Dusmet M. Chest and lungs. In: Henry MM, Thompson JN, editors. Clinical surgery. 2nd ed. Edinburgh: Elsevier Saunders; 2005. p. 264.
Jiang J, Zhu F, Jin F, Jiang Q, Wang L. Retroperitoneoscopic renal pedicle lymphatic disconnection for chyluria. Chin Med J (Engl). 2003;116:1746–8.
Ji YZ, Zheng JH, Chen JN, Wu ZD. Microsurgery in the treatment of chyluria and scrotal lymphangial fistula. Br J Urol. 1993;72:952–4.
Kanetkar AV, Karanjawalla DK, Deshmukh SM, Sen PK. Initial experience in the management of chyluria. Indian J Surg. 1966;28:381–8.
Karanjavala DK. Technique of clearance (or disconnection) of dilated lymphatics in the renal hilum and lower ureter and bladder in cases of intractable chyluria or haematochyluria. Br J Urol. 1979;51:440–2.

Katamine D. Studies on the pathogenesis of chyluria in filariasis I. The entrance of chyle in urine. Nagasaki Igakkai Zasshi. 1952;27(4):195–200.

Kaufman JJ, Goodwin WE. Renal lymphatics. III. Clinical implications and experiments of nature. Ann Intern Med. 1958;49(1):109–19. PMID:13545737.

Klousia JW, Mcclennan BL, Semerjian HS. Chyluria: a case report and brief literature review. J Urol. 1977;117:393–4.

Kumar M, Bhat HS. Chyluria: treatment with silver nitrate instillation. Indian J Surg. 1975;37:335–8.

Koga S, Arakaki Y, Matsuoka M, Ohyama C. Remission of filarial chyluria after treatment of coexistent conditions. Lymphology. 1990;23:164–6.

Maged A. Renal chyluria. Br J Urol. 1967;39:555–9.

Mandhani A, Kapoor R, Gupta RK, Rao HS. Can silver nitrate installation for the treatment of chyluria be fatal? Br J Urol. 1998;82:926–7.

Manson-Bahr PEC, Apted FIC. Filariases. In: Manson's tropical diseases. 18th ed. London: Bailliere Tindal; 1982. p. 148–80.

Mehta VK, Lohar H, Banerjee GK, Reddy MV, Harinath BC. Surgical filariasis: immuno screening for filarial IgG antibodies using Wuchereria bancrofti microfilarial excretory-secretary antigen. J Commun Dis. 1999;31:35–40.

Nandy PR, Dwivedi US, Vyas N, Prasad M, Dutta B, Singh PB. Povidone iodine and dextrose solution combination sclerotherapy in chyluria. Urology. 2004;64:1107–10.

Ngan H, Leong CH. A lymphographic study of chyluria. Br J Radiol. 1977;50(600):863–70.

Nutman TB, Weller PF. Filarial and related infections. In: Longo DL, Fauci AS, Kasper DL, Hauser SL, Jameson JL, Loscalzo J, editors. Harrison's internal medicine. 18th ed. New York: McGraw Hill; 2012. p. 1745–8.

Ohyama C, Saita H, Miyasato N. Spontaneous remission of chyluria. J Urol. 1979;121:316–7.

Okamoto K, Ohi Y. Recent distribution and treatment of filarial chyluria in Japan. J Urol. 1983;129:64–7.

Pandey AP. Chyluria: Oxford Textbook of Surgery; 1985. Desai R. Complications and precautions of sclerotherapy for chyluria. Indian J Urol 2005; 21: 30–3.

Pandey AP. Chyluria. In: Morris PJ, Malt RA, editors. Oxford textbook of surgery, vol. 2. New York: Oxford University Press; 1994. p. 2567–8.

Pecquet J. Experimentia nova anatomica. Paris; 1951. Kinmonth JB. The lymphatics. London: Edward Arnold 1982. p 267.

Pool MO, van der Hem KG, Stel HV, Luth WJ, Rasker FM, Gans RO. Bilateral excision of perinephric fat and fascia (Gerota's fasciectomy) in the treatment of intractable chyluria. J Urol. 1991;146:1374–6.

Pope, 1909: Quoted by Maged A. Renal chyluria. Brit J Urol. 1967;39:555.

Prasad PB, Choudhary DK, Barnwal SN, Jha S, Bharthuar A. Periureteric lymphovenous stripping in cases of chylohaematuria – report of 15 cases. Indian J Surg. 1977;39:607–12.

Punekar SV, Kelkar AR, Prem AR. Surgical dissection of lymphorenal communication for chyluria: a 15 year experience. Br J Urol. 1997;80:858–63.

Ravichandran R, Desai S, Acharya VN. Lymphuria (a case report). Indian J Surg. 1982;44:602–3.

Sabnis RB, Punekar SV, Desai RM, Bradoo AM, Bapat SD. Instillation of silver nitrate in the treatment of chyluria. Br J Urol. 1992;70:660–2.

Sen SB, Ellapan S. Chylous manifestations of filariasis: a clinical and lymphographic study. Part I. Filarial chyluria. Indian J Med Res. 1968;56:1535–45.

Shanmugam TV, Prakash JV, Sivashankar G. Povidone iodine used as a sclerosing agent in the treatment of chyluria. Br J Urol. 1988;82:557–8.

Sharma G, Chitale V, Karva R, Sharma A, Durug AB. Fluoroscopy-guided instillation therapy in chyluria using povidone iodine with contrast agent. Is a single instillation sufficient? Int Braz J Urol. 2008;34:270–6.

Sharma S, Hemal AK. Chyluria – an overview. Int J Nephrol Urol. 2009;1:14–26.

Singh KJ, Srivastava A. Nonsurgical management of chyluria (sclerotherapy). Indian J Urol. 2005;21:55–8.

Srivasta DN, Yadav S, Hemal AK, Berry M. Arterial hemorrhage resulting in massive hematuria following $AGNO_3$ instillation. Austral Radiol. 1998;42:234–5.

Suri A, Kumar A. Chyluria – SGPGI experience. Indian J Urol. 2005;21:59–62.

Tan IB, Chiang CP, Huang CH, Chou YH, Wang CJ. Experiences in the treatment of chyluria in Taiwan. J Urol. 1990;144:710–3.

Tanagho EA, Kane CJ. Specific infections of the genitourinary tract. In: McAninch JW, Lue TF, editors. Smith & Tanagho's general urology. 18th ed. New York: McGraw Hill Medical; 2013. p. 234–5.

Tang L, Yu D, Feng W, Shi H. Modified technique of renal pedicle disconnection for chyluria through laparoscopic surgery. Int J Clin Exp Med. 2014;7:2916–20.

Tuck J, Pearce I, Pantelides M. Chyluria after radical nephrectonry treated with N-butyl-2-cyanoacrylate. J Urol. 2000;164:778–9.

Xing C, Xing XM, Xing L. Immunological observation on chyluric patients with heat clearing and hemostatic drugs. Z hongguo Zhong Xi Yi Jie He Za Zhi. 1994;14:601–3.

Xu YM, Ji RJ, Chen JD, Qiao Y, Jin NT. Microsurgical treatment of chyluria: a preliminary report. J Urol. 1991;145:1184–5.

Yagi S, Goto T, Kawamoto K, Miyawaki I, Tanaka I, Mori K, et al. Endoscopic treatment of refractory filarial chyluria: a preliminary report. J Urol. 1998;159:1615–8.

Yamauchi S. Chyluria: clinical, laboratory and statistical study of 45 personal cases observed in Hawaii. J Urol. 1945;54:318.

Yu HHY, Ngan H, Leong CH. Chyluria: a 10-year follow up. Br J Urol. 1978;50:126–33.

Zhao WP, Hou LQ, Shen JL. Summary and prospects of fourteen year's experience with treatment of chyluria by microsurgery. Eur Urol. 1988;15:219–22.

31 Chylous Ascites: Chyloperitoneum

It is an accumulation of lipid-rich lymph or chyle in the peritoneal cavity due to the leak of chyle from chyle-bearing lymphatics.

31.1 Etiology

The most common cause of chylous ascites is abdominal malignancy. However, the classified list of causes of chylous ascites is as follows (Tavakkolizadeh et al. 2010):

31.1.1 Most Common Causes

(a) In eastern and developing countries
  1. Tuberculosis
  2. Lymphatic filariasis

(b) In western and developed countries
  1. Abdominal malignancies, especially lymphoma and metastatic lymph nodes of adenocarcinoma of pancreas or stomach (Kinmonth, 1982)
  2. Cirrhosis of liver

Foschi et al. (2008) reported a 43-year-old HIV-positive male who presented with chylous ascites secondary to B-cell non-Hodgkin lymphoma. Sharma et al. (2013) has described about a woman of 61 years of age who presented with perforated gall bladder with gall bladder stones and chylous ascites. The postoperative histology of gall bladder revealed an adenocarcinoma of gall bladder.

T.C. Goel, A. Goel, *Lymphatic Filariasis*, DOI 10.1007/978-981-10-2257-9_31

31.1.2 Other Causes

1. Abdominal and thoracic operations, e.g., abdominal aortic aneurysm repair, retroperitoneal lymph node dissection, inferior vena cava resection, liver transplantation
2. Congenital lymphatic abnormalities, e.g., primary lymphatic hyperplasia, megalymphatics
3. Radiation
4. Pancreatitis
5. Right-sided heart failure

Spence et al. (1977) described a 32-year-old man who developed chylous ascites following retroperitoneal lymph node dissection for a testicular tumor.

31.2 Pathogenesis

The collection of chyle in the peritoneal cavity occurs from one of the following mechanisms (Turnage and Badgwell 2012):

1. Obstruction of the major lymph channels at the root of mesentery or the cisterna chyli with exudation of chyle from dilated mesenteric lymphatics (lacteals)
2. Direct leakage of chyle through a lymphatico-peritoneal fistula caused by abnormal (megalymphatics) or injured retro-peritoneal lymphatics
3. Exudation of chyle through the walls of retro-peritoneal megalymphatics without a visible fistula or thoracic duct obstruction

In the filarial chylous ascites, it is the first factor which is responsible for peritoneal chylous accumulation.

31.3 Pathology

In lymphatic filariasis, the obstruction to the lymphatic flow occurs at the level of cisterna chyli or above or in the root of mesentery. The obstruction results in chylous reflux, congestion and exudation of chyle from the peritoneal surface. A well-defined lymphatico-peritoneal fistula as seen in primary lymphatic disease (megalymphatics) is not seen in filarial chylous ascites. Distended milky white lacteals may be seen on the surface of the small bowel, especially the jejunum.

31.4 Clinical Features

The patient presents with gradually increasing distension of abdomen with a past history of recurrent attacks of fever with rigors (Fig. 31.1). The patient may be lean and thin with protuberant abdomen.

There are signs of free fluid in the peritoneum which vary from mild to massive accumulation. Other manifestations of filariasis may be present.

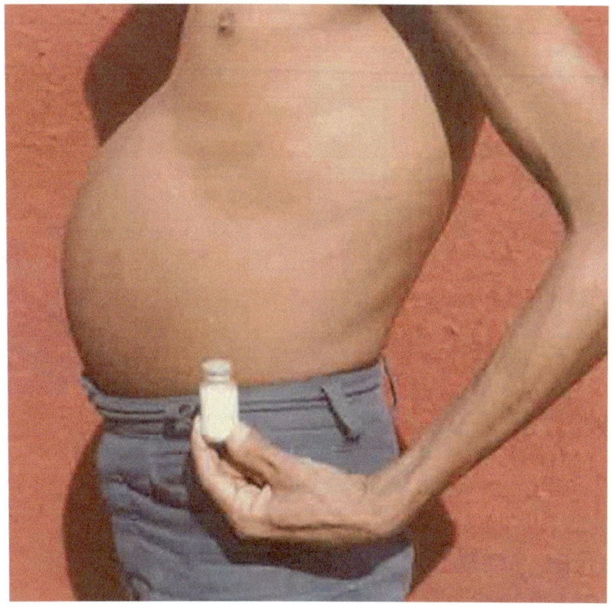

Fig. 31.1 Left lateral view of a chylous ascitic patient holding chylous peritoneal aspirate in his left hand

31.5 Investigations

- *Paracentesis abdominis* – The peritoneal aspirate is milky white in color (Fig. 31.1). It has chylomicrons with triglyceride level more than 110 mg/dL (more than that of plasma); it may be up to 1500 mg/dL (Doherty 2010). The serum-ascites albumin gradient (SAAG) is less than 1.1 mg/dL. Its leukocyte count is more than 1000/μL, and they are mostly lymphocytes.
- *Blood* examination shows anemia, hypoalbuminemia and lymphocytopenia (Doherty 2010). In filarial chylous ascites, the blood may show eosinophilia and elevated ESR. The immunological tests for filariasis may be positive.
- *Lymphography* shows the site of lymphatic obstruction high up in the retroperitoneum with diffusion of dye in the peritoneal cavity following peritoneal massage. Free dye is present in the pelvic peritoneum 12–24 h after injection.
- *CT scan* may show the cause and effect of this manifestation. It is not of much help in filarial chylous ascites. It helps in ruling out other causes of obstruction of chyle-bearing pathways.

31.6 Treatment

The cause of this manifestation is treated or removed, e.g., in filarial chylous ascites, a course of diethylcarbamazine 100 mg three times daily orally is given for 3–4 weeks. A low-fat diet supplemented with medium-chain triglycerides (MCTs) and high protein content is very helpful in reducing the loss of fat in the peritoneal cavity. The fatty acids with less than 10 carbon atoms in the chain are absorbed directly into the portal venous system (Moncure 1994) bypassing the intestinal lymphatic

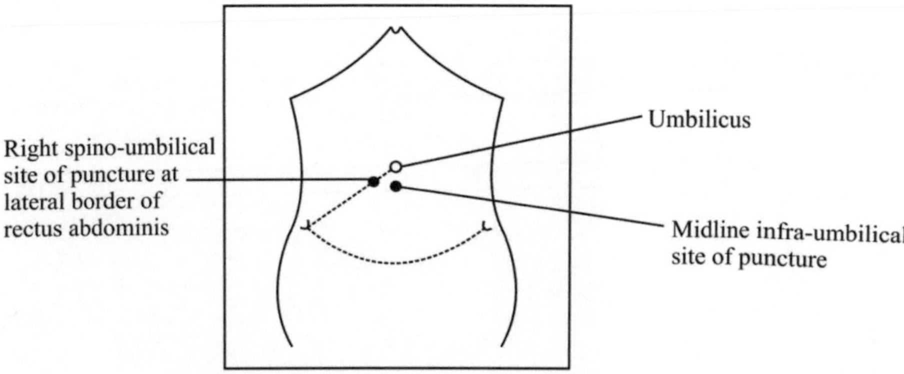

Fig. 31.2 Sites of paracentesis abdominis (●); *midline* infraumbilical or *right* spinoumbilical at the lateral border of the rectus abdominis

system. The diet should be rich in vitamins and minerals, especially calcium. Intravenous magnesium in addition to calcium helps in correcting hypocalcemia (Skyring 1967).

The patients who do not respond to the above measures should be put to fasting and given total parenteral nutrition (TPN). Somatostatin or octreotide may be of help by reducing the lymph flow. Overall, 60 % of patients respond to the above therapeutic measures.

- *Peritoneal tapping* – The symptoms of distension can be relieved by tapping the ascitic fluid but it refills rapidly adding to deficiency of nutrition and weakness. Hence, it is usually not recommended.
  The urinary bladder is emptied by a catheter and, under local anesthesia, the peritoneum is punctured with a trocar and cannula in the midline just below the umbilicus, or at the right spino-umbilical line just lateral to the lateral border of rectus abdominis (Fig. 31.2). The trocar is removed and a catheter is passed into the peritoneal cavity and the cannula is removed. The catheter is fixed to the abdominal wall with adhesive tape and connected to a sterile collecting bottle.
- *Peritoneo-venous shunting* (LeVeen et al. 1974)—If the patient does not respond to the conservative treatment, he/she may be treated with peritoneo-venous shunting for continuous or permanent drainage of peritoneal fluid into the venous blood.
  It is done with subcutaneous placement of a silicon catheter connecting the peritoneal cavity with a large vein, e.g., superior vena cava. This catheter has a small chamber approximately in the middle which has a unidirectional valve. It is put in the subcutaneous plane with one end inserted into the peritoneal cavity up to the pelvis and the other in the internal jugular vein and thence into the superior vena cava after removing air of the catheter (Fig. 31.3). The chamber may be compressed intermittently manually to drain the fluid rapidly.
  It is an effective method of treatment of ascites containing serous fluid. However, in chylous ascites, it is associated with a high occlusion rate. The other complications include overloading of the right side of the heart, sepsis and dis-

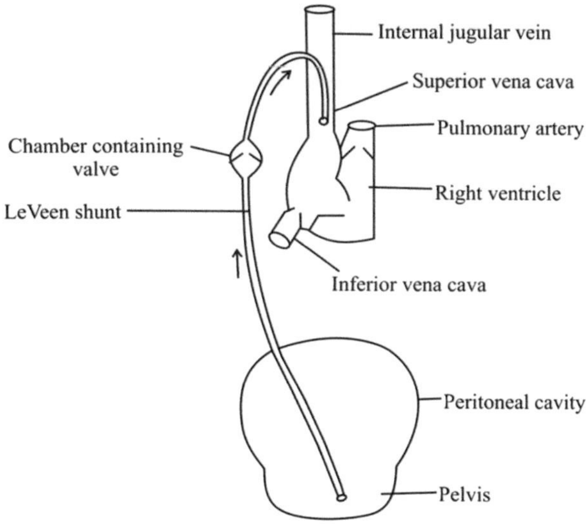

Fig. 31.3 Peritoneo-venous shunt (LeVeen et al. 1974)

seminated intravascular coagulation. The incidence of these complications can be reduced by evacuating the chylous ascitic fluid and partially substituting it with normal saline at the time of placement of the shunt. Postoperatively, the patient is given prophylactic antibiotics for 5 days and diuretics.

The venous end of the shunt may be inserted into the long saphenous vein and through that into the inferior vena cava.

The senior author (TCG) has done peritoneo-long saphenous venous anastomosis in a case of chylous ascites shown in Fig. 31.1. The immediate result was good but the long-term result is not known.

Following reinfusion of chylous ascitic fluid, several mortalities have occurred owing to anaphylaxis or more likely from fat embolism (Klippel and Hardy 1971). The latter may be obviated by the use of infusion filters.

- *Laparotomy* – Surgical exploration of peritoneal cavity and retro-peritoneum is generally reserved in patients who fail to improve with nonoperative treatment (Turnage and Badgwell 2012).

  In filarial chylous ascites, internal fistulae are usually not seen but may be seen in primary lymphatic disease when the closure of the fistula has its advocates (Clain 1971; Turnage and Badgwell 2012), but it is not always successful (Klippel and Hardy 1971) and is not without risk. Lipophilic dye markers, e.g., Sudan black, Sudan III, and Evans blue, which combine with ingested fat, may be placed in the intestine to facilitate identification of the fistula.

  A solitary fistula may be electrocoagulated, or the segment of the bowel containing the fistula/fistulae may be resected if it is a small segment. In some cases, application of fibrin glue may be of help (Turnage and Badgwell 2012).

  Sen et al. (1971) reported a case of chylous ascites following blunt injury of the abdomen where the site of leakage and the filarial pathology of the lymphatic system were demonstrated by preoperative lymphography. It was successfully treated by repair of rent by pedicle omental graft.

References

Clain A. Chylous ascites following vagotomy. Br J Surg. 1971;58:312–4.

Doherty GM. Peritoneal cavity. In: Doherty GM, editor. Current diagnosis & treatment – surgery. 13th ed. New York: McGraw Hill Medical; 2010. p. 474.

Foschi D, Rizzi A, et al. Chylous ascites secondary to B-cell non-Hodgkin's lymphoma in a patient with acquired immune deficiency syndrome (AIDS). Dig Liver Dis. 2008;40:481–2.

Kinmonth JB. The lymphatics. 2nd ed. London: Edward Arnold; 1982. p. 239.

Klippel AP, Hardy DA. Postoperative chylous ascites. Case reports. Mo Med. 1971;68:253–5.

LeVeen HH, Christoudias G, Moon IP, et al. Peritoneo-venous shunting for ascites. Ann Surg. 1974;180:580–91.

Moncure AC. Chylothorax. In: Morris PJ, Malt RA, editors. Oxford textbook of surgery, vol. 1. New York: Oxford University Press; 1994. p. 1933–5.

Sen SB, Chatterjee H, Pillai NK. Chylous ascites precipitated by rupture of pathological thoracic duct: a rare complication of filarial chylous reflux. J Indian Med Assoc. 1971;56:44–6.

Sharma BK, Pareek P, et al. Cholelithiasis with perforated gall bladder presenting as chylous ascites – a case report. IJRRMS. 2013;3:59–61. http://www.ijrrms.com/pdf/2013/jun-oct/17.pdf.

Skyring AP, 1967. Quoted by Kinmonth JB. The lymphatics. 2nd edn. London: Edward Arnold; 1982.

Spence CR, Solomon MD, Agee RE, Gangai MP. Chylous ascites: an unusual complication following retro-peritoneal lymphadenectomy for testis tumor. J Urol. 1977;117:676–7.

Tavakkolizadeh A, Whang EE, Ashley SW, Zinner MJ. Small intestine. In: Brunicardi FC, Andersen DK, Billiar TR, Dunn DL, Hunter JG, Matthews JB, Pollock RE, editors. Schwartz's principles of surgery. 9th ed. New York: McGraw Hill Medical; 2010. p. 1008–9.

Turnage RH, Badgwell B. Chylous ascites. In: Townsend Jr CM, Beauchamp RD, Evers BM, Mattox KL, editors. Sabiston textbook of surgery. 19th ed. Philadelphia: Elsevier Saunders; 2012. p. 1100.

Chylocele

32

It is a collection of chylous fluid in the tunica vaginalis of scrotum which presents clinically as hydrocele without translucency. It is a clinical manifestation of long-standing lymphatic filariasis (DeVries 2002). Sen et al. (1969) described four cases of chylocele with bilateral disease in two patients.

32.1 Etiology

It is a manifestation of filarial obstruction of chyle-bearing pathways in the retro-peritoneum resulting in ilio-inguinal backflow leading to dilatation and rupture of lymphatics of the cord. Sometimes, it is due to rupture of a chyle-containing cyst of spermatic cord into the cavity of tunica vaginalis.

32.2 Clinical Features

The patient presents with a scrotal swelling of insidious onset which has all the signs of a hydrocele except that translucency is absent (Fig 32.1). The swelling is relatively heavy. The scrotal skin may be more vascular with visible veins. A past history of recurrent attacks of fever with rigors is usually available.

32.3 Investigations

- *Blood* is usually normal. It may show eosinophilia and sometimes microfilariae especially if the patient had a recent attack of filariasis.
- *Ultrasonography* of the scrotum shows the fluid accumulation in the tunica with normal testis. The chylous accumulation cannot be differentiated from serous accumulation of scrotal hydrocele by this method of imaging.

T.C. Goel, A. Goel, *Lymphatic Filariasis*, DOI 10.1007/978-981-10-2257-9_32

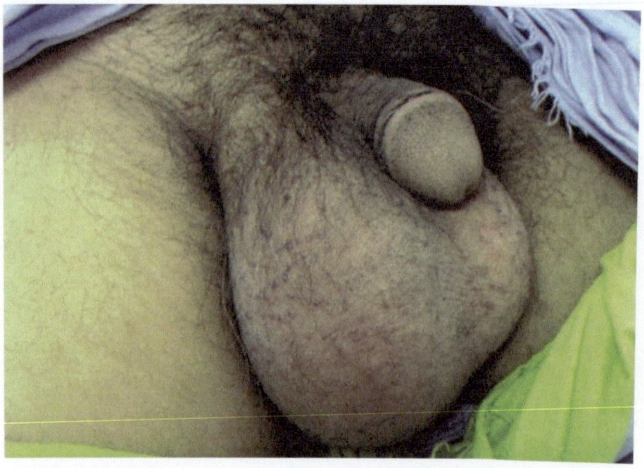

Fig. 32.1 Right-sided scrotal hydrocele which was found to be chylocele at operation

- *Needle aspiration* confirms the presence of chyle. The aspirate contains liquid fat which is rich in cholesterol. If this fluid is stored in a tall glass for some time, a film of liquid fat floats on the surface. It may be frankly milky. It often has leukocytes (DeVries 2002) and may have microfilariae. Sen et al. (1969) found microfilariae in one out of four patients with chylocele.
  The diagnostic needle aspiration is not done as a rule, as it is not of much practical advantage and may result in some complications, e.g., infection and bleeding. Hence, most of the time, the diagnosis of chylocele is made during surgery for 'hydrocele' when a hydrocele turns out to be chylocele.
- *Lymphography* is usually not done in these cases. However, Sen (1974) described the lymphographic findings in chylocele. It showed dilated spermatic cord lymphatics going into the retro-peritoneum with chylous reflux known as obstructive lymphangiopathy of spermatic cord.

32.4 Treatment

- A course of diethylcarbamazine is given and further mosquito bites are prevented.
- The scrotal swelling is operated as a scrotal hydrocele. After removal of the fluid, the tunica vaginalis is excised as it is too thick for eversion. It may be difficult in long-standing chylocele as there are dense adhesions between the scrotum and its contents. Sometimes, removal of the testis and spermatic cord is required.
- The overall results of treatment are good. However, filarial elephantiasis supervenes in a small number of patients after operation on a chylocele. Sometimes, devastating lymph scrotum may supervene (DeVries 2002).
- Kinmonth (1982) suggested extensive ligation of retro-peritoneal lympathatics to prevent recurrence.

References

DeVries CR. The role of the urologist in the treatment and elimination of lymphatic filariasis worldwide. BJU Int. 2002;89 Suppl 1:37–43.

Kinmonth JB. The lymphatics. 2nd ed. London: Edward Arnold; 1982. p. 219.

Sen SB, Chatterjee H, Ramprasad S. Chylous manifestations of filariasis: a clinical and lymphographic study. II. Lymphadenovarix, chylocoele and chylous lymph scrotum. Indian J Med Res. 1969;57:1738–44.

Sen SB. Chyluria and chyle reflux. In: Gooneratne BWM, editor. Lymphography: clinical and experimental. 1st ed. London: Butterworths; 1974. p. 123–45.

Chylothorax 33

It is the accumulation of lymphatic fluid or chyle in the pleural cavity due to leakage of chyle from the thoracic duct.

33.1 Etiology

A chylothorax occurs when the chyle from the thoracic duct empties or leaks into the pleural space (Nair et al. 2007), the causes of which are described below (DeMeester and Lafontaine 1990; Cohen et al. 1996).

- *Congenital*
  1. Atresia of thoracic duct
  2. Thoracic duct-pleural space fistula
  3. Birth trauma
- *Traumatic, including iatrogenic trauma*
  1. Blunt/penetrating thoracic trauma including hyperextension injury
  2. Surgical procedures
     (a) Cervical, e.g., radical cervical lymph node dissection
     (b) Thoracic, e.g., correction of patent ductus arteriosus, repair of coarctation of aorta, vascular procedures involving origin of left subclavian artery, esophagectomy, cervico-dorsal sympathectomy, resection of thoracic aneurysm, resection of mediastinal tumors, left pneumonectomy
     (c) Abdominal, e.g., lumbar sympathectomy, aortic aneurysm repair, radical retro-peritoneal lymph node dissection
  3. Diagnostic procedures, e.g., translumbar aortography, subclavian vein catheterization
- Sendama and Shipley (2015) reported a patient with right-sided chylothorax following traumatic burst fracture of lumbar one vertebra.
- *Tumors of mediastinum and neck*, especially lymphoma and metastatic lymph nodes

T.C. Goel, A. Goel, *Lymphatic Filariasis*, DOI 10.1007/978-981-10-2257-9_33

- *Infections*
  1. Tuberculous lymphadenitis
  2. Nonspecific mediastinitis
  3. Ascending lymphangitis
  4. Lymphatic filariasis
- *Other causes*
  1. Venous thrombosis of left subclavian-jugular vein or superior vena cava
  2. Pulmonary lymphangiomatosis

The lymphatic filariasis is a rare cause of chylothorax. The most common cause is trauma which includes iatrogenic injury, accidental trauma to the neck or chest (Kumar et al. 2005) including hyperextension injury. Strahberger and Scheuba (1958) described seven cases of chylothorax due to trauma, operation or tumor, and none due to lymphatic filariasis.

33.2 Pathology

In filarial chylothorax, the thoracic duct is blocked in its upper part due to fibrous scarring caused by filarial infection. The obstructed duct is reduced to an impermeable fibrous structure or a string (Kinmonth 1982). The chyle accumulates in the pleural cavity due to transudation of chyle from the pulmonary surface. It is more common on the right side as the thoracic duct has a longer course through the right chest (Fig. 33.1).

In traumatic chylothorax, the mediastinal pleura of one side is injured. If the pleura of both sides are injured, it may cause bilateral chylothorax.

Servelle et al. (1963) found definitive evidence of structural abnormality of thoracic duct in patients with chylous manifestations.

The chyle accumulates more commonly on the right side as compared to the left, and varies in volume. It contains 0.4–5 gm% total fat, 65–220 mg% total cholesterol, 1.2–4.1 gm% albumin, 1.1–3.6 gm% globulin and electrolytes similar to those

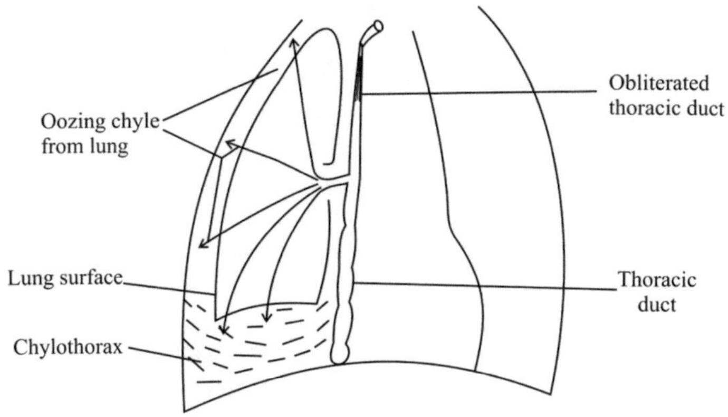

Fig. 33.1 Pathogenesis of filarial chylothorax: transudation of chyle from the pulmonary surface

of plasma. It also contains 400–6800 lymphocytes and 50–600 erythrocytes/mm^3 (Moncure 1994).

The pleura is usually normal but may show some thickening and adhesions.

33.3 Clinical Features

The patient usually presents with shortness of breath or exertional dyspnea. In filarial chylothorax, there may be a history of recurrent attacks of fever with rigors. Other clinical manifestations of filariasis may be present.

The patient may be weak and anemic and there are signs of pleural effusion on one or both sides, e.g., stony dullness on percussion and absence of breath sounds at the base of lungs. Many of these patients have genital manifestations such as epididymo-orchitis (Kanetkar et al. 1966).

33.4 Investigations

- *Blood* shows anemia, lymphocytopenia and may be hypoproteinemia. The eosinophils are usually more than 10 %. The night blood smear may be positive for microfilariae.
- *Imaging of chest* shows opacified hemithorax due to pleural effusion (Fig. 33.2), which may be further confirmed by ultrasonography. CT scan is required to rule out mediastinal tumors.
- *Pleural aspiration* results in recovery of non-clotting milky fluid containing chylomicrons which are relatively large particles. On lipoprotein analysis, a triglyceride level of more than 110 mg/dL is diagnostic (Putnam 2012). It has a high

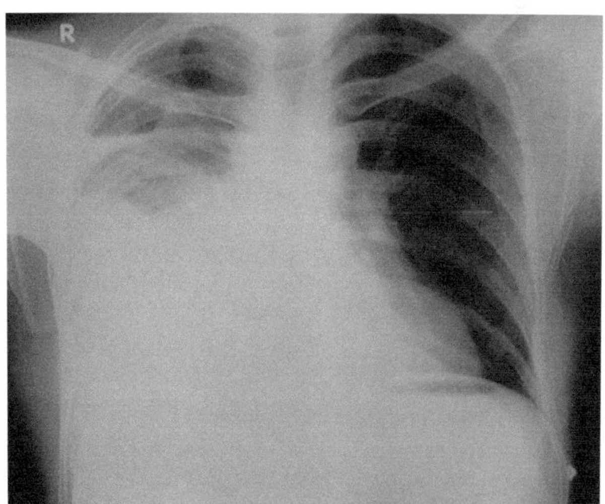

Fig. 33.2 Right-sided pleural effusion which turned out to be chylous on needle aspiration

lymphocyte count. It fills up rapidly after tapping. It must also be examined for *Mycobacterium tuberculosis* and malignant cells (Sriram Bhat 2013).

- The chylothorax must be differentiated from cholesterol pleural effusion (pseudochyle), which contains only a trace of fat and is associated with tumors and infections, e.g., tuberculosis.
- *Lymphography* shows the changes in the retro-peritoneal and thoracic lymphatic system including the dilatation and tortuosity of lymphatics, obstruction and the site of the leak.
- In filarial chylothorax, the dye passes into the lower part of the thoracic duct without hindrance. There is usually a complete block in the upper part of the thoracic duct (Kinmonth 1982). The dye runs outwards into the peribronchial lymphatics below the block and towards the periphery of the lungs. There is no localized lymphatic pleural fistula.
- *The immunological tests for filariasis* including the complement fixation test and skin test are positive (Ridley and Scott 1961).

33.5 Treatment

The basic treatment is removal of the cause. Thus, in filarial chylothorax, the patient is given diethylcarbamazine 100 mg three times daily orally after meals for 3–4 weeks and a fat-free, high-carbohydrate and high-protein diet. Medium-chain triglycerides, e.g., coconut oil, may be given to meet the fat requirements of the body.

If the fluid is abundant and causing significant symptoms, it may be tapped for immediate relief, but it refills rapidly. Repeated tapping is not advised as it results in significant loss of fluid and nourishment.

Some patients are relieved by the above measures. If there is no relief, the patient is given nothing orally, an intercostal tube is inserted to drain the chyle continuously and completely and he/she is put on lipid-free total parenteral nutrition (TPN). Use of octreotide or somatostatin may be of help (Roehr et al. 2006). Tube thoracostomy allows complete expansion of the lung.

The irritating nature of chyle promotes pleurodesis. Hence, in half of the patients, the leak stops spontaneously. Therefore, the instillation of sclerosing agents has also been advocated (Theodore and Jablons 2010).

Surgical treatment If the daily chyle loss exceeds 1500 mL for 5 successive days or persists after 2–3 weeks of conservative treatment, surgical treatment is indicated (Theodore and Jablons 2010).

The dilated thoracic duct proximal to the obstruction may be anastomosed to the azygos vein.

Pleurodesis is the most effective measure but the pleura must be stripped completely. The abrasive measures alone are insufficient. Postoperative suction drainage must be continued for at least 3 weeks to produce firm adhesion of the lung to the chest wall that resists separation by subsequent oozing of fluid (Kinmonth 1982). The chyle is now drained by parietal lymphatics.

The results of this procedure are very good (Romero 2000). Rarely, the drainage of chyle into the parietal lymphatics is not sufficient or fails when it may kill the patient from chyle-logged lungs as the excess chyle has nowhere to drain (Homer-Vanniasinkam and Russell 2013).

Other causes Traumatic chylothorax is treated by surgical ligation of thoracic duct both above and below the leak which may be done endoscopically (VATS), if the pleural fluid loss exceeds 1500 mL/day (from intercostal tube). Placement of olive oil or ice cream by a nasogastric tube into the stomach at the time of surgery may increase the chyle leakage into the operative area and may help in identifying the site of thoracic duct disruption (Putnam 2012). Percutaneous techniques with needle cannulation and duct occlusion, e.g., thoracic duct embolization have been proposed (Cope 2004). Laslett et al. (2012) reported chronic diarrhea and lower extremity swelling as a delayed complication of thoracic duct embolization.

In patients with malignancy as the cause of chylothorax irradiation of the tumor is useful.

Shunting of fluid into the peritoneal cavity or other hemithorax is also described (Moncure 1994).

33.6 Therapeutic Techniques

Pleural aspiration (thoracentesis) It is done with a large bore needle under local anesthesia (lignocaine 1 %) injected from the skin down to the parietal pleura with a fine-needle in the eighth or ninth intercostal space along the upper border of lower rib in the posterior axillary line. Introduction of some contrast medium into the pleural cavity helps in the location of the lower limit of the cavity on radiography and permits accurate placement of aspirating needle. The patient is made to sit with arms abducted so as to displace the scapula. All the chylous fluid is removed and sent for examination.

Tube thoracostomy It is done under local anesthesia with the patient seated. A catheter is inserted in the eighth or ninth intercostal space between the posterior axillary line and the scapular line depending upon the contrast study of pleural space. A stab incision is made and the trocar with the cannula is inserted into the chest with a steady thrusting movement accompanied by rotation. The instrument is kept in close touch with the upper border of the rib below to prevent injury to the intercostal vessels. The trocar is withdrawn and a stretched self-retaining catheter on an introducer is passed through the cannula. The cannula is removed, followed by the catheter introducer, so that the end of the catheter expands to make it self-retaining. The catheter is gently pulled until its

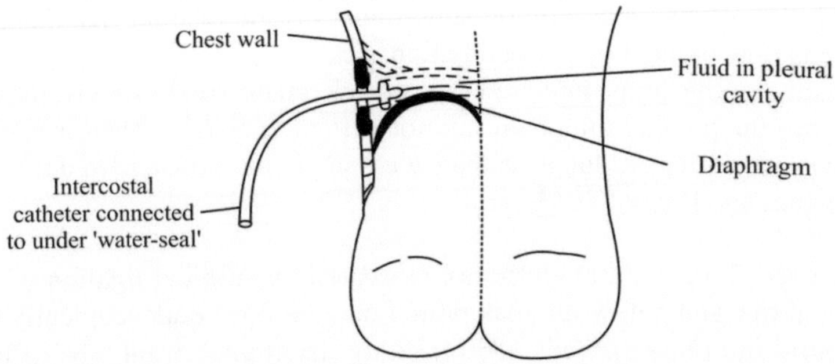

Fig. 33.3 Intercostal tube thoracostomy as viewed from the *back* in a seated patient with a self-retaining catheter inserted through the eighth or ninth intercostal space

Fig. 33.4 Under "water-seal" for closed drainage of chylothorax

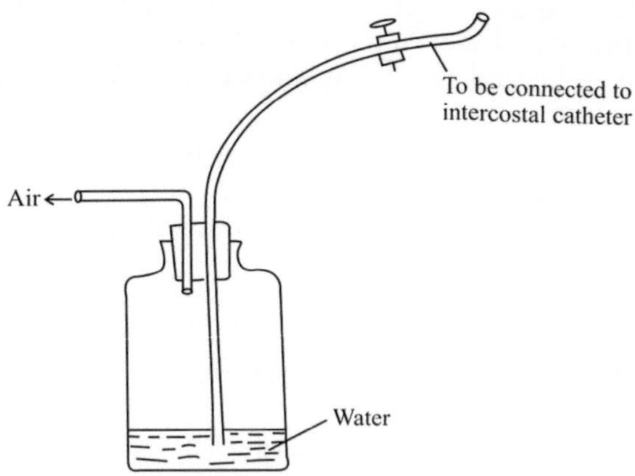

flange comes to lie against the chest wall and is fixed with dressing. The external end of the catheter is connected to an under "water-seal" for continuous drainage (Figs. 33.3 and 33.4).

33.7 Pseudochylothorax

It is a chyliform effusion in the pleural cavity of long duration with thickened and occasionally calcified pleura. Its fluid is negative for chyle when stained with Sudan III. It has high cholesterol content, sometimes more than 1000 mg/dL. The causes of pseudochylothorax include rheumatoid arthritis, tuberculosis, and idiopathic. The treatment includes removal of the cause. Occasionally, decortication of pleura is required (Dowdeswell 1994).

References

Cohen N, Dishi V, Alon I, Golik A, Modai D, Zaidenstein R. Chylothorax following median sternotomy. Clin Cardiol. 1996;19(11):910–2. PMID: 8914788.

Cope C. Management of chylothorax via percutaneous embolization. Curr Opin Pulm Med. 2004;10:311–4.

DeMeester TR, Lafontaine E. The pleura. In: Sabiston DC, Spencer FC, editors. Surgery of the chest. 5th ed. Philadelphia: WB Saunders; 1990. p. 455–8.

Dowdeswell IRG. Pleural diseases. In: Stein JH, Sande MA, editors. Internal medicine. 4th ed. St. Louis: Mosby; 1994. p. 1760.

Homer-Vanniasinkam S, Russell DA. Lymphatic disorders.In: Williams NS, Bulstrode CJK, O'Connell PR. editors. Bailey & Love's Short Practice of Surgery. 26th Edition. London: CRC Press; 2013. p. 938

Kanetkar AV, Karanjawalla DK, Deshmukh SM, Sen PK. Initial experience in the management of chyluria. Indian J Surg. 1966;28:381–8.

Kinmonth JB. The lymphatics. 2nd ed. London: Edward Arnold; 1982. p. 250–7.

Kumar A, Aggarwal S, Chumber S. Lungs, pleura and chest wall. In: Chumber S, editor. Essentials of surgery. New Delhi: Jaypee Brothers; 2005. p. 1437.

Laslett D, Trerotola SO, Itkin M. Delayed complications following technically successful thoracic duct embolization. J Vasc Interv Radiol. 2012;23:76–9.

Moncure AC. Chylothorax. In: Morris PJ, Malt RA, editors. Oxford textbook of surgery, vol. 1. New York: Oxford University Press; 1994. p. 1933–5.

Nair SK, Petko M, Hayward MP. Aetiology and management of chylothorax in adults. Eur J Cardiothorac Surg. 2007;32:362–9.

Putnam JB. Chylothorax. In: Townsend Jr CM, Beauchamp RD, Evers BM, Mattox KL, editors. Sabiston textbook of surgery. 19th ed. Philadelphia: Elsevier Saunders; 2012. p. 1598–9.

Ridley DS, Scott GJ. The skin test for filariasis. J Trop Med Hyg. 1961;64:297–9.

Roehr CC, Jung A, Proquitte H, et al. Somatostatin or octreotide as treatment options for chylothorax in young children: a systematic review. Intensive Care Med. 2006;32:650–7.

Romero S. Nontraumatic chylothorax. Curr Opin Pulm Med. 2000;6:287–91.

Sendama W, Shipley M. Traumatic chylothorax: a case report and review. Respir Med Case Rep. 2015;14:47–8.

Servelle M, Turiaf J, Rouffilange H, et al. Chyluria in abnormalities of the thoracic duct. Surgery. 1963;54:536–49.

Sriram Bhat M. SRB's manual of surgery. 4th ed. New Delhi: Jaypee; 2013. p. 271.

Strahberger E, Scheuba G. Therapy of chylothorax. Thoraxchirurgie. 1958;5:514–9.

Theodore PR, Jablons D. Thoracic wall, pleura, mediastinum, and lung. In: Doherty GM, editor. Current diagnosis and treatment: surgery. 13th ed. New York: McGraw Hill Medical; 2010. p. 323.

Chylous Diarrhea

34

Chylous diarrhea in lymphatic filariasis is very rare. It is characterized by loose frequent stools that contain fat, protein, and other nutrients of the diet. These products are not present in the stool due to malabsorption but due to regurgitation of digested fat into the lumen of small bowel due to obstruction in chyle-bearing pathway at the root of the mesentery (Fig. 34.1).

Another cause of chylous diarrhea is intestinal lymphangiectasia, which is a rare autosomal dominant disorder that leads to lymphatic obstruction, poor chyle transport, and concomitant problems (Vardy et al. 1975; Rodriquez 2006).

34.1 Pathology

In filariasis, this manifestation occurs due to lymphatic obstruction at the base of the mesentery leading to burst of dilated lacteals into the lumen of the bowel. The intestinal wall is swollen due to edema, and numerous dilated lymphatics are visible on its external surface, especially the jejunum. If the bowel lumen is opened, the intestinal mucosa looks like a spectacular carpet of dilated white chyle-filled villi (Kinmonth 1982).

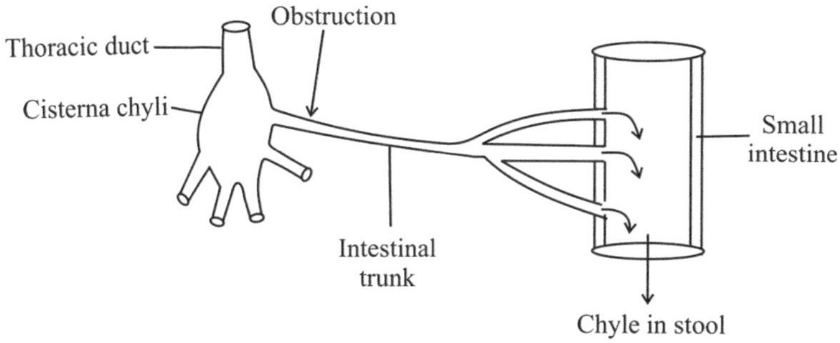

Fig. 34.1 Pathogenesis of chylous diarrhea

T.C. Goel, A. Goel, *Lymphatic Filariasis*, DOI 10.1007/978-981-10-2257-9_34

34.2 Clinical Features

The patient presents with chronic diarrhea and passes whitish loose stools (steatorrhea). A history of recurrent attacks of fever with rigors may be present.

Because of nutritional loss, the patient suffers from anemia, hypoproteinemia, and hypocalcemia resulting in edema, especially of external genitalia, asthenia, and tetany (Kinmonth and Cox 1975). It may be associated with chylous ascites.

34.3 Investigations

- Stool is pale whitish in color, very offensive, and has excessive amounts of fats and proteins.
- Blood shows eosinophilia, lymphopenia, anemia, hypoproteinemia, and hypogammaglobulinemia (Freeman and Nimmo 2011). It may be positive for microfilariae. The serum calcium level is low as the calcium is lost in the small bowel due to linkage with protein and partly as calcium soaps with the lost fat.
- Barium follow-through study may show thickening of valvulae conniventes of the small intestine.
- The radioisotope study consisting of injecting radioactive chromium ($^{51}CrCl_3$) intravenously may be done. This isotope is fixed to plasma proteins. Hence, the stools are seen for radioactivity for 5 consecutive days, indicating the amount of protein loss during this period. Normally, the loss in less than 15%.
- CT scan/MRI—the dilated lacteals may be imaged by these techniques.
- Endoscopy—upper gastro-intestinal endoscopy may show the presence of chyle in the duodenum.

Push–pull enteroscopy and capsule endoscopy are other investigations which can be done to discover the causative lesion (Huber et al. 2015). Intestinal biopsy will reveal dilated lacteals in the mucosa.

34.4 Treatment

The patient is given a course of diethylcarbamazine and advised high-protein and low-fat diet supplemented with medium-chain triglycerides. It will minimize the chyle production and flow. Coconut oil is a good natural source of medium-chain triglycerides which are absorbed by intestinal mucosa and transported to the liver through the portal vein. They do not contribute to chylomicron formation. Many patients are relieved by these measures.

The patients who do not respond to the above treatment should be put on nothing orally and total parenteral nutrition (TPN). Somatostatin or octreotide may help by decreasing the lymph flow.

Surgical treatment may be indicated in patients with severe chylous diarrhea not controlled by the above measures. The abdomen is opened and explored and the affected segment of the small bowel is resected if the lesions are localized. If there is a definite fistula, as evidenced by a bunch of dilated lymphatics on the surface of the bowel and entering into it, it may be ligated or that segment of the bowel may be resected.

References

Freeman HJ, Nimmo M. Intestinal lymphangiectasia in adults. World J Gastrointest Oncol. 2011;3(2):19–23.

Huber T, Paschold M, Eckardt AJ, et al. Surgical therapy of primary intestinal lymphangiectasia in adults. J Surg Case Rep. 2015;2015(7). pii: rjv081. doi:10.1093/jscr/rjv081.

Kinmonth JB, Cox SJ. Protein-losing enteropathy in lymphedema. Surgical investigation and treatment. J Cardiovasc Surg. 1975;16:111–4.

Kinmonth JB. The lymphatics. 2nd ed. London: Edward Arnold; 1982. p. 241–8.

Rodriquez LG. Intestinal lymphangiectasia: a forgotten cause of chronic diarrhea. Rev Gastroenterol Mex. 2006;71:55–8.

Vardy PA, Lebenthal E, Shwachman H. Intestinal lymphangiectasia: a reappraisal. Pediatrics. 1975;55(6):842–51.

[illegible] to make sure that elements of the novel may be [illegible]

References

[illegible]

Chylous Arthritis (Filarial Arthropathy) 35

Synovial effusion is defined as chylous when it contains greater than 800mg/100 mL of lipids in it (Borges et al. 2015). The creamy aspect of fluid results from intra-articular fat emulsification caused by lysosomal enzymes and other synovial proteins (White et al. 1985).

35.1 Etiology

Chylous arthritis is a rare clinical manifestation of lymphatic filariasis. Servelle (1963) reported one such case. Das and Sen (1968) from Pondicherry (India) reported 25 patients of chylous arthritis of knee joint and described its clinical features and investigative findings. In the subsequent year, they (Sen and Das 1969) reported eight more patients of chylous arthritis of the knee.

Arthritis involving the large joints, mainly the knee joint, has been described from Papua New Guinea in which the joint effusion was creamy. Microfilaremia was demonstrated in every patient and a rapid cure followed treatment with diethylcarbamazine (Salfield 1975).

Apart from lymphatic filariasis, other causes of chylous arthritis include trauma (Soojian and Tejwani 2004; Borges et al. 2015), nephrotic syndrome and pancreatitis (Soojian and Tejwani 2004).

Trauma causes chylous arthritis probably due to an occult fracture with bone marrow leakage or intra-articular fat pad injury.

35.2 Pathogenesis

The changes in the retroperitoneal lymphatic system are identical with the pattern observed in other manifestations of filariasis associated with chylous reflux (Servelle 1963; Kanetkar et al. 1966). Thus, chylous reflux into the joint is the basic cause of this manifestation.

T.C. Goel, A. Goel, *Lymphatic Filariasis*, DOI 10.1007/978-981-10-2257-9_35

The presence of chyle, having protein-containing chylomicrons in the joint cavity, acts as an irritant (Dole and Hamlin 1962) and sets up an allergic reaction to produce acute arthritis. This acute inflammatory response produces systemic manifestations such as fever and toxemia, and local response with signs of acute inflammation with muscle spasm (Das and Sen 1968).

35.3 Why Disease of the Knee Joint?

The ilio-inguinal backflow of chyle occurs towards the lower extremity in chylous arthritis, but it involves the knee joint only and no other joint. The cause of this selective involvement is not known. However, Das and Sen (1968) have described the following conjectures:

1. The knee joint has the largest synovial surface and the lymphatics draining it are constantly subjected to forces of gravity
2. Greater mobility of joint during walking
3. The lymphatics of knee drain only into the deep system
4. Its association with hypoplasia of the superficial system

However, these explanations do not answer this question clearly. Hence, further studies are required.

35.4 Clinical Features

It is commonly seen in patients of 20–25 years of age and more commonly in males. All the patients so far reported had the lesion in the knee joint, mostly on one side. In Das and Sen (1968) series of 25 cases, both knees were involved in only one patient.

The disease starts with high fever accompanied by rigor and chill. After 2–3 days of fever, the knee joint becomes painful, swells up and has limitation of movements. The patient looks toxic and has fever varying from 100 to 103 °F. The affected joint is held semiflexed, markedly swollen, red, hot and very tender. All the joint movements are restricted or lost due to pain and muscle spasm. The ipsilateral inguinal lymph nodes are enlarged and tender.

35.5 Course of Disease

The fever subsides within 3–5 days with reduction of other symptoms and signs. The swelling persists for 7–10 days after remission of fever but reduces completely by pressure bandaging. The joint returns to normal within 2–4 weeks of the first attack.

Das and Sen (1968) followed 12 out of 25 patients for 1–2 years after successful initial treatment. They had repeated effusions into the joint without signs of acute inflammation. After three to four such attacks, the synovial membrane of the joint gets thickened and becomes nodular and the joint became painful.

Chylous arthritis may be followed by fibrous ankylosis or synovitis that may proceed to pus formation (Manson-Bahr and Apted 1982).

35.6 Investigations

Blood it shows mild to moderate leukocytosis with 8000–12,000 total leukocytes/mL. Eosinophilia is usually present and the blood culture is negative.

Night blood smear may be positive for microfilariae. Das and Sen (1968) found it positive in 8 out of 25 patients and none in a second series of 8 patients (Sen and Das 1969).

Arthrocentesis the joint aspirate is thin, creamy and yellowish and looks like pus. It is negative for microfilariae and sterile on culture. It has high lipid content. Das and Sen (1968) found it to be 1.5–3 times the normal, i.e., 0.9–2 gm percent with an average of 1238 mg/mL.

Synovial biopsy Das and Sen (1968) did synovial biopsy in 10 patients with chylous arthritis, of which 6 had acute arthritis and 4 had arthritis with subsidence of acute symptoms.

In acute disease, the micro-picture looked like acute suppurative synovitis with predominant polymorphonuclear infiltration with many lymphocytes and macrophages, and a few eosinophils and plasma cells.

In late disease, the synovium was lined by chronic inflammatory granulation tissue with focal hyperplasia of covering epithelium. It was infiltrated with lymphocytes, plasma cells and eosinophils.

Plain radiography the radiographs of the knee joint show increased soft tissue shadow, and increased joint space without any change in the bones.

Lymphography Sen and Das (1969) tried to do lymphography in eight patients with chylous arthritis by cannulating a lymphatic channel behind the lateral malleolus and injecting 5 mL of ultrafluid lipiodol, but could do it successfully in five patients only. The findings are described below.

1. A single normal-looking afferent lymphatic vessel accompanying the short saphenous vein terminating in one to four popliteal lymph nodes
2. Normal or enlarged and spongy popliteal lymph nodes
3. Lymphangiectasia, stasis and backflow in the efferents of popliteal lymph nodes
4. A short truncated blind (aberrant) channel or channels leading towards the knee joint and terminating abruptly
5. Abnormal collateral channels along the synovial refection, some of them running forwards along the margin of the suprapatellar pouch

6. Localized streaks and specks of contrast at periphery of joint, especially in delayed films
7. Stasis in abnormally dilated lymphatics in films taken several days later
8. Tortuous and dilated thigh lymphatics with segmental beading
9. Normal or enlarged and spongy inguinal lymph nodes
10. Absent or fewer in number and often enlarged and spongy pelvic and retroperitoneal lymph nodes
11. Dilated and vermiform pelvic lymphatic channels

35.7 Differential Diagnosis

This condition has to be differentiated from septic arthritis, which is not easy clinically (Das and Sen 1968). Hence, estimation of lipids in the joint aspirate is a safe, simple and quick method of identifying it with a sufficiently high degree of accuracy. Further, in filaria-endemic areas, the possibility of this condition must be kept in mind.

35.8 Treatment

The patient is given bed rest, analgesics, e.g., NSAIDs, and a full course of diethylcarbamazine. A pressure bandage tied on the joint is helpful in reducing pain, inflammation and swelling. With this treatment, most of the patients recover completely with normal joint function.

Every effort should be made to prevent the recurrence of this manifestation as it leads to joint stiffness and loss of joint function.

35.9 Filarial Arthropathy

Filarial arthopathy is a rare clinical manifestation of lymphatic filariasis (Manson-Bahr and Apted 1982). It includes acute synovitis, arthritis, myositis and tendinitis (Pani 2013).

A joint includes the bones taking part in its formation, joint capsule and ligaments, synovial membrane, and muscles and tendons working on the joint or in its vicinity. Any (or many) of these structures may be involved in this infection resulting in its (or their) inflammation. It may affect one or more joints, the first one being the more common. The joints of the lower extremity are commonly affected, especially the knee and ankle.

35.10 Acute Synovitis

This is an acute inflammation of the synovial membrane of the joint with effusion into it. The patient presents with acute pain and swelling of the joint associated with fever with rigors. The pain occurs at the beginning of the movement are becomes less and less as the joint is moved more and more. The joint is red, hot and tender.

As soon as there is effusion into the joint, it takes the position of function, i.e., the knee is slightly flexed (Pani 2013).

The blood shows leukocytosis and eosinophilia and may be microfilariae. Radiography of the joint shows the soft tissue shadow of swollen synovial membrane and normal bones.

35.11 Arthritis

It is the involvement of all the structures constituting the joint in filarial infection, i.e., the synovium, the articular ends, joint capsule and ligaments.

- *Acute arthritis*: it is the acute inflammation of the joint. The patient presents with acute pain and swelling with loss of function associated with fever with rigors. The most common joints which may be affected include ankle, elbow, wrist and rarely the shoulder joint. The joint is swollen, red, hot and tender. Red streaks of associated lymphangitis are usually present.
  Radiography shows swelling of the joint with hazy articular surfaces. Microfilariae may be present in the blood and joint aspirate.
- *Recurrent arthritis*: in the obstructive phase of disease, inflammation may recur in the same joint. Occasionally, it may affect the other joints. Usually unilateral, it may sometimes be bilateral. It may subside spontaneously specially in patients with good antifilarial immunity in endemic areas.
- *Chronic arthritis*: a chronic form of arthritis occurs in the lower extremity joints in patients with obstructive lymphatic disease. The affected joint may develop fibrous ankylosis associated with elephantiasis of the lower extremity (Pani 2013).
- *Polyarthritis*: bancroftian filariasis may present with polyarthritis, which simulates rheumatism.

35.12 Myositis and Tendinitis

As the joints of the lower extremity, i.e., knee and ankle, are involved in lymphatic filariasis, the related muscles, e.g., quadriceps femoris, gastrocnemius, soleus and tendo-Achilles, may be involved in the inflammatory process and contribute or add to the pain, swelling, redness and tenderness (Pani 2013).

35.13 Treatment

The patient is given symptomatic treatment including analgesics and anti-inflammatory drugs, antihistaminics, antibiotics and rest to the joint in functional position. The tetracyclines or chloramphenicol are the antibiotics of choice (Pani 2013). Diethylcarbamazine is added to the treatment 2–3 days after the start of the treatment to avoid adverse reactions.

In the patients presenting with effusion in the joint, aspiration may be done for the purposes of diagnosis and treatment. It may reveal microfilariae and it should be sent for culture. It relieves pain by reducing the stretching of joint capsule and ligaments. If pus is encountered, the joint should be opened (arthotomy) to remove pus and necrotic tissue and to irrigate with sterile normal saline. After closure of the wound, may be with a drain, the joint is immobilized in the functional position, i.e., knee in 5–10° flexion and the ankle at a right angle to the leg (Pani 2013).

References

Borges PE, Franco MC, Recuero S, Sanchez Pernaute O. Chylous joint effusion: a rare entity that mimics septic arthritis. Case Rep Int Med. 2015;2(3):13–17. http://www.sciedupress.com/journal/index.php/crim/article/viewFile/6575/4226.

Das GC, Sen SB. Chylous arthritis. Br Med J. 1968;2(5596):27–9.

Dole VP, Hamlin JT. Particulate fat in lymph and blood. Physiol Rev. 1962;42:674–701.

Kanetkar AV, Karanjawalla DK, Deshmukh SM, Sen PK. Initial experience in the management of chyluria. Indian J Surg. 1966;28:381–8.

Manson-Bahr PEC, Apted FIC. Filariases. In: Manson's tropical diseases. 18th ed. London: Bailliere Tindal; 1982. p. 148–80.

Pani S. Pani's filariasis. 3rd ed. New Delhi: Jaypee Brothers; 2013. p. 53.

Salfield S. Filarial arthritis in the Sepik District of Papua New Guinea. Med J Aust. 1975;1(9):264–7.

Sen SB, Das GC. Chylous complications in filariasis, chylous arthritis. 3. A clinical and lymphographic study. Indian J Med Res. 1969;57(9):1745–50.

Servelle M. Pathology of the thoracic duct. (17 case reports). J Cardiovas Surg (Torino). 1963;4:702–27.

Soojian MG, Tejwani N. Chylous knee effusion: is it septic arthritis? A case report and review of literature. J Trauma. 2004;57:1121–4.

White RE, Wise CM, Agudelo CA. Post-traumatic chylous joint effusion. Arthritis Rheum. 1985;28:1303–6.

Chylo-Lymphatic Cyst 36

It is a distension cyst of chyle-bearing lymphatics that is a result of lymphatic obstruction and chylo-lymphatic backflow. Hence, it occurs in the areas of chylo-lymphatic backflow most commonly in the spermatic cord.

36.1 Chylous Cyst of the Spermatic Cord

Chylous cyst may occur in the spermatic cord due ilio-inguinal backflow of chyle. It occurs due to localized dilatation of a lymphatic vessel. Hence, it is a thin-walled cyst. It presents as a smooth, nontender nodule in the cord. It may rupture to produce a chylocele. Kinmonth (1982) has described it as inguinal chylocele. It should be excised (Fig. 36.1).

36.2 Chylo-lymphatic Cyst of Mesentery

It is the most common cyst of the mesentery which occurs due to a collection of chyle in a sequestered lymphatic of the mesentery. It may occur in patients with filariasis due to chylous reflux into the peritoneum as seen in chylous diarrhea and chylous ascites due to accumulation of chyle in an obstructed lymphatic. Hence, some of the chylo-lymphatic cysts of mesentery seen in filarial-infested regions may be due to filariasis.

Pathology The wall of the cyst in thin and consists of connective tissue lined by flat endothelium. It is filled with chyle of varying consistency from watered milk to cream. It is usually solitary and unilocular; its blood supply is independent from that of the adjacent bowel. Hence, the cyst can be enucleated easily without compromising the blood supply of the adjacent bowel (Homer-Vanniasinkam and Russell 2013).

T.C. Goel, A. Goel, *Lymphatic Filariasis*, DOI 10.1007/978-981-10-2257-9_36

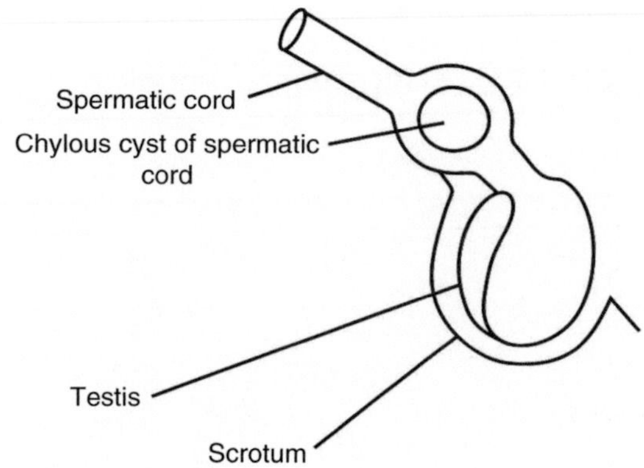

Fig. 36.1 Chylous cyst of right spermatic cord

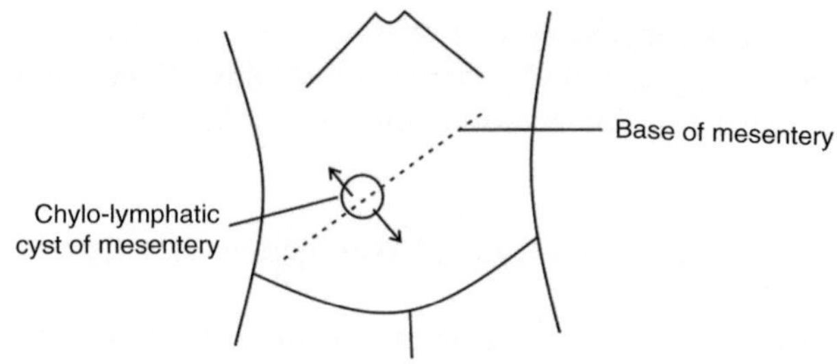

Fig. 36.2 Signs of a chylo-lymphatic cyst of mesentery

Clinical features The patient is usually a male of about 45 years of age who is present with a painless abdominal swelling with the following features (Fig. 36.2):

1. A fluctuating swelling in the abdomen near the umbilicus
2. Moving freely to the right angle of attachment of small bowel mesentery
3. A zone of resonance around and classically a belt of resonance across the cyst

These three signs are collectively known as Tillaux's triad after Paul Tillaux (1834–1904) Tillaux Paul (2013).

A past history suggestive of filariasis may be available.

The complications of the cyst include recurrent temporary impaction of food bolus in the segment of bowel narrowed by the cyst, torsion of the portion of mesentery containing the cyst, rupture of the cyst, intra-cystic hemorrhage and infection of the cyst. They all are characterized by acute abdominal pain.

Investigations Ultrasonography and/or CT scan may be done to image the lesion (Fig. 36.3). The blood may show eosinophilia and the immunological tests for filariasis may be positive.

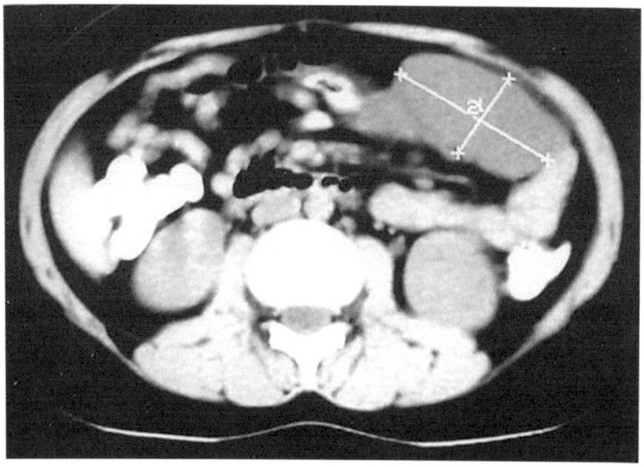

Fig. 36.3 Axial CT scan of abdomen showing a chylo-lymphatic mesenteric cyst, which is thin-walled and homogeneous (Courtesy of Dr. P.R. Gupta)

The second common cyst of the mesentery is an enterogenous cyst which must be differentiated from a chylo-lymphatic cyst. The differences between these two cysts are given in the following table:

Features	Chylo-lymphatic cyst	Enterogenous cyst
Origin	From sequestered or obstructed lymphatics of the mesentery	From the diverticulum or duplication of small bowel
Wall	Thin stretched wall of a lymphatic	Thick as it contains all the layers of the bowel wall
Contents	Chyle or lymph	Thick mucus
Blood supply	Independent of blood supply of the bowel	Blood supply common with blood supply of the bowel
Treatment	Enucleation of cyst	Excision of cyst with excision of adjacent bowel

Treatment The cyst is removed by enucleating from its capsule without endangering the blood supply of bowel. If there is a doubt regarding the blood supply of adjacent bowel, it may be resected with the cyst provided it is not a significant length of bowel.

If the cyst is too big or situated deep in the mesentery, it is partially excised with marsupialization of the remaining cyst into the peritoneal cavity. The cyst lining of the left-over cyst is sclerosed with 10 % glucose solution, diathermy or tincture of iodine to reduce the chances of recurrence. Even then, it may recur in up to 13 % of patients (Homer-Vanniasinkam and Russell 2013).

References

Homer-Vanniasinkam S, Russell DA. Lymphatic disorders. In: Williams NS, Bulstrode CJK, O'Connell PR, editors. Bailey & love's short practice of surgery. 26th ed. London: CRC Press; 2013. p. 923–40.

Kinmonth JB. The lymphatics. 2nd ed. London: Edward Arnold; 1982. p. 229–63.

Tillaux Paul. Quoted by Bhat S. SRB's Manual of Surgery. 4th ed. New Delhi: Jaypee Brothers; 2013. p. 611.

Eosinophilia in Lymphatic Filariasis 37

One of the most common findings in patients with lymphatic filariasis is elevated eosinophil count (eosinophilia), which is of two types

1. Eosinophilia associated with clinical manifestations of filariasis such as funiculitis, epididymo-orchitis, chronic lymphedema and filarial chyluria. Ghooi and Khanna (1976) found eosinophilia more than 10 % in 70 cases out of 90 patients of various filarial manifestations. In our study (Goel 1986), an eosinophil count of more than 10 % was present in 80 % of patients of filariasis. The eosinophils are more in acute filarial manifestations, e.g., acute funiculitis than in chronic manifestations. This type of eosinophilia may be labelled as secondary eosinophilia.
2. Eosinophilia occurring with no other clinical manifestation of filariasis called as occult filariasis or tropical pulmonary eosinophilia. It is a separate clinical entity and needs detailed description.

37.1 Tropical Pulmonary Eosinophilia (TPE)

37.1.1 Synonyms

Tropical eosinophilia, eosinophilic lung, tropical febrile eosinophilic asthma, Weingarten's syndrome, Meyers–Kouwenaar syndrome and occult filariasis.

37.1.2 Definition

Tropical pulmonary eosinophilia is a syndrome of immunological hyper-responsiveness to the microfilariae in the lungs (Ottesen and Nutman 1992; Dreyer et al. 1999) characterized by bronchial asthma-like symptoms and signs and hypereosinophilemia.

T.C. Goel, A. Goel, *Lymphatic Filariasis*, DOI 10.1007/978-981-10-2257-9_37

Tropical pulmonary eosinophilia was recognized as a clinical entity in the thirties of the last century. It was described as occult filariasis by Meyers and Kouwenaar (1982) in Indonesia in 1939. The same year, Vishwanathan from India reported this entity as eosinophilic bronchitis in the Annual Report of the Medical College where he was working (Vishwanathan and Jaggi 1981). Frimodt-Moller and Barton (1940) reported the same condition under the title, 'pseudotuberculosis of the lung with massive eosinophilia'. Later, Weingarten (1943) gave the name tropical eosinophilia and employed arsenic injections in the treatment.

37.1.3 Etiology

This syndrome is etiologically related to *Wuchereria bancrofti* and *Brugia malayi* infection typically without microfilaremia, i.e., cryptic filarial infection (Rosenthal 2015). Its filarial etiology is proved by the following facts:

1. Its geographic distribution closely parallels that of lymphatic filariasis.
2. This manifestation has been produced experimentally in man with full clinical features by inoculation with *Brugia pahangi* (filarial parasite of monkey) and *B. malayi* (Buckley 1958).
3. The microfilariae have been found in the areas of eosinophilic infiltration in the lungs (at autopsy or biopsy) in patients with this syndrome (Danaraj 1959; Webb et al. 1960).
4. It responds remarkably to diethylcarbamazine, a drug used almost exclusively for treating filarial infection (Donohugh 1963).
5. Jaggi and Sadana (1972) demonstrated bancroftian microfilariae in the peripheral blood of a patient of tropical eosinophilia 4 days after administration of prednisolone 10 mg three times daily which were absent before the administration of cortisone.
6. It is a hypersensitivity reaction to filarial worms as suggested by hypereosinophilemia, high filarial antibody titer and marked increase in total IgE levels.

Thus, this syndrome is the result of altered immune response in which the microfilariae are destroyed in tissues (lungs) without reaching the peripheral circulation. The altered immune response may have a genetic origin as most of the patients are of Indian origin.

The eosinophils infiltrate the lungs to produce bronchial asthma-like symptoms.

37.1.4 Pathology

In this syndrome, the pathological changes are seen in the lungs (Danaraj 1959; Udwadia and Joshi 1964), lymph nodes (Bras and Lie 1951), liver (Webb et al. 1960) and spleen.

Lungs The microfilariae and the parasitic antigens are rapidly cleared by the lungs from the bloodstream leading to allergic inflammatory reaction in the lungs.

The lungs have changes suggestive of eosinophilic bronchitis and bronchiolitis. There are tubercle-like small nodules, yellowish grey in color and up to 5 mm in diameter with groups of giant cells in the centre and clusters of surrounding monocytes and eosinophils. Microfilariae may be found in these lesions, which may be surrounded by hyaline material and known as Meyers–Kouwenaar bodies.

A prominent eosinophil-enriched intra-alveolar cytotoxic infiltrate is often seen with the release of cytotoxic proinflammatory eosinophil granular proteins that may mediate some of the pathologic changes seen in this clinical manifestation of filariasis.

Danaraj et al. (1966) have found microfilariae in lung biopsies of four out of five cases of tropical pulmonary eosinophilia. However, Udwadia and Joshi (1964) found microfilariae in only 1 out of 26 biopsies.

These lesions fade out spontaneously in 3–4 weeks in most of the patients without any residual lesion or calcification.

If it is not treated, in some cases, it may be followed by interstitial fibrosis, which may result in progressive pulmonary damage.

Many Meyers–Kouwenaar bodies are found scattered throughout the lymph node. Epitheloid granulomas with foreign body giant cells are occasionally seen.

Liver The liver shows eosinophilic infiltration along the portal tracts and in the sinusoids with formation of yellowish grey nodules. There are often areas of focal necrosis with numerous multinucleated giant cells (Webb et al. 1960).

The spleen may show similar changes.

37.1.5 Clinical Features

Age Most of the patients are of 20–30 years of age, but this disease is reported to occur in all ages from infancy to old age.

Sex Males are affected more commonly than females (4:1). In a series of 25 patients described by Gupta and Menon (1984), there were 19 males and 6 females.

Racial and geographic distribution Most of the patients have been reported from India, Pakistan, Sri Lanka, Brazil, Guyana and Southeast Asia (Nutman and Weller 2012); and 90 % of patients are of Indian origin.

Onset Usually, the onset is gradual with lassitude and low-grade fever. In some cases, the disease may have sudden onset.

Symptoms The typical symptoms include episodic nocturnal coughing (usually dry cough), wheezing, debility, malaise, anorexia, loss of weight and occasional hemoptysis.

Breathlessness is a major complaint and varies from shortness of breath with a sense of suffocation (a feeling of 'smoke' in the lungs) to expiratory dyspnea. It occurs following bouts of coughing.

The other symptoms include debility, malaise, anorexia, loss of weight, headache, constricting type of chest pain and occasional hemoptysis.

Signs The physical signs are those of bronchial asthma with hyper-resonant chest, bilateral rhonchi and a few crepts more marked on the bases of lungs. The apical zones are clear, opposite to tuberculosis. Poor expansion of chest is present in all the patients (Gupta and Menon 1984). In addition, the patient may have lymphadenopathy and splenomegely in 30–50 % cases. There may be other manifestations of filariasis.

Our experience About 25 patients with tropical eosinophilia were admitted every year in the medical wards of King George's Medical College, where I worked till retirement in 1999, and 1 out of 100 patients attending medical outpatients used to be a patient of tropical eosinophilia. Recurrences were common.

37.1.6 Investigations

Blood It shows extreme eosinophilia (20–90 %) with more than 3,000 eosinophils/μL of blood. The level of eosinophilia is not related to the extent or severity of symptoms. Premature eosinophils may be seen in the peripheral blood as well as bone marrow.

The filarial antibody titers are markedly elevated. The serum IgE is elevated and varies from 10,000 to 100,000 ng/mL (Nutman and Weller 2012).

Radiography or CT scan of the chest may be normal or may show hilar congestion and increased broncho-vascular markings. Diffuse miliary lesions or mottled opacities may be present in the middle and lower lung fields. It may be confused with miliary tuberculosis but the sputum is negative for mycobacteria.

Sputum Sputum shows excess of eosinophils without acid-fast bacilli (Pani 2013).

Microfilariae are not present in the blood but the lung biopsies have shown microfilariae in some patients.

Lung function tests They show restrictive abnormalities in most of the patients and the obstructive defects in half.

37.1.7 Treatment

Ganatra et al. (1958) were the first to report the successful use of diethylcarbamazine, which is the drug of choice, in this syndrome. It is given 4–6 mg/kg of body weight for 14 days. The symptoms usually resolve within 3–7 days from the start of the treatment (Nutman and Weller 2012).

In some patients, there may be exacerbation of symptoms during the first 3–4 days with diethylcarbamazine therapy. They soon disappear with continuation of therapy. Hence, the patient must be informed about them; otherwise, he/she may stop the treatment. Therefore, some experts initially relieve the symptoms with the use of antibiotics, anti-histaminics and bronchodilators, e.g., aminophylline, as required (Pani 2013). Corticosteroids may be used in a refractory case. As soon as the acuteness subsides, diethylcarbamazine is started.

Recurrence Relapse of this syndrome occurs in about 12–25 % of patients; sometimes after several years. It is treated with another course of diethylcarbamazine (Nutman and Weller 2012).

37.1.8 Prognosis

Overall, this syndrome has a good prognosis. However, if the condition becomes chronic or recurrent the patient will be left with some pulmonary fibrosis resulting in restrictive ventilation and impaired diffusion. In extreme cases, cor pulmonale may supervene.

References

Buckley JJC. Occult filarial infections of animal origin as a cause of tropical pulmonary eosinophilia. East Afr Med J. 1958;35:492–500.

Bras G, Lie Kan Joe. Documenta neerl. indones. Morp Trop 1951; 3: 289. Quoted by Manson-Bahr & Apted, 1982

Danaraj TJ. Pathologic studies in eosinophic lung (tropical eosinophilia); case reports. AMA Arch Pathol. 1959;67:515–24.

Danaraj TJ, Pacheco G, Shanmugaratnam K, Beaver PC. The etiology and pathology of eosinophilic lung (tropical eosinophilia). Am J Trop Med Hyg. 1966;15:183–9.

Donohugh DL. Tropical eosinophilia. An etiologic inquiry. N Engl J Med. 1963;269:1357–64.

Dreyer G, Dreyer P, Piessens WF. Extralymphatic disease due to bancroftian filariasis. Braz J Med Biol Res. 1999;32:1467–72.

Frimodt-Moller C, Barton RM. A pseudo-tuberculosis condition associated with eosinophilia. Ind Med Gaz. 1940;75:607.

Ganatra RD, Sheth UK, Lewis RA. Diethylcarbamazine (hetrazan) in tropical eosinophilia. Indian J Med Res. 1958;46(2):205–22.

Ghooi AM, Khanna T. Surgical manifestations of filariasis. Indian J Surg. 1976;38:150.

Goel TC. Clinical manifestations of lymphatic filariasis. In: Sen AB, Katiyar JC, editors. Perspectives of parasitology vol I. Lucknow: Print House; 1986. p. 89–123.

Gupta S, Menon V. Clinical and immunological studies in tropical eosinophilia. J Indian Med Assoc. 1984;82:429–32.

Jaggi OP, Sadana GS. Microfilaria detected in peripheral blood in tropical eosinophilia (a preliminary report). Indian J Chest Dis. 1972;14:197–201.

Meyers FM, Kouwenaar W. Geneesk Tijdschr. Ned-Indie 1939; 79: 853. Quoted by Manson-Bahr & Apted. 1982; 179

Nutman TB, Weller PF. Filarial and related infections. In: Longo DL, Fauci AS, Kasper DL, Hauser SL, Jameson JL, Loscalzo J, editors. Harrison's internal medicine. 18th ed. New York: McGraw Hill; 2012. p. 1745–8.

Ottesen EA, Nutman TB. Tropical pulmonary eosinophilia. Annu Rev Med. 1992;43:417–24.

Pani S. Pani's filariasis. 3rd ed. New Delhi: Jaypee Brothers; 2013. p. 86.
Rosenthal PJ. Lymphatic filariasis. In: Papadakis MA, McPhee SJ, editors. Current medical diagnosis & treatment. 54th ed. New York: McGraw Hill; 2015. p. 1513–4.
Udwadia FE, Joshi VV. A study of tropical eosinophilia. Thorax. 1964;19:548–54.
Vishwanathan R, Jaggi OP. Tropical eosinophilia. In: Ahuja MMS, editor. Progress in clinical medicine in India. 2nd ed. New Delhi: Arnold-Heinemann; 1981. p. 75–91.
Webb JKG, Job CK, Gault EW. Tropical eosinophilia:demonstration of microfilariae in the lung, liver and lymph nodes. Lancet. 1960;1(7129):835–42.
Weingarten RJ. Tropical eosinophilia. Lancet. 1943;1:103.

38 Filarial Hematuria

In tropical countries, especially in areas where lymphatic filariasis is endemic, hematuria may be caused by filariasis (Narasanagi et al. 1970; Mahadevan 1974; Ghooi and Khanna 1976; Clarks 1981). Narasanagi et al. (1970) reported 32 patients with hematuria due to filariasis out of 50 cases of recurrent gross hematuria. Ghooi and Khanna (1976) encountered three cases of filarial hematuria out of 90 patients with filariasis. Das and Dandapat (1979) reported 3 patients with hematuria amongst 200 patients with filariasis.

38.1 Etiopathogenesis

Lymphatic filariasis can cause hematuria due to the following changes in the kidneys:

1. Renal lymphatics are often dilated due to lymphatic obstruction resulting in rupture into the renal pelvis.
2. The small veins in the vicinity of lymphatics are obstructed leading to congestion and rupture into the pelvis (Mahadevan 1974).

Melrose (2002) demonstrated changes in renal parenchyma in filariasis and labelled them collectively as filarial nephropathy.

The pathogenesis of hematuria can be postulated on the same basis as that of hematochyluria (Narasanagi et al. 1970). Mason-Bahr and Apted (1982) thought that the latter is probably caused by the rupture of small blood vessels into the dilated lymphatics in the vicinity that rupture into the renal pelvis.

T.C. Goel, A. Goel, *Lymphatic Filariasis*, DOI 10.1007/978-981-10-2257-9_38

38.2 Clinical Features

The patient is usually an adult who presents with painless hematuria of varying degrees. It is very rare during childhood. However, Chari (1981) reported a case of filarial hematuria in the infant son of a doctor coming from a highly endemic area. The blood was positive for microfilariae and the patient responded to diethylcarbamazine.

Other manifestations of filariasis are commonly present. Among patients with filarial hematuria reported by Narasanagi et al. (1970), 75 % had one or many filarial manifestations, orchitis and funiculitis being the most common.

38.3 Investigations

- *Blood*: It shows leukocytosis, eosinophilia and usually microfilaremia. In 32 cases of filarial hematuria reported by Narasanagi et al. (1970), the blood smear was positive for microfilariae in all the patients.
- *Urine*: Apart from blood and/or chyle, the urine may also have microfilariae. In Narasanagi et al. (1970) series of 32 cases, 8 patients had microfilariae in the urine. Sapico and Baltazar (1967) reported a case of gross hematuria in which live microfilariae were present in the urine.
- *Radioimaging* of urinary tract including intravenous or CT urography is usually normal. They are usually not required in filarial hematuria but may be required to rule out other causes of hematuria especially the malignant lesions of urinary tract. They may show a retained hematochylous clot in the urinary bladder.

38.4 Treatment

The patient is given plenty of fluids and a 3–4 weeks' course of diethylcarbamazine 6 mg/kg in three divided doses after meals. Majority of patients respond to this therapy. However, Narasanagi et al. (1970) reported that 10 % of patients do not respond to the generally accepted therapy described above, but respond to a continuous therapy of 10 mg/kg body weight in divided doses for up to 10 weeks.

In case of gross hematuria, blood replacement may be required as well as the evacuation of hematochylous clots from the urinary bladder by endoscopic or open methods.

Previously, some of these cases were subjected to nephrectomy with a diagnosis of so-called essential hematuria (Mahadevan 1974). In 1966, the senior author (TCG) has assisted in the renal exploration of such a case that had essential hematuria with left renal pain (ultrasound/CT scan, etc., were not available at that time). The kidney was mildly enlarged and congested. The renal pelvis was opened which had clotted blood. The clots were removed and nephrostomy was done. In the postoperative phase, silver nitrate irrigation was done daily. The patient recovered completely and the nephrostomy tube was removed on the 10th day.

References

Chari MV. Progress in filariasis. In: Ahuja MMS, editor. Progress in clinical medicine in India. 2nd ed. New Delhi: Arnold-Heinemann; 1981. p. 28–48.

Clarks J. Parasites and piranhas: a journey round Guyana. Br Med J (Clin Res Ed). 1981;282(6263):554–5.

Das S, Dandapat MC. Management of acute manifestations of filariasis. J Indian Med Assoc. 1979;73:215–9.

Ghooi AM, Khanna T. Surgical manifestations of filariasis. Indian J Surg. 1976;38:150.

Mahadevan R. A text-book of surgery. London: Asia Publishing House; 1974. p. 362–3.

Manson-Bahr PEC, Apted FIC. Filariases. In: Manson's tropical diseases. 18th ed. London: Bailliere Tindal; 1982. p. 148–80.

Melrose WD. Lymphatic filariasis, new insights into an old disease. Int J Parasitol. 2002; 32: 947–60.

Narasanagi SS, Antani JA, Krishnamurthy, Colabawalla BN. Recurrent hematuria of filarial etiology. Indian J Surg. 1970;32:485–9.

Sapico FC, Baltazar RF. Filariasis presenting as a case of gross hematuria. Acta Med Philipp. 1967;3:273–5.

39 Very Rare Manifestations

39.1 Pericardial Filariasis

Pericardial involvement in filariasis is very rare. Two types of pericardial lesions have been reported, i.e., pericardial effusion and constrictive pericarditis (Mukherji 1963; Chakravarty and Gupta 1966; Sinha and Charan 1971; Charan and Sinha 1973; Reddy and Balsunderan 1977).

39.1.1 Pericardial Effusion

Reddy and Balasunderan (1977) described a patient who had hemorrhagic pericardial effusion containing microfilariae. The effusion cleared rapidly following diethylcarbamazine therapy.

The effusion may be chylous if there is a filarial obstruction of the thoracic duct in the upper part with chylous backflow into the pericardium. The symptoms and signs of pericardial effusion include breathlessness, cough and dysphagia. The neck veins are engorged and the pulse is paradoxical. The patient prefers to lie prone while made to sit (Mohammadan prayer attitude). The apex beat is not visible and area of cardiac dullness is increased. The heart sounds are distant and feeble. The diagnosis can be confirmed by chest X-ray, which shows the enlarged and near-round shadow of the heart. CT scan confirms the presence of pericardial effusion. Pericardiocentesis is done for microbiologic and cytologic studies. It may show microfilariae.

It is treated with diethylcarbamazine. Sinha and Charan (1971) treated a case of pericardial filarial effusion successfully with diethylcarbamazine The fluid may require removal.

T.C. Goel, A. Goel, *Lymphatic Filariasis*, DOI 10.1007/978-981-10-2257-9_39

39.1.2 Constrictive Pericarditis

Charan and Sinha (1972) reported two patients with constrictive pericarditis due to filarial infection, where the pericardial aspirate contained microfilariae. They were treated with pericardiectomy with permanent relief.

The symptoms and signs of constrictive pericarditis include engorged neck veins, enlarged tender liver, edema over feet, low systemic blood pressure, paradoxical pulse, systolic retraction of lower chest, invisible cardiac activity and a loud third heart sound. Echocardiography shows a septal 'bounce'. Cardiac CT or MRI may show pericardial thickening if it is >4 mm.

It is treated with diuretics, diethylcarbamazine and excision of thickened pericardium between the phrenic nerves of both sides.

39.2 Filarial Gangrene

It is a manifestation of filariasis which can occur in the scrotum or lower extremity (Das 1976).

In endemic areas, the filarial infection of the scrotum may progress to cause gangrene which looks very much like Fournier's gangrene of the scrotum. It is probably due to sudden transient plugging of capillaries of the scrotum by microfilariae (Gradwhol et al. 1951). Chincholkar (1957) described eight cases of Fournier gangrene of the scrotum of which four patients were considered to be filarial in origin as they came from the areas where filariasis was endemic. Das and Dandapat (1979) described 11 cases of gangrene of the scrotum (with abscess) out of 200 patients with filariasis.

It is treated by symptomatic and supportive treatment and broad spectrum antibiotics. Two to three days after the start of treatment, a course of diethylcarbamazine is given. The gangrenous tissue needs excision.

39.3 Filarial Salpingo-Oophoritis

Similar to epididymo-orchitis in a male, filarial infection may involve the fallopian tube and/or ovary in a female and cause their inflammation (salpingitis, oophoritis or salpingo-oophoritis).

The patient presented with fever with rigor and paramedian pain (pelvic pain) just above the symphysis pubis (Das 1976). Local tenderness is usually present. On the right side, it has to be differentiated from acute appendicitis. The blood shows leukocytosis, eosinophilia and microfilaremia. The lesion can be visualized by ultrasonography or CT scan. A pelvic abscess may occur as a complication.

It is treated by analgesics, antibiotics and diethylcarbamazine. An abscess may require the removal of pus, which may be done percutaneously.

Das and Dandapat (1979) described a patient who was diagnosed as ectopic pregnancy. On exploration, apart from normal pregnancy, tortuous dilated lymphatics were seen on both ovaries. The tubes were normal. This patient had microfilaremia and responded to antifilarial treatment.

39.4 Chylometrorrhea

It is one of the very rare manifestation of chylous reflux (Kinmonth 1982) and is characterized by chylous discharge per vaginum.

39.5 Cutaneous Manifestations of Chylous Reflux

Chylous reflux in the skin can produce a variety of lesions described below (Kinmonth 1982):

1. Vesicles with rupture and fistula formation: the discharge of chyle from the fistulae may continue intermittently or continuously for many years.
2. White vesicles discharging chyle only when injured.
3. Solid and semisolid warts and plaques of cream yellow color (xanthoma). Microscopy of these lesions shows histiocytic absorption of lipids.

These lesions are the most common in the perineum and thighs but may occur at any level including the knee, ankle and toes (Hunter et al. 1970).

39.6 Intra-ocular Filariasis

Intra-ocular filariasis is very rare. So far, 42 such cases have been reported in the world literature. Mathai and David (2000) have reported a case from Vellore (India) in which a 2-cm-long adult male *W. bancrofti* was removed surgically from the anterior chamber of the eye. The patient had redness, irritation and diminution of vision for a week. As the eye has no lymphatics, the entry of the worm was presumed to be hematogenous.

39.7 Cystic Lump in Axilla

Bedi et al. (1984) reported a case: a male 26 years of age who presented with a cystic swelling in the right axilla. The aspirate of the swelling revealed live microfilariae which were identified as those of *W. bancrofti*.

References

Bedi VP, Singh A, Patnaik S. Cystic swellings in axilla. J Indian Med Assoc. 1984;82:448–9.

Chakravarty SN, Gupta HB. Filarial pericarditis. J Indian Med Assoc. 1966;46:503–4.

Charan A, Sinha K. Constrictive pericardilis following filarial effusion. Indian Heart J. 1972;25:213–5.

Chincholkar VS. Idiopathic gangrene of scrotum. Indian J Surg. 1957;19:270.

Das K. Clinical methods in surgery. 9th ed. Calcutta: Published by the Author; 1976. p. 344–6.

Das S, Dandapat MC. Management of acute manifestations of filariasis. J Indian Med Assoc. 1979;73:215–9.
Gradwhol, et al. Clinical tropical medicine. St. Louis: CV Mosby Co. 1951. Quoted by Chincholkar VS. Idiopathic gangrene of scrotum. Indian J Surg. 1957;19:270.
Hunter JA, Morley WN, Peterkin GA. Xanthomatosis secondary to lymphedema. Trans St Johns Hosp Dermatol Soc (Lond). 1970;56:143.
Kinmonth JB. The lymphatics. 2nd ed. London: Edward Arnold; 1982. p. 265–6.
Mathai E, David S. Intraocular filariasis due to Wuchereria bancrofti. Trans R Soc Trop Med Hyg. 2000;94(3):317–8.
Mukherji BB. Pericardial effusion of filarial origin. J Indian Med Assoc. 1963;40:459.
Reddy GS, Balsunderan S. Filarial pericardial effusion. J Indian Med Assoc. 1977;68:125–6.
Sinha K, Charan A. Successful treatment of filarial pericardial effusion with diethylcarbamazine. Indian Heart J. 1971;23:157–8.

Brugia timori Filariasis

40

David and Edeson (1965) recognized *Brugia timori* as a distinct type of filarial worm from *Brugia malayi*. This type of lymphatic filariasis occurs on the island of Timor at the eastern end of the Indonesian Archipelago (Timor filaria). The adult worms of this disease were recovered from the experimentally infected jirds and described by Partono (1987).

40.1 Parasitology

Adult worm The male adult worm measures 2 cm × 70 μm. The female adult worm is larger and measures 3 cm × 100 μm. The anterior end of both worms is expanded into a bulb-like structure (head). The tail is long, tapered and smoothly rounded.

Microfilariae They are like those of *Wuchereria bancrofti* and *B. malayi* and show nocturnal periodicity. They are ensheathed and the sheath extends beyond the anterior and posterior ends. The microfilariae of B timori can be differentiated from those of *B. malayi* by the failure of the sheath to stain with Giemsa stain, a long cephalic space larger in size (average size, 310 μ × 6 μm) and a greater number of contiguous nuclei (five to eight) in the tail and smaller nuclei in the distal portion of tail.

Life cycle Man is the definitive host and the adult worms inhabit the lymphatic system where the adult male fertilizes the female worm who gives birth to a large number of microfilariae who find their way into the blood stream to produce microfilaremia.

Anopheles barbirostris is the intermediate host. It breeds in rice fields and bites at night and transmits infection.

T.C. Goel, A. Goel, *Lymphatic Filariasis*, DOI 10.1007/978-981-10-2257-9_40

40.2 Clinical Features

This type of lymphatic filariasis is limited to the Lesser Sunda Islands extending from Wallace's line on the west of Weber's line beyond Timor in the east.

The clinical features of *B. timori* filariasis are few and mild and very much like those of *B. malayi*. They include lymphadenitis, lymphangitis, abscess and elephantiasis.

The infection with *B. timori* appears to result in more abscesses than infection with *B. malayi* (Edesen 1962) or *W. bancrofti* (Okon et al. 2010). The abscess formation may occur at the site of lymph nodes or anywhere along a distal lymphatic vessel (Chandy et al. 2011).

The elephantiasis is confined to the leg below the knee joint in the lower extremity, and forearm below the elbow joint in the upper extremity.

The scrotal lesions including hydrocele are almost absent.

The main differences between clinical manifestations of bancroftian filariasis and *B. timori* filariasis are given in the following table:

Features	Bancroftian filariasis	*Brugia timori* filariasis
Clinical manifestations	More and may be severe	Few and mild
Hydrocele and other genital manifestations	Common	Almost absent
Abscesses	Fewer abscesses	More abscesses
Elephantiasis		
Lower extremity	Involves leg and thigh	Involves leg only
Upper extremity	Involves forearm and upper arm	Involves forearm only

The investigations, treatment and the preventive measures are same as for the other two filarial infections.

References

Chandy A, Thakur AS, Singh MP, Manigauha A. A review of neglected tropical diseases: filariasis. Asian Pac J Trop Med. 2011;4:581–6.

David HL, Edeson JF. Filariasis in Portuguese timor, with observations on a new microfilaria found in man. Ann Trop Med Parasitol. 1965;59:193–204.

Edesen JF. The epidemiology and treatment of infection due to Brugia malayi. Bull World Health Organ. 1962;27(4–5):529–41.

Okon OE, Iboh CI, Opara KN. Bancroftian filariasis among the Mbembe people in Cross River State, Nigeria. J Vector Borne Dis. 2010;47(2):91–6.

Partono F. The spectrum of disease in lymphatic filariasis. Ciba Found Symp. 1987;127:15–31.

Index

T.C. Goel, A. Goel, *Lymphatic Filariasis*, DOI 10.1007/978-981-10-2257-9

MIX
Papier aus verantwortungsvollen Quellen
Paper from responsible sources
FSC® C105338

FSC
www.fsc.org

If you have any concerns about our products,
you can contact us on
ProductSafety@springernature.com

In case Publisher is established outside the EU,
the EU authorized representative is:
Springer Nature Customer Service Center GmbH
Europaplatz 3, 69115 Heidelberg, Germany

Printed by Libri Plureos GmbH
in Hamburg, Germany